Regis'   N   f   C ll
Acce

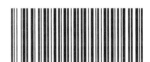

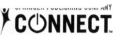

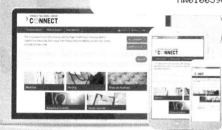

our print purchase of *Physical Medicine and Rehabilitation
'ocketpedia,* **includes online access to the contents of your
ook**—increasing accessibility, portability, and searchability!

\ccess today at:

ttp://connect.springerpub.com/content/book/978-1-6170-5293-4
**r scan the QR code at the right with your smartphone
nd enter the access code below.**

ΓG8YK9R

*Scan here for
quick access.*

LS

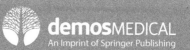

demosMEDICAL
An Imprint of Springer Publishing
View all our products at springerpub.com/demosmedical

PHYSICAL MEDICINE AND REHABILITATION POCKETPEDIA

Third Edition

Editors

Matthew Shatzer, DO
Residency Program Director
Assistant Professor
Department of Physical Medicine and Rehabilitation
Donald and Barbara Zucker School of Medicine at
    Hofstra-Northwell
Hempstead, New York

Howard Choi, MD
Assistant Clinical Professor of Rehabilitation Medicine
Icahn School of Medicine at Mount Sinai
New York, New York

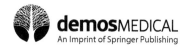

demosMEDICAL
An Imprint of Springer Publishing

Visit our website at springerpub.com

ISBN: 9781620701164
ebook ISBN: 9781617052934

Acquisitions Editor: Beth Barry
Compositor: Exeter Premedia Services Private Ltd.

Medicine is an ever-changing science. Research and clinical experience are continually expanding our knowledge, in particular our understanding of proper treatment and drug therapy. The authors, editors, and publisher have made every effort to ensure that all information in this book is in accordance with the state of knowledge at the time of production of the book. Nevertheless, the authors, editors, and publisher are not responsible for errors or omissions or for any consequences from application of the information in this book and make no warranty, expressed or implied, with respect to the contents of the publication. Every reader should examine carefully the package inserts accompanying each drug and should carefully check whether the dosage schedules mentioned therein or the contraindications stated by the manufacturer differ from the statements made in this book. Such examination is particularly important with drugs that are either rarely used or have been newly released on the market.

Library of Congress Cataloging-in-Publication Data

Names: Shatzer, Matthew M., editor. | Choi, Howard, editor.
Title: Physical medicine and rehabilitation pocketpedia / Matthew Shatzer, Howard Choi, editors.
Other titles: Physical medicine & rehabilitation pocketpedia.
Description: Third edition. | New York : Demos Medical Publishing/Springer Publishing Company, [2018] | Preceded by: Physical medicine & rehabilitation pocketpedia. 2nd ed. / [edited by] Matthew M. Shatzer. | Includes bibliographical references and index.
Identifiers: LCCN 2017035590 | ISBN 9781620701164
Subjects: | MESH: Physical Therapy Modalities | Rehabilitation—methods | Handbooks
Classification: LCC RM701 | NLM WB 39 | DDC 615.8/2—dc23
LC record available at https://lccn.loc.gov/2017035590

Printed in the United States of America by McNaughton & Gunn.
17 18 19 20 21/5 4 3 2 1

CONTENTS

CONTRIBUTORS

Hilary Berlin, MD, Clinical Assistant Professor, Departments of Physical Medicine and Rehabilitation, and Pediatrics, Donald and Barbara Zucker School of Medicine at Hofstra-Northwell, Hempstead, New York

Adrian Cristian, MD, MHCM, Chair, Department of Physical Medicine and Rehabilitation, Glen Cove Hospital, Glen Cove, New York

Renee Enriquez, MD, RMSK, Attending Physician, Assistant Professor, Interventional Pain Management, Department of Physical Medicine and Rehabilitation, UT Southwestern Medical Center, Dallas, Texas

Katie Gibbs, DO, Resident Physician, Department of Physical Medicine and Rehabilitation, Donald and Barbara Zucker School of Medicine at Hofstra-Northwell, Hempstead, New York

Emily Gray, MD, Chief Resident, Department of Physical Medicine and Rehabilitation, Donald and Barbara Zucker School of Medicine at Hofstra-Northwell, Hempstead, New York

Diane Horowitz, MD, Assistant Professor, Department of Medicine, Divison of Rheumatology, Donald and Barbara Zucker School of Medicine at Hofstra-Northwell, Hempstead, New York

Natalie A. Hyppolite, DO, MBS, Former Resident Physician, Department of Physical Medicine and Rehabilitation, Donald and Barbara Zucker School of Medicine at Hofstra-Northwell, Hempstead, New York

Navdeep Singh Jassal, MD, Attending Physician and Assistant Clinical Professor, Department of Pain Medicine and Neurology, Florida Pain Medicine and University of South Florida, Wesley Chapel, Florida

Sylvia John, MD, Vice Chair, Department of Physical Medicine and Rehabilitation, Northwell-Southside Hospital, Bay Shore, New York

Sarah Khan, DO, Assistant Professor, Department of Physical Medicine and Rehabilitation, Donald and Barbara Zucker School of Medicine at Hofstra-Northwell, Hempstead, New York

Cosmo Kwok, MD, Resident Physician, Department of Physical Medicine and Rehabilitation, Donald and Barbara Zucker School of Medicine at Hofstra-Northwell, Hempstead, New York

Thomas Lione, DO, Former Chief Resident, Department of Physical Medicine and Rehabilitation, Donald and Barbara Zucker School of Medicine at Hofstra-Northwell, Hempstead, New York

Susan Maltser, DO, Director, Cancer Rehabilitation, Department of Physical Medicine and Rehabilitation, Donald and Barbara Zucker School of Medicine at Hofstra-Northwell, Hempstead, New York

Fergie-Ross Montero-Cruz, DO, Former Resident Physician, Department of Physical Medicine and Rehabilitation, Donald and Barbara Zucker School of Medicine at Hofstra-Northwell, Hempstead, New York

Anthony Oreste, MD, Assistant Professor, Department of Physical Medicine and Rehabilitation, Donald and Barbara Zucker School of Medicine at Hofstra-Northwell, Hempstead, New York

Edward Papa, DO, Assistant Clinical Professor, Department of Pain Medicine, Stony Brook University Hospital, Stony Brook, New York

Komal Patel, DO, Resident Physician, Department of Physical Medicine and Rehabilitation, Donald and Barbara Zucker School of Medicine at Hofstra-Northwell, Hempstead, New York

Shaheda A. Quraishi, MD, Assistant Professor, Departments of Physical Medicine and Rehabilitation and Neurosurgery, Donald and Barbara Zucker School of Medicine at Hofstra-Northwell, Hempstead, New York

Craig Rosenberg, MD, Eastern Region Regional Director and Chairman, Department of Physical Medicine and Rehabilitation, Northwell Health-Southside Hospital, Bay Shore, New York

Rosanna C. Sabini, DO, Assistant Professor, Department of Physical Medicine and Rehabilitation, Northwell Health-Southside Hospital, Bay Shore, New York

Julie Schwartzman-Morris, MD, Associate Professor, Donald and Barbara Zucker School of Medicine at Hofstra-Northwell, Hempstead; Attending Physician, Northwell, Department of Medicine, Division of Rheumatology, Northwell, Great Neck, New York

Adam Stein, MD, Chairman and Professor, Department of Physical Medicine and Rehabilitation, Donald and Barbara Zucker School of Medicine at Hofstra-Northwell, Hempstead, New York

Dana Sutton, MD, Former Resident Physician, Department of Physical Medicine and Rehabilitation, Donald and Barbara Zucker School of Medicine at Hofstra-Northwell, Hempstead, New York

Dana Vered, PT, DPT, Physical Therapist, Department of Physical Therapy, Northshore University Hospital, Manhasset, New York

Jennifer Weidenbaum, MS, CCC-SLP, Speech-Language Pathologist, Department of Rehabilitation, North Shore University Hospital, Manhasset, New York

Lyn D. Weiss, MD, Chair and Residency Program Director, Department of Physical Medicine and Rehabilitation, Nassau University Medical Center, East Meadow, New York

PREFACE

The third edition of *Physical Medicine and Rehabilitation Pocketpedia* expands upon the first two editions, with new evidence-based data and updated references on topics relevant to the field of physical medicine and rehabilitation. New chapters covering topics of increasing importance in the field have been incorporated, including Quality Improvement, Cancer Rehabilitation, Acupuncture, and Ultrasound.

We hope that this new edition will continue to provide readers with a concise, handy, and up-to-date reference for ongoing education and clinical practice in our field.

Matthew Shatzer, DO
Howard Choi, MD

CHAPTER 1

NEUROLOGIC EXAMINATION

MENTAL STATUS

Mental status is based on numerous aspects of cognitive functioning. Orientation is necessary for basic cognition and is based on person, place, time, and situation. Attention is the ability to address situations without distraction and can be tested with serial 7s. Concentration is the ability to pay attention for a longer period of time. The three components of memory include learning, retention, and recall. Ask the patient to repeat three objects initially and recall them after 5 minutes. Recent and remote memory can be tested by asking questions pertaining to the past 24 hours and major events over the patient's lifetime. Mood can be determined by asking, "How are you feeling?" or "Are you feeling sad or depressed?" Insight is the patient's ability to understand awareness of impairment, need for treatment, and attribution of symptoms. Judgment can be determined by assessing one's ability to solve everyday problems. Speech and language are analyzed by monitoring rate, articulation, fluency, naming, word comprehension, repetition, writing, and reading. Higher cognitive functions include calculation, abstract thinking, and drawing a clock. Mini Mental Status Examination is a screening tool for cognitive function; a score of 24 or greater out of 30 is normal.

CRANIAL NERVES

Cranial nerve (CN1), the olfactory nerve, can be tested by using aromatic nonirritating products to evaluate the sense of smell. The optic nerve (CN2) is examined by testing visual fields and acuity. The three nerves involved in eye movement are oculomotor (CN3), trochlear (CN4), and abducens (CN6). The oculomotor nerve is involved in pupillary constriction, opening the eye, and all muscles of eye movement except lateral rectus and superior oblique. The lateral rectus in innervated by the abducens nerve and allows for lateral deviation of the eye. The trochlear nerve innervates the superior oblique and causes downward and inward movement of the eye. The trigeminal nerve (CN5) provides both motor and sensory innervation. Motor innervation is provided to the temporalis and masseter muscles, which cause jaw clenching and lateral movement of the jaw. Sensory innervation to the face is broken into three divisions: ophthalmic (V1), maxillary (V2), and mandibular (V3). The facial nerve (CN7) provides motor innervation to the facial muscles allowing for facial movements, including facial expression, closing the eye, and closing the mouth. Sensory innervation allows for the taste of salty, sweet, sour, and bitter substances on the anterior two thirds of the tongue.

Vestibulocochlear (CN8) has two actions: hearing (cochlear division) and balance (vestibular division). Glossopharyngeal (CN9) provides motor innervation to the pharynx and sensory innervation to the posterior portions of the eardrum and ear canal, the pharynx, and the posterior tongue, including taste (salty, sweet, sour, and bitter). The vagus nerve (CN10) provides motor innervation to the soft palate (elevation), pharynx, and larynx. Sensory innervation to the pharynx and larynx are also vagus mediated and are represented by the gag reflex. Motor innervation to the sternocleidomastoid and upper portion of the trapezius are via the spinal accessory nerve (CN11). Hypoglossal nerve (CN12) provides pure motor innervation to the muscles of the tongue.

MUSCLE TONE

Muscle tone is the resistance to muscle stretch through passive elongation. Muscle tone is flaccid in the absence of resistance to muscle stretch. Clinical indication of lower motor neuron involvement is observed in Guillain-Barré syndrome, acute phase of stroke, and spinal cord injury. Spasticity is increased resistance to muscle stretch that is velocity dependent. Clinical indication of upper motor neuron involvement is seen in multiple sclerosis, chronic phase of stroke, and spinal cord injury. It is measured using the modified Ashworth Scale. Rigidity is increased resistance to muscle stretch that is independent of velocity. It is a clinical indication of basal ganglia involvement and often observed in parkinsonism.

MUSCLE STRENGTH GRADING

Grade	Description
0	No muscular contraction
1	Trace contraction that is visible or palpable
2	Full active range of motion with gravity eliminated
3	Full active range of motion against gravity
4	Full active range of motion against gravity with minimal to moderate resistance
5	Full active range of motion against gravity with maximal resistance

MUSCLE STRETCH REFLEXES ARE TESTED BY TAPPING THE TENDON WITH A HAMMER TO ELICIT MUSCLE CONTRACTION

Upper extremity reflexes include biceps reflex (C5, C6); brachioradialis reflex (C5, C6); and triceps reflex (C6, C7). The lower extremity reflexes include patella or knee-jerk reflex (L2–L4); medial hamstrings L5–S1 tibial portion of the sciatic nerve; Achilles or ankle-jerk reflex (S1); and plantar reflex (L5, S1). To optimize the response, distract the patient by asking him or her to interlock flexed fingers (Jendrassik maneuver).

Grade	Description
0	No response
1+	Diminished response—hypoactive
2+	Normal response
3+	Brisk response—hyperactive without clonus
4+	Hyperactive with clonus

SENSORY TESTING SHOULD INCLUDE SUPERFICIAL AND DEEP SENSATION AND COMPARE DERMATOME DISTRIBUTIONS ON EACH SIDE WITH THE PATIENT'S EYES CLOSED

- Light touch: Use a cotton tip applicator
- Pain: Use a safety pin
- Temperature: Use two different test tubes of hot and cold liquids
- Joint position or proprioception: Move the patient's finger or toe holding the digit on the medial and lateral margins and test the ability to distinguish between the upward and downward movements
- Vibration: Use a 128-Hz or 256-Hz tuning fork over a bony prominence and ask the patient when the stimulus ends
- Point localization: Lightly touch the patient and ask for identification of the area
- Two-point discrimination: Ask the patient to distinguish between one point and two points of stimulus on the fingertips or palm
- Stereognosis: Place a common object in the patient's hand for identification
- Graphesthesia: Draw a number or letter on the patient's palm for identification

COORDINATION, STANCE, AND GAIT ASSESSMENT CAN REVEAL CEREBELLAR INVOLVEMENT THROUGH CLUMSY MOVEMENTS, ATAXIA, AND IMPAIRED BALANCE

- Finger-to-nose test and heel-to-shin test
- Rapid alternating movements
- Pronator drift: Ask the patient to keep arm held up with eyes closed; if there is a downward drift, it indicates a positive sign
- Romberg test: Ask the patient to stand with feet together and close the eyes; if there is any swaying, it indicates a positive sign and lack of position sense

- Observe the individual walk down hallway, do a tandem walk, walk on the heels/toes, hop on each foot, and perform shallow knee bend

SUGGESTED READING

Bickley L. *Bates' Guide to Physical Examination and History Taking*. 8th ed. Philadelphia, PA: Lippincott Williams & Wilkins; 2003.

Daroff RB, Jankovic J, Mazziotta JC, & Pomeroy SL. *Bradley's Neurology in Clinical Practice*, 2 Vol., 7th ed. Philadelphia, PA: Elsevier; 2016.

CHAPTER 2

GAIT AND GAIT AIDS

GAIT CYCLE

The normal gait cycle has two primary components: *stance phase,* which represents the duration of foot contact with the ground, and *swing phase,* which represents the period in which the foot is in the air (Figure 2.1). Stance phase makes up 60% of the typical gait pattern, whereas the swing phase makes up 40%. A *step* is defined as the time measured from an event in one foot to the same event occurring in the *contralateral* foot. A *stride* is defined as the time measured from an event in one foot to the same event occurring in the *same* foot.

THE SIX DETERMINANTS OF GAIT

Saunders et al. (1) assumed that gait is most efficient when the vertical and lateral excursions of the body's center of gravity (COG) are minimized. They identified six naturally occurring "determinants" in normal gait that reduced these excursions and suggested that pathologic gait could be identified when these determinants were compromised.

1. **Pelvic Rotation in the Horizontal Plane –** The pelvis rotates 4° to each side, which occurs maximally during double support, elevating the nadir of the COG pathway curve by about 3/8".

2. **Pelvic Tilt in the Frontal Plane –** The pelvis drops 5° on the side of the swinging leg controlled by the hip abductors, shaving 3/16" from the apex of the COG pathway curve.

3. **Knee Flexion (KF) –** Lowers the apex of the COG by 7/16" at mid-stance (10°–15°).

4. **Knee and Ankle Motion –** Rotation over the calcaneus in early stance with rotation over the metatarsal heads in late stance combined with KF in late stance produces a smooth sinusoidal pathway for the COG.

5. **Lateral Pelvic Displacement –** Normal anatomic valgus at the knee and varus at the hip decreases lateral sway, reducing total horizontal excursion from about 6" to <2".

MUSCLE ACTIVITY DURING UNIMPAIRED GAIT

Ankle Dorsiflexors – These muscles (primarily the tibialis anterior, but also the extensor digitorum longus and the extensor hallucis longus) eccentrically contract to smoothly lower the foot from heel strike to foot flat. They also concentrically contract during the swing phase to

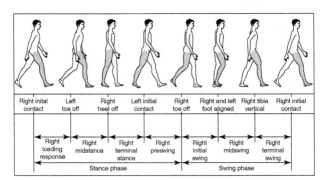

| Right inital contact | Left toe off | Right heel off | Left initial contact | Right toe off | Right and left foot aligned | Right tibia vertical | Right initial contact |

| Right loading response | Right midstance | Right terminal stance | Right preswing | Right initial swing | Right midswing | Right terminal swing |

Stance phase | Swing phase

FIGURE 2.1 Components of the gait cycle.

dorsiflex the ankle and effectively shorten the swinging limb in order to clear the ground.

Ankle Plantar Flexors – The triceps surae act eccentrically during midstance to control ankle dorsiflexion caused by the body's forward momentum. At push-off, they act concentrically to lift the heel and toes off the ground (see Figure 2.2).

Hip Abductors – The gluteus medius and minimus contract eccentrically during stance phase to limit pelvic tilt of the swing phase leg. Maximum contraction occurs after heel strike.

Hip Flexors – The hip flexors (primarily the iliopsoas) contract eccentrically after midstance phase to slow truncal extension caused by the ground reactive force (GRF) passing behind the hip. The tensor fasciae latae, pectineus, sartorius, and iliopsoas contract concentrically to flex the hip and shorten the limb for effective ground clearance during swing phase.

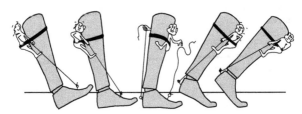

FIGURE 2.2 The actions of the ankle dorsiflexors/plantar flexors in normal gait.
Source: Adapted from Ref. (2).

Hip Extensors/Hamstrings – The gluteus maximus and hamstrings start to eccentrically contract just before heel strike to maintain hip stability and slow down the forward momentum of the trunk, since the GRF is anterior to the hip at this stage. They become essentially inactive after foot flat, once the GRF passes posterior to the hip. The hamstrings may weakly contract during the swing phase to flex the knee for ground clearance. The hamstrings have a double peak of activity prior to and after heel strike. The first peak occurs during swing phase when there is an open kinetic chain (foot not in contact with ground). This activation decelerates the forward swing of the leg by eccentrically contracting during hip extension and flexing at the knee. At the moment of heel strike, the open kinetic chain is converted to a closed kinetic chain (foot in contact with ground), while the hamstrings act predominantly as hip extensors preventing both hip and knee buckling. There is a less consistent peak of activity during late stance phase when hip extension by the gluteus maximus propels the COG forward.

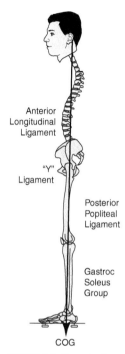

FIGURE 2.3 The center of gravity line.
Source: Adapted from Ref. (3).

Knee Extensors – The quadriceps act primarily to absorb shock as they eccentrically contract during heel strike to keep the knees stable. They are also active just before toe-off to help initiate the forward swing of the limb.

Standing – The gastroc-soleus complex (primarily the soleus) is the only muscle normally active during quiet standing. Ligaments and bony articulations maintain the stability of the other joints. The COG is located ~2″ anterior to S2 (Figure 2.3).

GAIT DEVIATIONS AND PRESCRIPTIONS

Muscle-Deficit Gait

Antalgic Gait – To reduce pain, there is avoidance of weight bearing (WB) on the affected limb. The examiner may note a decrease in the stance phase, a reduced step length on the unaffected side, and a prolonged period of double support.

Gastrocnemius Gait – Weak plantar flexors during terminal stance and toe-off prevent adequate heel lift. To limit the drop in the COG that occurs without heel lift during terminal stance, the step length of the contralateral leg is shortened. *Treatment*: A solid or semisolid ankle–foot orthosis (AFO) with a full-length footplate simulates plantar flexion during terminal stance.

Chronic Gastrocnemius Gait ("Go Backward Before You Go Forward" Gait) – Chronic weakness of the gastrocnemius muscles causes the calcaneus to become more vertical, and a cavus foot may develop with a large rubbery bursa over the heel. At heel strike, the body's movement tends to roll the foot forward over the bursa. As the GRF passes in front of the ankle and the thrust of the leg is directed backward, the foot will roll backward over the bursa. This rocking movement makes it look as though one is taking a step backward prior to moving forward. Additionally, the lack of push during the stance phase may eliminate the heel-off-to–touch-off phase, leading to a lift-off from foot flat stance. There is also a tendency for a shortened stance phase on the affected leg to avoid unstable collapse of the ankle into dorsiflexion.

Gluteus Medius–Minimus (Trendelenburg) Gait – In an uncompensated Trendelenburg gait (Figure 2.4A), there is contralateral pelvic drop secondary to the inability of the hip abductors to stabilize the pelvis during stance. In a compensated Trendelenburg gait (Figure 2.4B), weak abductors are compensated by a lateral lurch over the affected side to reduce the stress on the weak muscles. *Treatment*: A cane used in the contralateral hand widens the base of support and decreases the hip abductor strength needed to keep the pelvis level. In bilateral

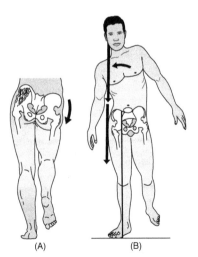

(A)   (B)

FIGURE 2.4 Uncompensated (A) and compensated (B) Trendelenburg gait.

abductor weakness, bilateral canes with a four-point gait may be used.

Gluteus Maximus (Extensor Lurch) Gait – This may be seen following injury to the inferior gluteal nerve or a subtrochanteric hip fracture. Weakened hip extensors are unable to decelerate the forward momentum of the body (hip flexion moment) at heel strike. To compensate, the subject adopts a prominent posterior lean and locks the hip joint in extension against the iliofemoral ligament, which keeps the body's COG behind the hip. *Treatment*: Two crutches or canes are used for a three-point gait (Figure 2.5).

Quadriceps (Back Knee) Gait – With weakness or inhibition of the quadriceps (e.g., distal femoral fracture), measures will be adopted to prevent buckling of the knee. One compensation is the use of the

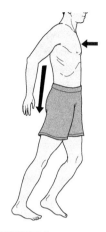

FIGURE 2.5 Gluteus maximus (extensor lurch) gait.

hand(s) to force the knee into extension. The trunk may also lurch forward at initial contact and the ankle plantar flexors strongly contract in order to bring the COG in front of the knee and force it into extension. Another compensatory technique is external rotation of the leg at initial contact and early stance to bring the medial collateral ligament anteriorly to prevent knee buckling. *Treatment*: A knee brace may be used to provide knee stability at heel strike (Figure 2.6). Also, the use of a rolling walker promotes trunk flexion to bring COG in front of the knee.

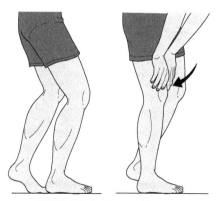

FIGURE 2.6 Quadriceps (back knee) gait.

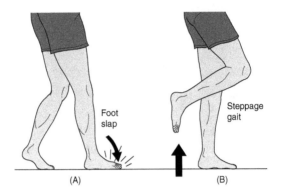

FIGURE 2.7 Tibialis anterior gait. (A) Foot slap. (B) Steppage gait.

Tibialis Anterior Gait – Pretibial muscle weakness that is at least antigravity (≥3/5 grade) may cause *foot slap* after heel strike. If the muscles are <3/5 grade, foot slap is generally *not* heard because a steppage gait is more likely. The hip and knee are hyperflexed in a steppage gait to clear the foot during swing phase, which may otherwise drag (Figure 2.7). The affected limb may alternatively be circumducted during swing phase. *Treatment*: A standard posterior leaf spring orthosis (PLSO), which allows plantar flexion and assists in dorsiflexion. An AFO is often used both to prevent foot slap and to allow clearance of the foot during swing phase. Note, however, that ankle plantar flexion stabilizes the knee. Thus, a standard hinged AFO (with plantar flexion posterior stop) may destabilize the knee.

Central Nervous System Gait Deviations

Hemiplegic Gait – Persons with extensor synergies will typically ambulate independently. The typical extensor synergy pattern has a predilection for knee extension, ankle plantar flexion, and inversion. Therefore, extensor tone effectively makes the plegic limb longer than the nonplegic side. A circumduction gait compensates via exaggerated hip abduction to allow for toe clearance and ends with toe strike. Despite the circumduction, there is a decreased step length and swing phase on the plegic side. Gait speed will be reduced in order to maintain an acceptable rate of energy expenditure. *Treatment:* A solid AFO or a hinged AFO with a posterior stop to decrease effective limb length may be helpful. A small degree of plantar flexion, however, should be maintained to promote knee stability when there is quadriceps weakness. With genu recurvatum, providing additional plantar flexion at the ankle via the addition of a heel lift (Figure 2.8D), and/or cutting the footplate just proximal to the metatarsal heads (Figure 2.8E),

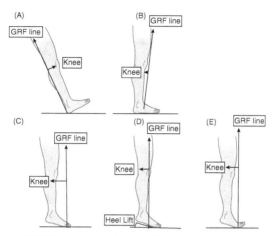

FIGURE 2.8 Ground reactive force (GRF) in relation to ankle mobility.
Source: Adapted from Ref. (4).

moves the COG posteriorly at the knee level, reducing the knee extension moment compared to the untreated state (Figure 2.8C; 4).

Parkinsonian Gait – The classic triad of Parkinson's disease is tremor, bradykinesia, and instability, with at least the last two affecting gait. While standing, the knees, trunk, and neck are typically flexed and the body appears stiff. When there is ambulation, there is a characteristic shuffling gait with short quickening steps, as if the patient were racing after the COG (festination). Turns are made "en bloc." Decreased arm swing further compromises balance. *Treatment:* Heel lifts and assistive devices may help reduce the tendency to fall backward. Walkers with added weight may provide additional stability. Physical therapy to address postural issues can be helpful (Figure 2.9).

Spastic Paraplegia or Diplegia/Crouched Gait – Often seen in persons with cerebral palsy. While standing, the hip and knees are flexed and internally rotated and the foot is held in equinovarus. With

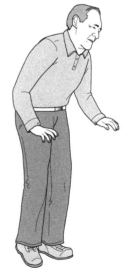

FIGURE 2.9 Parkinsonian gait.

ambulation, the increased adductor tone at the thighs causes the knees to scissor in front of each other with each step. Hip adduction causes short step lengths, making the feet seem like they are sticking to the floor. Balance may be impaired as a result of a narrowing base of support. To compensate for this, there is a tendency to lean forward and toward the supporting side. The upper extremities tend to be semiflexed with elbows held out to the sides. Diagnostic nerve blocks may help establish whether or not a contracture is present. *Treatment:* AFOs can be used to address equinovarus. Botulinum toxin injection therapy may be helpful for addressing adductor scissoring and equinovarus. Use of an assistive device (e.g., a walker) may provide additional stability.

GAIT AIDS

Cane Basics

Cane length should be from the bottom of the shoe's heel to the upper border of the greater trochanter with the user standing. The shoulders should be level and the arm holding the cane should be flexed ~20° to 30° at the elbow, to provide proper push-off. A cane can unload up to 20% of body weight off the affected lower limb, depending on cane design and the user's level of training.

In general, a cane should be held in the hand opposite to the lower limb with neuromuscular weakness or joint pathology. It is advanced together with the affected limb in a three-point gait pattern. Stairs are usually ascended with the stronger lower limb first, then the cane and affected limb. The affected lower limb and cane proceed down first during stair descent. ("Up with the good, down with the bad.") In practice, however, there are no hard-and-fast rules.

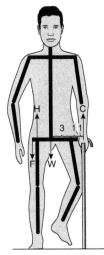

The basis for holding a cane on the opposite side of hip joint pathology is elegantly described in detail in Kottke's textbook (5). In essence, the cane provides a rotatory moment (**C**; see Figure 2.10) that counteracts the weight of the body (**W**) and reduces the force of the gluteus medius (**F**) necessary to maintain equilibrium at the hip fulcrum (**H**) when the affected lower limb is in single-support stance phase.

FIGURE 2.10 The basis for holding a cane on the opposite side of the affected hip.

Crutch Basics

Crutches have two points of contact with the body and are thus more stable than canes. The shoulder depressors (latissimus dorsi and pectoralis major) are the primary muscles used during ambulation with crutches. Other muscles include the triceps brachii, biceps brachii, quadriceps, hip extensors, and hip abductors. These various muscles may benefit from strengthening for optimal and better tolerated crutch use.

Axillary Crutch (Figure 2.11A) – Length is 1" to 2" plus the distance from the anterior axillary fold to a point on the ground 6" lateral to the bottom of the heel while standing. The handpiece is placed with the elbow flexed 30°, the wrist in extension, and the fingers forming a fist. The user should be able to raise the body 1" to 2" by complete elbow extension. Use of heavy padding on the axillary area of the crutch, although a popular practice, should be discouraged. This encourages the habit of resting the body on the crutches, which increases the risk of *compressive radial neuropathies*. When used properly, bilateral crutches can provide total WB relief to a lower limb.

Forearm Crutches (Lofstrand, Canadian; Figure 2.11B) – These provide less trunk support than axillary crutches but may be indicated if pressure in the axilla is contraindicated, for example, an open wound or compression neuropathy. A single forearm crutch can relieve up to 40% to 50% of body weight off a lower limb. B/1 forearm crutches, used properly, can provide total WB relief to a lower limb.

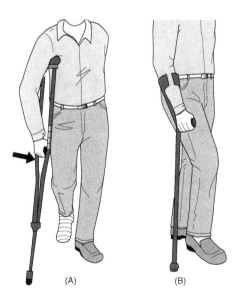

FIGURE 2.11 Crutches. (A) Axillary crutch. (B) Forearm crutch.

Crutch Gaits (Figure 2.12A) – The crutches and involved limb serve as point 1, while the uninvolved limb is point 2 in the *two-point* (or *"hop-to"*) *gait*. In a *three-point gait* (i.e., the involved limb is partial WB), the crutches (1 point) and the two limbs (points 2 and 3) are advanced separately, with any two of the three points maintaining contact with the ground at all times. In a *four-point gait*, each individual crutch and lower limb is advanced separately. Efficiency is forsaken for increased stability or balance. When negotiating stairs without a banister, one method might be stronger limb → weaker limb → crutch → crutch for ascent and crutch → weaker limb → stronger limb for descent. A rail or banister, if present, replaces one of the crutches in this method (Figure 2.12B).

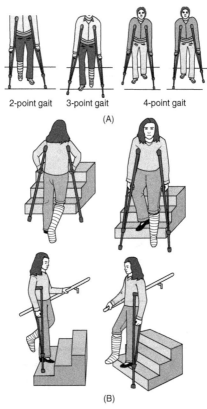

FIGURE 2.12 Crutch gaits. (A) Two-, three-, and four-point gaits. (B) Negotiating stairs using a banister for support.

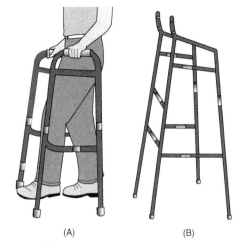

(A)   (B)

FIGURE 2.13 (A) Basic walker. (B) Platform walker.

Walker Basics

Walkers (Figure 2.13A) provide a wider base of support and a generally safer gait than canes or crutches. They allow up to 100% WB relief from an affected lower limb, depending on how they are used. A walker is fitted by placing it about 10" to 12" in front of the user. The proper height is set with the user standing straight, shoulders relaxed, and the elbows flexed about 20°. The main disadvantages are that they cause a slow and awkward gait and in the long term, can promote bad posture.

Rolling walkers are indicated for persons who lack the coordination or strength in the upper limbs to lift and advance a standard walker. These are preferred, because of the smoother gait, in the rehabilitation of patients who have undergone total joint replacement.

A *hemiwalker* is used by a person affected by hemiplegia. It is wide based, provides more lateral support than a quad cane, and is advanced on the nonplegic side.

Platform walkers (Figure 2.13B) are used in a variety of situations including distal upper extremity joint deformities, grip weakness, and flexion contractures of the elbow. They allow WB at the elbow, bypassing the hand, wrist, and part of the forearm, and may be useful for persons who have sustained injuries that preclude the use of a conventional walker.

REFERENCES

1. Saunders JB, Inman VT, Eberhart HD. The major determinants in normal and pathological gait. *J Bone Joint Surg Am.* 1953;35:543–548.

2. Inman V. *Human walking*. Philadelphia, PA: Williams & Wilkins; 1981.
3. Cailliet R. *Low back pain syndromes*. 5th ed. Philadelphia, PA: FA Davis; 1995
4. Appasamy M, De Witt ME, Patel N, et al. Treatment strategies for Genu Recurvatum in adult patients with Hemiparesis: A case series. *PM R*. 2015;7(2):105–112.
5. Kottke FJ, Lehmann JF, eds. *Krusen's Handbook of Physical Medicine and Rehabilitation*. 4th ed. Philadelphia, PA: WB Saunders; 1990.

SUGGESTED READING

Blount WP. Don't throw away the cane. *J Bone Joint Surg Am*. 1956;38:695–698.

Deathe AB. The biomechanics of canes, crutches, and walkers. *Crit Rev Phys Med Rehab*. 1993;5:15–29.

CHAPTER 3

WHEELCHAIRS

MANUAL WHEELCHAIRS

A comprehensive wheelchair (WC) and seating evaluation includes assessment of the medical history, cognition/communication, special sensory skills (vision and hearing), motor and sensory function, skin integrity, current seating/mobility device(s), WC skills, home environment/barriers, method(s) of available transportation, and level of community function (e.g., employment or school). A mat evaluation, which includes supine and sitting evaluations, helps to determine postural deformities (e.g., joint contractures, pelvic obliquities, spinal kyphosis, or scoliosis), trunk/postural control, and pertinent range of motion findings. Important patient measurements include hip/trunk/shoulder width, knee-to-seat depth, knee-to-heel length, shoulder height, and axilla height (Figure 3.1).

Typical Measurements

Back height	Self-propeller, good trunk control	2″ below inferior angle of scapula
	Self-propeller, poor trunk control	2″ below scapular spine
	Poor upper limb strength, poor trunk control	Standard (typically 16.5″)
Seat width	Widest point, usually hip, plus 1″	18″
Seat depth	Buttock to popliteal fossa, minus 2″	16″
Seat height	Popliteal fossa to floor, plus 2″	19″
WC width	18″ seat width usually corresponds to 27″ WC width. (Doorways need to have a clearance that is ≥32″ wide to be ADA compliant)	
WC weight	Standard (no set definition)	~43–50 lb.
	Lightweight	<35 lb.
	Ultralightweight (e.g., sports chairs)	<28 lb.
	Heavy duty (for users >250 lb)	45–60 lb.
Wheel size	Standard	24″
	"Hemichair"	20″

ADA, Americans With Disabilities Act; WC, wheelchair.

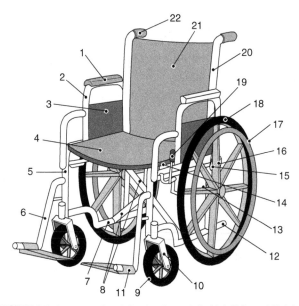

FIGURE 3.1 Components of a typical outdoor sling-seat wheelchair. (1) Arm pad; (2) desk-style removable armrest; (3) clothes guard; (4) sling seat; (5) down tube; (6) footrest; (7) bottom rail; (8) cross brace, X bar, or X frame; (9) caster; (10) caster fork; (11) footplate; (12) tipping lever; (13) axle; (14) seat rail; (15) armrest bracket or hole for non-wraparound armrest; (16) armrest bracket or hole for wraparound arm rest; (17) handrim; (18) wheel; (19) wheel lock; (20) back post; (21) sling back; (22) push handle.

Prescription Considerations

Frame and Weight – Folding frames are easier to transport but may be heavier, less durable, and require more energy to propel. Rigid frame chairs are more durable and energy efficient during propulsion, but may be more difficult to transport. Rigid frame WCs are not particularly useful for ambulatory persons because they do not typically come with swing-away footrests, making it difficult for them to perform sit-to-stand transfers. Decreasing the weight of a manual WC reduces rolling resistance, but does not necessarily reduce work of propulsion on level surfaces to a clinically significant degree. A difference, however, is appreciable on uphill grades. Lighter WCs are also easier for a user or caregiver to lift into vehicles for transport. Research has demonstrated statistically similar propulsion efficiencies for titanium, aluminum, and carbon fiber WC frames, although carbon fiber frames reduce vibration transmission in comparison to titanium and aluminum (1).

Axle – Posterior placement is advantageous for users with poor trunk control, amputees, and reclining/posterior tilt WCs, but increases turning radius, rolling resistance, and the difficulty in doing wheelies. Anterior placement decreases rolling resistance and improves maneuverability (decreased turning radius and easier wheelies), but also increases the risk of tipping over backward.

Molded Plastic (Mag) Versus Wire-Spoked Wheels – Mag wheels are slightly heavier but more durable than spoked wheels. Spoked wheels are preferred in most sports chairs, but require more maintenance and are less safe for some individuals whose fingers may get caught in the spokes.

Pneumatic Versus Rubber Tires – Pneumatic (air-filled inner tube) tires offer a comfortable ride on uneven terrain but are susceptible to going flat and have a higher resistance to propulsion. Solid rubber tires are generally preferred due to the easier propulsion and lower maintenance, especially if the WC is mostly used indoors (e.g., office work, hospitals) where the difference in comfort versus pneumatic tires is negligible.

Camber (Typically Ranges 3°–5°) – Increasing camber decreases turning radius, improves side-to-side and forward stability, decreases rolling resistance at high speeds (no effect at typical speeds), and protects user hands during sports. Disadvantages include difficulty in tight spaces due to increased overall WC width, increased tire/wheel-bearing wear, and decreased rear stability.

Handrims – Small-diameter handrims (sports WCs) increase the distance covered with each stroke, but require greater force. Pegged handrims ("quad knobs") improve ease of use for tetraplegics and users with hand deformities, but increase risk of trauma during attempts to stop and may reduce accessibility.

Casters – Small (≤5″ diameter), narrow casters are appropriate for smooth, level surfaces and are less likely to shimmy. Smaller casters, however, are more likely to get caught in sidewalk cracks and elevator thresholds. Large (≥6″ diameter), wide casters are advantageous in rougher, outdoor terrain, but have increased rolling resistance on smooth surfaces and are more likely to shimmy.

Cushions – *Foam cushions* are lightweight and inexpensive, but are not washable and dissipate heat poorly. These cushions do not offer adequate pressure relief. They are appropriate for ambulatory persons or users who are able to perform pressure relief independently with intact sensation.

Gel/foam combo cushions (e.g., Jay J2 and J3) consist of a firm gel emulsion on a contoured foam base, enclosed in a nonbreathable plastic. They provide good postural stability, are durable and easy to maintain and clean, and dissipate heat well. They are, however, expensive and heavy, and the contouring can interfere with transfers. The new Jay J3 has a customizable base for better stability and can accept a ROHO insert instead of a gel insert. *Air-filled villous cushions,* such as the ROHO, consist of multiple balloon-like air cells that assure maximum skin contact and provide the best pressure relief. The design is favorable for pressure ulcer prevention or healing. These cushions are lightweight, good at heat dissipation, and easy to clean and transport, but expensive and poor at providing postural stability. User vigilance is required to maintain optimal air pressure in each of the cells and to identify and repair punctures as needed.

Recline/Tilt-in-Space – Reclining and tilt-in-space WCs may be necessary for persons who lack the ability to otherwise achieve adequate pressure relief and for persons with orthostatic instability. Reclined positioning may also be beneficial for spasticity/spasm management and performing activities such as bladder catheterization or lower body dressing without having to transfer out of the WC. Users of reclining WCs may, however, be susceptible to increased spasms and shear forces during the actual reclining motion. Tilt-in-space WCs offer pressure relief without shear and also reduce the likelihood of triggering a spasm during the tilt. Backflow of urine in the tilted position, however, may be an issue in users with indwelling catheters. Manual recline/tilt-in-space positioning requires caregiver assistance. These WCs are often prescribed as backups for persons who primarily use power WCs.

Special WCs

"Hemichair" – This may be an option for some users with hemiplegia due to stroke. The seat height is lowered ≈2" and a footrest is removed to allow the user to employ the neurologically intact foot for propulsion and steering.

Lower Limb Amputee – The rear axle is moved posteriorly ≈2" to compensate for the rearward displacement of the patient's center of gravity. Turning radius is increased. A leg rest can be replaced by a residual limb support on the involved side.

One-Arm Drive – This is an option for persons with hemiplegia or unilateral arm amputation. Both handrims are on one side. Turning both rims propels the WC; one rim turns the WC. WC width and weight are increased. Good strength and coordination are required.

Power-Assisted WC – This is a manual WC that operates by combining the force of the user and electrical power from a motor on the wheel of the chair. It is indicated for users who are able to propel a manual WC, but have poor endurance, shoulder issues, or difficulty propelling on uneven surfaces. Power-assisted wheels increase the width of a WC and may reduce the precision of maneuvers in the WC (2).

Standing WC – These WCs have frames that allow the user to passively assume a standing position. The standing position provides pressure relief and weight bearing, may improve bowel/bladder function, and increases some accessibility (e.g., reaching cabinets). Standing WCs may also provide a psychological benefit for users. These potential benefits must be weighed against the additional componentry that increases the size of the WC, increases the work of propulsion, and reduces some accessibility due to increased WC dimensions.

POWER MOBILITY DEVICES

Scooters

Indications – For persons who can ambulate and transfer but have poor endurance or poor tolerance for prolonged manual WC use secondary to arthropathy or other conditions. Scooters are typically used for community mobility because their large turning radii often limit maneuverability within a household environment.

User Requirements – Good sitting balance, intact cognitive and visuo-perceptual skills, good hand–eye coordination, and adequate function of at least one upper limb to operate the controls are needed.

Caution – Some models tip over fairly easily, especially at high speeds. Scooters are not generally recommended for persons with progressive diseases such as multiple sclerosis. Functional decline may soon preclude safe use of the scooter, but it may be pragmatically difficult to fund and procure a more suitable power mobility device in a timely fashion.

Power WCs

Indications – Power WCs are for users with physical limitations incompatible with manual WC propulsion (e.g., users with Cl-to-C4–level SCI and many with C5-to-C6–level SCI) and for those with strength or endurance deficits (e.g., severe chronic obstructive pulmonary disease [COPD] and cardiac failure) who may not otherwise be candidates for a power scooter. Users may not have the postural stability/truncal control to use a power scooter and may require supportive features (e.g., custom seating and tilt-in-space functionality) not available in scooters.

User Requirements – Users must have at least one reliably reproducible movement to access the control system, adequate cognitive and visuo-perceptual function, proper judgment, and motivation. Candidates should undergo trials to determine if they can adequately and safely control a power WC.

REFERENCES

1. Chénier F, Aissaoui R. Effect of wheelchair frame material on users' mechanical work and transmitted vibration. *Biomed Res Int*. 2014;2014:609369.
2. Kloosterman MG, Snoek GJ, van der Woude LH, et al. A systematic review on the pros and cons of using a pushrim-activated power-assisted wheelchair. *Clin Rehabil*. 2013;27(4):299–313.

CHAPTER 4

MODALITIES

ESSENTIAL POINTS OF PRESCRIPTION OF MODALITIES

The key components of a modality prescription include diagnosis, impairments/disabilities, precautions, modality and settings (e.g., intensity and temperature range), area to be treated, frequency of treatment, duration of treatment, goals/objectives of treatment, and reevaluation date.

SELECTED MODALITIES

Heat (Thermotherapy) – The therapeutic temperature range is 40°C to 45°C. Superficial heat penetrates up to 1 cm; deep heat, 3 to 5 cm. Heat should be maintained for 5 to 30 minutes. Excessive exposure to heat, for example, >30 minutes of topical heat with <1-hour recovery can cause tissue congestion and reflex vasoconstriction, counteracting the intended effects of heat application. Appropriately applied, heat can be helpful during the postacute phase for pain relief, muscle relaxation, and facilitation of tissue healing.

Conduction is the transfer of heat by contact, for example, paraffin baths and hot packs. Although paraffin bath temperatures are ~52°C to 54°C, poor heat conductivity and low specific heat allows tolerance. Moist heat (e.g., hydrocollator packs) has traditionally been favored, compared to dry heat (e.g., electric heating pads) because water is more efficient at heat transfer than air and because moist heat draws less moisture out of treated tissue, that is, it avoids desiccation of the treatment area and promotes better capillary blood flow. Research, however, has not borne out that moist heat is clinically more effective than dry heat. *Convection* involves the flow of heat, for example, fluidotherapy, whirlpool, and moist air. *Conversion* is the transformation of nonthermal energy to heat (e.g., infrared, ultrasound [US], shortwave diathermy [SWD], and microwave diathermy [MWD]). Infrared penetrates 1 cm deep and may be used on skin with defects, since it is applied from a distance. US penetrates 3.5 to 8 cm. The greatest heating is at the bone–tissue interface due to high attenuation of bone. US parameters include a frequency of 0.8 to 3 MHz; treatment area of 25 cm^2; duration of 5 to 10 minutes; and intensity (measured in W/cm^2) adjusted to just below pain threshold. SWD penetrates 4 to 5 cm. Fat is heated more than muscle. The most commonly used frequency is 27.12 MHz. Treatment sessions last 20 to 30 minutes. MWD penetration is not as deep as SWD. MWD is rarely used.

Contraindications to heat therapy include acute hemorrhage or bleeding dyscrasia, inflammation, malignancy, insensate skin, inability to respond to pain, atrophic skin, infection, and ischemia.

Contraindications for US also include treatment over fluid-filled cavities (e.g., eyes and uterus) or near a pacemaker, laminectomy site, malignancy, or joint prosthesis with plastics (may use with metallic implants). SWD and MWD should not be used in children (due to immature epiphyses) and persons with metallic implants, contact lenses, or menstruating/pregnant uteri.

Cryotherapy – Cold, unlike heat, is limited to superficial applications only. Modalities include ice packs and cold sprays (e.g., fluoromethane). The physiological effects of cold include inhibition of histamines and other vasodilators (resulting in vasoconstriction) and decrease in nerve conduction velocity by prolonging Na+ channel opening (causing a sensation of numbness and diminishing the transmission of pain signals). Maximum vasoconstriction occurs at about 10°C to 15°C of skin temperature, generally at about 15 to 30 minutes of cold application. Further exposure to cold causes rebound vasodilation, which is the body's protective response to rewarm the area. This negates the intended effects of cold therapy. Skin erythema to cold exposure is a reflection of increased oxyhemoglobin levels due to decreased O_2 dissociation and is not necessarily a reflection of vasodilation. Cold is contraindicated in the setting of ischemia, insensate skin, severe HTN, or cold sensitivity syndromes (e.g., Raynaud's syndrome, cryoglobulinemia, and cold allergy).

Traction – Traction may increase the intervertebral space up to 1 to 2 mm and widen the neural foraminae, but these effects are temporary. Traction is typically prescribed for nerve impingement from disc herniations, narrowed intervertebral foramen, discogenic pain, and muscle spasm, as well as for spondylolisthesis, spur formation, degenerative facets, and hypomobile joints. General contraindications for spinal traction include ligamentous instability, osteomyelitis, discitis, bone malignancy, spinal cord tumor, severe osteoporosis, and untreated HTN. Contraindications specific to cervical spine traction include vertebrobasilar artery insufficiency, rheumatoid arthritis, midline herniated disk, and acute torticollis. Contraindications specific to lumbar spine traction include restrictive lung disease, pregnancy, active peptic ulcers, aortic aneurysms, gross hemorrhoids, and cauda equina syndrome.

Cervical traction – About 25 to 30 lb. of force is recommended for cervical traction (of this, about 10 lb. is used to overcome the effects of gravity, i.e., the weight of the head). The intervertebral space is greatest at 30° of flexion; traction in extension is not recommended due to risk of vertebrobasilar insufficiency.

Lumbar traction – A force of 26% of body weight is needed to overcome the effects of friction when lying supine with the hips and knees flexed (1). An additional 25% of body weight is needed to achieve vertebral separation. A split lumbar traction table can essentially eliminate the frictional component. Although frequently prescribed for back pain (e.g., for herniated disks and radiculopathy), the efficacy of lumbar traction is not clear.

TENS – The "gate theory," introduced by Melzack and Wall (2) posits that stimulation of large myelinated fibers (A-β and A-γ) excites interneurons in the substantia gelatinosa. This, in turn, exerts an inhibitory influence on lamina V, where the small unmyelinated A-δ and C pain fibers synapse with spinal neurons. Other theories regarding the mechanism of action of TENS also have been proposed.

"Conventional" or high-frequency (>50 Hz) TENS uses barely perceptible, low-amplitude, short-duration signals that cause a tingling sensation. Periodic adjustments to the pulse width and frequency may be necessary due to accommodation to the settings. "*Acupuncture-like*" TENS uses larger amplitude, low-frequency (1–10 Hz) signals that may be uncomfortable (β-endorphin release may play a role in the analgesic effects). Studies have not shown that TENS is effective in treating chronic low back pain (LBP), but it has been shown to be effective for diabetic peripheral neuropathy. Contraindications to TENS include use near pacemakers or stimulators, gravid uteri, open incisions or abrasions, and carotid sinuses or sympathetic ganglia. Incorrectly applied devices may result in burns.

Massage – Classic Western techniques include effleurage (stroking), petrissage (kneading), tapotement (percussion), and Swedish massage (tapotement + petrissage + deep tissue massage). Deep friction massage is used to break up the adhesions seen in chronic muscle injuries. Myofascial release aims to release soft tissue entrapped in tight fascia through the prolonged application of light pressure in specific directions. Eastern techniques include acupressure and Shiatsu massage.

Absolute contraindications to massage include malignancy, DVT, atherosclerotic plaques, and infected tissues. Relative contraindications include incompletely healed scar tissue, anticoagulation, calcified soft tissues, and skin grafts.

Phonophoresis – Topical medications (e.g., steroids and anesthetics) are mixed with an acoustic coupling medium, which are then driven into the tissue by US. Common uses include osteoarthritis, bursitis, capsulitis, tendonitis, strains, contractures, scar tissue, and neuromas.

Iontophoresis – Electrical currents are used to drive medications across biological membranes directly into symptomatic areas, theoretically avoiding the side effects associated with systemic medications.

REFERENCES

1. Judovich BD. Lumbar traction therapy: elimination of physical factors that prevent lumbar stretch. *JAMA*, 1955;159:549–550.
2. Melzack R, Wall PD. Pain mechanisms: a new theory. *Science*. 1965;150: 971–979.

CHAPTER 5

THERAPEUTIC EXERCISE

MUSCLE FIBER CHARACTERISTICS

Type I muscle fibers are "slow-twitch," highly fatigue-resistant, grossly dark fibers ("dark meat" due to their rich vascular supply) that appear light on myosin ATPase (at pH 9.4) or periodic acid–Schiff (PAS) staining. *Type II* fibers comprise the "white meat" but are dark histologically with these stains (see Table 5.1 for characteristics of each type/subtype).

All fibers in a given motor unit are of the same type. According to the *Henneman size principle*, smaller motor units are recruited first. Progressively larger units are then sequentially recruited as contraction strength increases.

EMG predominately records type I fiber activity. Functional electrical stimulation (FES) preferentially recruits type II fibers but may turn type IIs into type Is after long-term use. Steroids predominately cause type IIb fiber atrophy. Both types decrease with aging.

STRENGTH TRAINING

Isometric Strengthening – Tension is generated without visible joint motion or appreciable change in muscle length (e.g., pushing against a wall). This exercise is most efficient when the exertion occurs at the resting length of the muscle and most useful when joint motion is contraindicated (e.g., s/p tendon repair) or in the setting of pain or inflammation (e.g., rheumatoid arthritis). Injury risk is minimized. Isometric exercise should be avoided in the elderly and in patients with HTN due to its tendency to elevate BP (Figure 5.1).

Isotonic Strengthening – This is characterized by constant external resistance but variable speed of movement. Examples include free weights, weight machines (e.g., Nautilus), calisthenics (e.g., pull-ups, push-ups, and sit-ups), and TheraBand. The equipment is readily available, but there is potential for injury with this type of exercise.

Isokinetic Strengthening – This is characterized by a relatively constant angular joint speed but variable external resistance. This exercise does not exist in nature; special equipment is required, for example, Cybex and Biodex. If the user pushes harder, the speed of the manipulated piece of equipment will *not* increase, but the resistance supplied by the machine will. This maximizes resistance throughout the length–tension curve of the exercised muscles and is beneficial in the early phases of rehabilitation. Injury risk is relatively low.

TABLE 5.1 Characteristics of Skeletal Muscle Fiber Subtypes

	Type I: Slow oxidative	Type IIa: Fast oxidative glycolytic	Type IIb: Fast glycolytic
Motor unit type	Slow fatigue resistant	Fast fatigue resistant	Fast fatigable
Oxidative capacity	High	Moderately high	Low
Glycolytic capacity	Low	High	Highest
Contractile speed	Slow	Fast	Fast
Fatigue resistance	High	Moderate	Low
Motor unit strength	Low	High	High

Concentric Contractions Versus Eccentric Contractions – Concentric contractions are characterized by active muscle shortening. The least amount of force is generated during fast concentric contractions. Eccentric contractions are characterized by active muscle lengthening, which generate high forces at low energy cost. The greatest amount of force is generated during fast eccentric, followed by isometric, slow concentric, and finally, fast concentric contractions (see Figure 5.2).

Plyometric Exercise – A plyometric movement is a brief, explosive maneuver that consists of an eccentric muscle contraction followed immediately by a concentric contraction (e.g., planting and jumping during sports). This produces a more powerful concentric contraction. Plyometric training is aimed at increasing power.

Progressive Resistive Exercise – The *DeLorme axiom* posits that high-resistance, low-repetition (rep) exercise builds strength, while low-resistance, high-rep exercise improves endurance (1). In the DeLorme method, a 10 repetition maximum (RM) is first determined. Ten reps of the exercise are performed in sets of 50%, 75%, and 100% of the 10 RM. The sessions are performed ~3 to 5 times/week and the 10 RM is

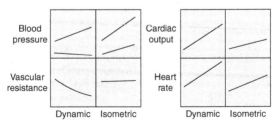

FIGURE 5.1 Acute hemodynamic responses to dynamic (isotonic) versus isometric exercise.

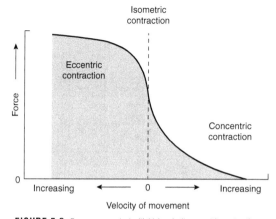

FIGURE 5.2 Forces are greatest with high-velocity eccentric contractions.

redetermined approximately each week. In the *Oxford technique,* the order of the sets is reversed, so that 10 reps at 100% of the 10 RM are performed first, followed by sets of 75% and 50%. DeLateur BJ later demonstrated that for the most part, strength and endurance gains are equivalent for the two types of exercise as long as muscles are exercised to fatigue (2). High-resistance, low-rep exercise, however, achieves its results more efficiently (i.e., fewer reps, less time). Moritani and de Vries (3) demonstrated that gains in the first few weeks of strength training were mostly due to neural factors (e.g., improved coordination of muscle firing) and not muscle hypertrophy.

The *Daily Adjusted Progressive Resistance Exercise* (DAPRE) method involves four sets of exercise per muscle group, where the first set is 10 reps at 50% of 6 RM, the second set is 6 reps at 75% of 6 RM, and the third set is as many reps as possible at 6 RM. The weight for the fourth set is based on the reps completed during the third set. If 5 to 7 reps of the 6 RM are completed, the weight remains the same. With fewer reps, the weight is decreased. With higher reps, the weight is increased. Adjustments to the working weight (6 RM) for the next training session are also made as needed.

AEROBIC EXERCISE

Regular aerobic exercise increases max oxygen consumption (VO_2max) and decreases resting BP, whereas strength training does *not* have an effect on either of these (Table 5.2). Other long-term cardiovascular adaptations/benefits of aerobic exercise include *increased* stroke volume (SV) with exercise, cardiac output (CO) during maximum exertion, work capacity, and high-density lipoprotein (HDL); and *decreased*

TABLE 5.2 Example of an Aerobic Exercise Program for a Presumably Healthy Individual

Program phase	Week no.	Exercise dur/freq (per week)	Intensity (%VO_2 max)	Program phase	Week#	Exercise dur/freq (per week)	Intensity (%Vo_2 max)
Initial	1	12 min/3x	40–50	Improvement	6–9	21 min/3–4x	70–80
	2	14 min/3x	50		10–16	24 min/3–4x	70–80
	3	16 min/3x	60		17–23	28–30 min/4–5x	70–80
	4	18 min/3x	60–70		24–27	30 min/4–5x	70–85
	5	20 min/3x	60–70	Maintenance	28+	30–45 min/3x	70–85

VO_2 is the body's rate of O_2 utilization (mL O_2/kg/min). Once VO_2 max is reached, further increases in work rate are powered by anaerobic (glycolytic) metabolism. VO_2 max can be calculated by the *Fick equation*: VO_2 max = max CO × (a-v O_2 difference), where CO = SV × HR.

VO_2max, max oxygen consumption.

Source: Adapted from Ref. (5).

resting heart rate (HR), HR response to submaximal workloads, myocardial O_2 consumption at rest and submaximal activities, low-density lipoprotein (LDL), and triglyceride levels. Maximum HR does not change. Historically, aerobic exercise was felt to have a negligible effect on skeletal muscle mass, but more recently, the mitigating effects of aerobic exercise on muscle mass loss and even hypertrophic/anabolic effects have been reported (4). Diabetic patients benefit from reduced obesity and insulin requirements. Improvements in mood, sleep, immune function, and bone density may also be observed.

Anaerobic threshold signifies the onset of metabolic acidosis during exercise, traditionally determined by serial measurements of blood lactate. It can be noninvasively determined by assessment of expired gases during exercise testing, specifically pulmonary ventilation (VE) and carbon dioxide production (Vco$_2$). The anaerobic threshold signifies the peak work rate or O_2 consumption at which energy demands exceed circulatory ability to sustain aerobic metabolism (5).

THE AMERICAN COLLEGE OF SPORTS MEDICINE (ACSM) GUIDELINES

At least 30 minutes/day on at least 5 days/week for at least 150 minutes/week of moderate intensity exercise is recommended.

Alternatively, at least 20 minutes/day on at least 3 days/week for at least 75 minutes/week of vigorous intensity exercise can be performed. In addition, resistance exercises 2 to 3 days/week and range of motion exercises at least 2 days/week are also recommended (6).

THE EXERCISE PRESCRIPTION

Preexercise Evaluation – The physician's evaluation should be comprehensive and include key elements of history, such as current and previous exercise patterns, motivations/barriers to exercise, discussion of risks/benefits of exercise, preferred types of activity, social support, and time and scheduling considerations. Special attention should be given to physical limitations, current and past medical problems, current medications, history of exercise-induced symptoms (shortness of breath, asthma, hives, and chest pain), and a thorough review of heart disease risk factors, including DM, HTN, smoking, hyperlipidemia, sedentary lifestyle, obesity, and family history of heart disease before age 50 years (5). Those in need of exercise stress testing and/or other formal testing should be identified as per the American Heart Association (AHA) and ACSM guidelines. The most recent ACSM recommendations (2015) seek to reduce unnecessary barriers to adopting and maintaining a structured exercise program and/or regular physical activity (7).

Components of an Exercise Prescription – These five components apply to exercise prescriptions for persons of all ages and fitness levels. Careful consideration should be given to the health status, medications, risk factors, behavioral characteristics, personal goals, and exercise preferences.

Mode is the particular form or type of exercise. Mode selection should be based on the desired outcomes and exercises that are most likely to be enjoyed and sustained on a long-term basis.

Intensity is the relative physiologic difficulty of the exercise. Intensity is calculated based on HR and rate of perceived exertion. The most commonly used scale is the Borg Scale of Perceived Exertion, which is scored from 6 (no exertion at all) to 20 (maximal exertion). A score of 9 is "very light" and consistent with a healthy person walking slowly. A score of 13 is "somewhat hard" and consistent with moderate intensity exercise; it feels okay to continue. A score of 17 is "very hard" and consistent with a healthy person who can go on, but really has to push himself/herself. Goal Borg scores are based on the goals of the exercise program. A goal of 12 to 14, for instance, would be consistent with a moderate intensity exercise program.

Duration (time) is the length of an exercise session. It may be continuous or intermittently accumulated during a day.

Frequency refers to the number of exercise sessions per day and per week.

Progression (overload) is the increase in activity during exercise training, which, over time, stimulates adaptation. This may be a change in frequency, intensity, and/or duration (5).

REFERENCES

1. DeLorme TL. Restoration of muscle power by heavy-resistance exercises. *J Bone Joint Surg Am*. 1945;27:645–667.

2. deLateur BJ. A test of the DeLorme axiom. *Arch Phys Med Rehabil*. 1968;49:245–248.

3. Moritani T, de Vries HA. Neural factors vs. hypertrophy in the time course of muscle strength gain. *Am J Phys Med Rehabil*. 1979;58:115–130.

4. Konopka AR, Harber MP. Skeletal muscle hypertrophy after aerobic exercise training. *Exerc Sport Sci Rev*. 2014;42(2):53–61.

5. Cifu DX. *Braddom's Physical Medicine and Rehabilitation*. 5th ed. Philadelphia, PA: Elsevier; 2016:321.

6. ACSM. Quantity and quality of exercise for developing and maintaining cardiorespiratory, musculoskeletal, and neuromotor fitness in apparently healthy adults: Guidance for prescribing exercise. *Med Sci Sports Exerc*. 2011;43(7):1334–1359.

7. Riebe D, Franklin BA, Thompson PD, et al. Updating ACSM's Recommendations for Exercise Preparticipation Health Screening. *Med Sci Sports Exerc*. 2015;47(11):2473–2479.

CHAPTER 6

ACUPUNCTURE

BRIEF HISTORY AND BASIC CONCEPTS

Acupuncture has been in use for thousands of years. Its use is described in detail in *Huangdi Neijing* ("The Yellow Emperor's Classic of Internal Medicine"), which is the fundamental doctrinal text of Traditional Chinese Medicine (TCM). TCM theory describes a vital energy called *qi* that circulates in the body through pathways called meridians. Each meridian typically corresponds to an organ (e.g., the heart, liver, or gall bladder) and extends peripherally (e.g., a limb and/or head). Disease and pain are thought to occur when *qi* flow through these meridians is disturbed. Acupuncture needles are used to stimulate points along the meridians to restore proper *qi* flow.

As Western influence grew in China during the Qing dynasty (1644–1912), its leadership felt the need to modernize. Acupuncture was removed from the medical academy syllabus, and its practice gradually declined. In 1929, the Kuomintang officially outlawed its practice. In 1949, there was a resurgence of acupuncture in China as the Communist government sought to provide low-cost basic health care to the general population. In 1971, James Reston, a *New York Times* reporter, wrote a column describing his personal successful experience with acupuncture for postoperative pain following an emergency appendectomy while visiting China. A surge of interest in acupuncture in the United States and the West followed. In 1997, a National Institutes of Health (NIH) consensus conference published positive conclusions concerning the clinical effectiveness of acupuncture, particularly with respect to postoperative and chemotherapy-related nausea and vomiting, as well as postoperative dental pain. Acupuncture was described to be a potential adjunct or acceptable alternative in the treatment of various conditions such as headache (HA), tennis elbow, carpal tunnel syndrome (CTS), low back pain (LBP), myofascial pain, and osteoarthritis (OA). In 2003, the WHO published a review of clinical trials and listed 28 symptoms, conditions, or diseases that had been shown through clinical trials to be effectively treated by acupuncture, including HA, dental pain, temporomandibular joint (TMJ) dysfunction, neck pain, periarthritis of the shoulder, tennis elbow, LBP, sciatica, knee pain, sprains, rheumatoid arthritis (RA), stroke, essential hypertension, depression, postoperative pain, morning sickness, nausea/vomiting, gastritis, renal colic, primary dysmenorrhea, and adverse reactions to radiation or chemotherapy.

Acupuncture's mechanism of action remains inadequately understood from a Western scientific standpoint. There is an absence of evidence to support the existence of *qi* or the meridians. Nevertheless, physiologic effects have been observed when acupuncture points are stimulated, such as the release of neurotransmitters, endorphins, enkephalins, nerve growth factor, and endogenous cannabinoids. Mechanical movements or electrical stimulation of the acupuncture needle may potentiate these effects. Acupuncture likely derives some benefit from the proximity of acupuncture points to local nerves. Pain messaging may be reduced via acupuncture-induced action potentials traveling in sensory afferents to depress dorsal horn activity, compatible with the gate control theory of Melzack and Wall (1). Melzack and Wall, reported a high correlation between acupuncture points and myofascial trigger points, which they felt could be explained by the same underlying neural mechanisms. Functional MRI studies have also revealed that parts of the brain are activated and deactivated during needling.

One of the inherent methodological challenges of modern clinical acupuncture research has been identifying an ideal placebo control, given that "sham" acupuncture (i.e., at sites not generally accepted to be acupuncture points) can elicit responses that may not differ significantly from treatment given at accepted acupuncture points. More recently, non-penetrating acupuncture needles that retract back into the handle of the acupuncture needle after an initial skin prick have been utilized as placebos. These devices, however, are not standardized, and each has been found to have its own limitations.

NEEDLING TECHNIQUES, SAFETY, AND LICENSING

Most modern acupuncture needles are made of stainless steel and are available in a variety of lengths and fine gauges (typically #30 to #40 gauge), often described to be approximately the thickness of a single human hair. Different needling techniques besides simple insertion have been described to offer a stronger stimulation, including needle rotation, vibration, pecking, and electroacupuncture.

Although generally considered safe, some adverse reactions have been reported, most commonly bleeding and needling pain. Other adverse reactions include bruising and drowsiness. The risk of presyncope and syncope can be mitigated by flat positioning, close monitoring during an initial visit, and post-procedural observation until full recovery. The use of disposable, sterile needles eliminates the risk of cross-contamination. Major adverse events are rare, with pneumothorax the most frequently reported serious complication.

The American Board of Medical Acupuncture has established guidelines and qualification requirements for physicians to practice medical acupuncture in the United States. Licensing guidelines for the practice of acupuncture are determined by each specific state.

CLINCAL APPLICATIONS

Headaches – Studies have suggested a benefit of acupuncture in migraine HA prophylaxis over no acupuncture, with an effect similar to some prophylactic drugs (with fewer adverse effects). Multiple studies have shown a therapeutic effect of acupuncture over sham acupuncture in the treatment of migraine HAs (2). Auricular acupuncture may be a consideration in the management of migraine HAs. There are less available data regarding the effectiveness of acupuncture for tension HAs and other types of HAs.

Neck Pain – Acupuncture has been reported to be useful for the treatment of neck pain. High-quality data informing the literature, however, are limited. A review by Fu, Li, and Wu (3) noted that pooled data supported a quantitatively significant benefit of acupuncture over sham acupuncture for short-term pain relief, but qualitative review of the trial data limited the support of this conclusion. More recent high-quality data are lacking.

Carpal Tunnel Syndrome and Peripheral Neuropathy – Acupuncture has been shown to be associated with improved sensory and motor nerve conduction study parameters and decreased hyperactivity in the contralateral sensorimotor cortex on functional MRI in patients with CTS. Acupuncture has been reported to alleviate CTS symptoms, with effects similar to steroid injection therapy and night splinting. A 2017 systematic review by Dimitrova, Murchison, and Oken (4) noted that the majority of trials meeting review criteria showed a benefit of acupuncture over control in CTS, diabetic neuropathy, and Bell's palsy.

Low Back Pain – Acupuncture is widely used by patients with LBP. Improvements reported in the literature have included decreased pain, sleep disturbance, psychological distress, disability, and use of analgesics. A systematic review by Liu et al. (5) concluded that for acute LBP, there is inconsistent evidence that acupuncture relieves pain better than sham acupuncture and consistent evidence that acupuncture does not improve function better than sham acupuncture. For chronic LBP, the review noted that acupuncture improves pain on short-term follow-up versus sham acupuncture, but does not marginally improve function. For chronic LBP, the review noted that there is consistent evidence of short-term, clinically relevant benefit of acupuncture for pain and function in comparison to no treatment or when added to other treatment for chronic LBP.

Knee Pain and Osteoarthritis – Acupuncture has been reported to be an adjunctive therapy option for OA. A review by Manyanga et al. (6) concluded that acupuncture provides significant improvements in pain intensity, functional mobility, and health-related quality of life. Subgroup analyses suggested that acupuncture is most effective for reducing OA pain when administered for more than 4 weeks. The reviewers concluded that acupuncture is an alternative for traditional analgesics in patients with OA. A 2014 randomized controlled trial (RCT) by Hinman et al. (7; not included in the Manyanga et al. review) reported that neither laser nor needle acupuncture (× 12 weeks) improved pain or function in patients older than 50 years with moderate or severe chronic knee pain versus sham acupuncture. Benefits versus the no-acupuncture group were noted. Some criticisms of the methodology of the Hinman et al. (7) RCT have been published in the literature.

Rheumatoid Arthritis – Acupuncture has been reported to improve RA symptoms such as pain, joint mobility/morning stiffness, fatigue, depression, and insomnia, as well as findings such as grasp strength and laboratory markers. A review by Macfarlane et al. (8), however, noted a lack of high-quality evidence to support the efficacy of acupuncture in RA.

Postoperative Pain – Acupuncture may be useful in predictable situations involving acute pain, such as dental procedures and postoperative pain. Electroacupuncture before lower abdominal surgery has been reported to reduce postoperative analgesic requirements and decrease the side effects of systemic opioids.

Cancer Pain – Given the common adverse effects of pharmaceutical analgesics, complementary interventions such as acupuncture are increasingly being employed in the management of cancer-related pain. A review by Hu et al. (9) concluded that acupuncture alone does not have superior analgesic effects compared to conventional drug therapy for cancer-related pain, but acupuncture plus drug therapy (compared to drug therapy alone) results in increased pain remission rate, shorter onset time of pain relief, longer pain-free duration, and better quality of life, without serious adverse effects.

Stroke – Acupuncture has been used to treat stroke patients for many years in Asian countries. It is theorized that the analgesic effect of acupuncture encourages muscle relaxation, which results in improved muscle movement, function, and ability to participate and benefit from rehabilitation. Multiple trials have reported a benefit of acupuncture on poststroke spasticity. A 2015 meta-analysis by Lim et al. (10) noted that acupuncture could be effective in treating poststroke spasticity, but many studies had low methodological quality. A 2016 Cochrane review noted that trials have shown benefits of acupuncture versus no acupuncture, including for cognition, depression, pain, swallowing function, specific neurological impairments, and dependency level for activities of daily living. The Cochrane review noted no benefit of acupuncture versus sham acupuncture in motor function and quality of life for patients with stroke in the convalescent stage. Overall, the available data were interpreted to be of insufficient quality to allow conclusions regarding the routine use of acupuncture for stroke treatment.

REFERENCES

1. Melzack R, Wall PD. Pain mechanisms: a new theory. *Science.* 1965;150(3699): 971–979.
2. Millstine D, Chen CY, Bauer B. Complementary and integrative medicine in the management of headache. *BMJ.* 2017;357:j1805.

3. Fu LM, Li JT, Wu WS. Randomized controlled trials of accupuncture for neck pain: systematic review and meta-analysis. *J Altern Complement Med.* 2009 Feb;15(2):133–145.

4. Dimitrova A, Murchison C, Oken B. Acupuncture for the Treatment of Peripheral Neuropathy: A systematic review and meta-analysis. *J Altern Complement Med.* 2017;23(3):164–179.

5. Liu L, Skinner M, McDonough S, et al. Acupuncture for low back pain: an overview of systematic reviews. *Evid Based Complement Alternat Med.* 2015;2015:328196.

6. Manyanga T, Froese M, Zarychanski R, et al. Pain management with acupuncture in osteoarthritis: a systematic review and meta-analysis. *BMC Complement Altern Med.* 2014;14:312.

7. Hinman RS, McCrory P, Pirotta M, et al. Acupuncture for chronic knee pain: a randomized clinical trial. *JAMA.* 2014;312(13):1313–1322.

8. Macfarlane GJ, Paudyal P, Doherty M, et al. A systematic review of evidence for the effectiveness of practitioner-based complementary and alternative therapies in the management of rheumatic diseases: rheumatoid arthritis. *Rheumatology (Oxford).* 2012;51:1707–1713.

9. Hu C, Zhang H, Wu W, et al. Acupuncture for pain management in cancer: A systematic review and meta-analysis. *Evid Based Complement Alternat Med.* 2016;2016:1720239.

10. Lim SM, Yoo J, Lee E, et al. Acupuncture for spasticity after stroke: a systematic review and meta-analysis of randomized controlled trials. *Evid Based Complement Alternat Med.* 2015:870398.

SUGGESTED READING

Chen L, Michalsen A. Management of chronic pain using complementary and integrative medicine. *BMJ.* 2017;357:j1284.

Lam M, Galvin R, Curry P. Effectiveness of acupuncture for nonspecific chronic low back pain: a systematic review and meta-analysis. *Spine.* 2013;38:2124–2138.

Yang A, Wu HM, Tang JL. Acupuncture fokr stroke rehabilitation. *Cochrane Database Syst Rev.* 2016;(8):CD004131.

Zhang CS, Tan HY, Zhang GS. Placebo devices as effective control methods in acupuncture clinical trials: A systematic review. *PLoS One.* 2015;10(11):e0140825.

CHAPTER 7

AMPUTATION/PROSTHETICS

EPIDEMIOLOGY, ETIOLOGY, AND LEVELS OF AMPUTATION

In the United States, an estimated 185,000 people undergo amputation of an upper or lower limb each year. It was estimated that 1.6 million people were living with the loss of a limb in 2005, and this is expected to increase to 3.6 million by 2050. Amputation due to dysvascular disease accounts for 54% of cases, and of these, two thirds have a diagnosis of DM. Trauma accounts for 45% of cases, and cancer for the remaining less than 2% (Figures 7.1–7.3; 1). *Major amputation* refers to an amputation above the ankle. The level is determined by the extent of disease, the potential for healing, and rehabilitation potential of the patient, with the goal of preserving limb length while ensuring complete removal of all affected tissues. Physical exam findings and objective tests (ankle-brachial index [ABI], arterial Doppler, angiography, skin perfusion pressure, presence of pressure ulcers) to evaluate for ischemia are employed, and palpation of a pulse proximal to the level of amputation is associated with ~100% healing rate. *Primary amputation* refers to an amputation without the attempt at limb salvage (revascularization, bony repair, or soft tissue coverage), whereas *secondary amputation* refers to amputation following an attempt at limb salvage (2,3). In the setting of limb-threatening lower extremity trauma, according to the Lower Extremity Assessment Project (LEAP), there is no good measure to predict limb salvage versus amputation (4).

LOWER EXTREMITY AMPUTATION

Preferred Mature Residual Limb Length and Shape

Transhumeral (TH) – Cylindrical appendage with retention of the deltoid tuberosity. Generally, the longer, the better (up to 90% of normal length).

Transradial (TR) – Ideal shape follows the contours of the natural limb. Longer appendages provide better lever arms and more pronation/supination, and are optimal for body-powered prostheses and heavy labor. Retention of the brachioradialis improves elbow flexion. Medium-length limbs are optimal for externally powered prostheses.

Transfemoral (TF) – Ideal shape is conical. Longer residual limbs improve seating balance and tolerance. For shorter limbs, maintaining the greater trochanter and its attachment to the hip abductors is key. Myodesis surgical technique provides increased stability in adduction, and increased hip flexion (HF) and extension. Myoplasty may be

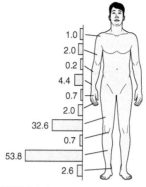

FIGURE 7.1 Percentage of amputations by site.

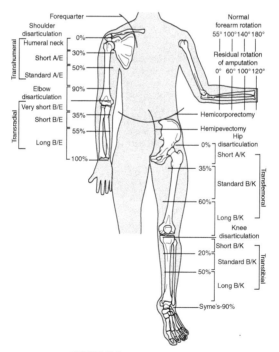

FIGURE 7.2 Amputation terminology.
A/E, above elbow; A/K, above knee; A/E, above elbow; B/K, below knee.

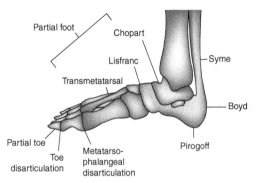

FIGURE 7.3 Foot amputation levels; mnemonic: The chopart is shorter, the *lisfranc* is longer.

preferable in severely dysvascular patients. In either technique, muscle mass tapering is required to avoid excess distal bulk, which may affect prosthesis fit.

Transtibial (TT) – This is the most common amputation and is the most proximal level at which near-normal function is available. Ideal shape and length is a cylindrical appendage about one third the original tibial length, with retention of the patellar tendon attachment to the tibial tuberosity. The fibula should be shorter than the tibia. In vascular disease, longer limbs may not have adequate circulatory supply, and fitting of the below-knee socket may be problematic. The ideal length recommended from medial tibial plateau to bony end is 5" to 7".

Postamputation Preprosthetic Care

Wound Care – Keep limb clean and protected and debride any nonviable tissue. Monitor for signs of infection especially in patients with fever or excessive residual limb pain (2).

Edema Control

- Elastic wraps: Most commonly Ace bandages using a *figure-of-eight elastic* wrapping technique and should begin immediately after surgery. May be time-consuming as ideally rewrapped qid and taught to patient. A residual limb (stump) shrinker may also be used.
- Elastic socks: Alternative to wraps. Not expensive and easy to apply.
- Rigid dressings: Protective. Allow for weight bearing to desensitize the limb. Examples include the *immediate postoperative-fitting prosthesis*, which is not removable and therefore inhibits ability to check and desensitize the skin. The *removable rigid dressing* is custom-made and allows for wound inspection and desensitization.

Scar Mobilization – Scar mobilization massage should be instituted as soon as tolerated to help prevent adherence of the scar to the underlying soft tissues and bone. Once the sutures are removed, massage can be performed more aggressively.

Anti-Contracture Management – Due to muscle imbalance. Above-knee amputations (AKAs) commonly develop HF, hip abduction, and hip external rotation contractures. In addition, below-knee amputations (BKA) develop knee flexion (KF) contractures. Prevent with a firm mattress, prone lying 15 minute tid, promoting knee extension while resting. A posterior splint to maintain knee extension can be considered for patients at higher risk.

Preprosthetic and Prosthetic Training – Hip active range of motion (AROM) and strengthening exercises are key. A good test to determine cardiovascular tolerance for prosthesis use is ambulation (hopping) with a walker (without a prosthesis). Prosthetic gait training should begin with parallel bars and progress to walkers or canes. Crutches should be avoided, since they promote poor gait patterns. The *preparatory prosthesis* is fitted while the residual limb is still molding, and *definitive prosthesis* is usually created at 3 to 6 months.

TT PROSTHETICS

TT Socket Designs
The socket connects the residual limb to the rest of the prosthesis and plays an important role in the transfer of body weight to the ground (Figure 7.4). For any socket, soft inserts made of polyethylene foam or silicone gel provide extra protection, for example, for cases of peripheral vascular disease (PVD) or extensive scarring. The inserts, however, reduce the intimacy of contact between the limb and prosthesis, which is important for proprioception. A soft foam distal end discourages verrucous hyperplasia formation.

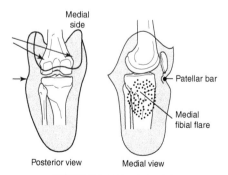

FIGURE 7.4 Total contact socket.

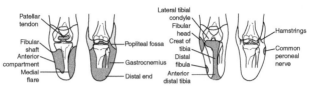

FIGURE 7.5 Pressure-tolerant/sensitive areas in the TT total contact socket.
TT, transtibial.
Source: Adapted from Ref. (5).

The *patellar tendon–bearing socket* uses the patellar tendon and soft tissues as partial weight-bearing surfaces to distribute weight over "pressure-tolerant areas" (Figure 7.5), but not over the bony prominences. The *total surface–bearing socket* (Figure 7.4) distributes pressure across the entire residual limb surface, in addition to bony areas sensitive to increased pressure. Additional socket options include the rigid external frame with flexible inner socket. Addition of socks may be used if fluctuating edema is present as well as silicone liners to protect skin.

Selected TT Suspension Options

Sleeve – An elastic sleeve can serve as a primary or secondary suspension via longitudinal tension, negative pressure during swing phase, and friction between the residual limb and socket. It can provide additional security for short residual limbs, when mediolateral knee stability is questionable or when hyperextension control is required.

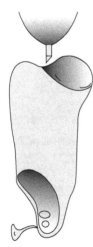

Silicone Locking Liner – A flexible, molded silicone liner is rolled directly onto the residual limb and secured to the socket with a pin. This provides optimal suspension, proprioception, and increased range of motion in flexion, but requires stable limb volumes and good hand dexterity for donning/doffing (Figure 7.6).

Supracondylar and Supracondylar–Suprapatellar Suspension – Includes a brim suspension as an extension of the socket over the medial and lateral femoral condyles, which provides increased mediolateral knee stability and may be useful for short residual limbs. A supracondylar cuff with fork strap and waist belt suspension provides additional stability for very active patients, for example, manual laborers.

FIGURE 7.6 Silicone locking liner.

Elevated Vacuum Suspension – Consists of a gel liner, suspension sleeve, and air evacuation pump, which creates a negative pressure and seal to anchor the liner tightly within the socket. Maintains limb volume throughout the day, which improves prosthetic control and proprioception, and avoids loosening within the socket and shear forces causing skin breakdown (Figure 7.7).

Selected Foot–Ankle Assembly Options

The prosthetic foot should serve as a simulation of the original foot-and-ankle joint and musculature to provide normal energy-efficient gait, shock absorption, and sufficient weight-bearing base of support.

Solid Ankle Cushioned Heel Foot – SACH feet are light, durable, inexpensive, and stable. The soft heel simulates plantar flexion (PF) during heel strike and provides good shock absorption (Figure 7.8A). It is most commonly used for children and most adult TT amputees or ankle disarticulations.

Single-Axis Foot – These feet are heavier but less durable than the SACH feet and are available for exo- and endoskeletal prostheses. They are most commonly used for TF amputees, that is, when knee stability is desired (a quick foot flat improves knee stability). Only sagittal axis movement is allowed.

Multiaxis Foot (Greissinger, Endolite Multiflex, SAFE II, TruStep) – The multiaxis foot provides significant ankle motion and improved balance

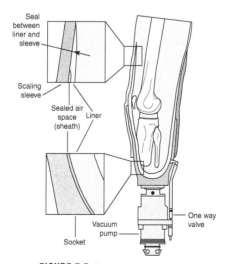

FIGURE 7.7 Elevated vacuum suspension.

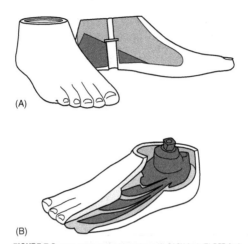

FIGURE 7.8 Foot–ankle assembly options. (A) SACH foot. (B) DER foot.
SACH, solid ankle cushioned heel.
Source: Adapted from Ref. (5).

and coordination by allowing PF/dorsiflexion (DF), inversion/eversion, and rotation. It provides good shock absorption and is good for uneven ground, but is heavy and costly, and needs relatively frequent adjustments or repairs.

DER Foot (Seattle Light, Carbon Copy II, Quantum Foot, Flex-Foot, SpringLite) – These feet were formerly called "energy-storing feet," but they have *not* demonstrated a reduction in the energy cost or rate of energy expenditure during level walking, compared with the SACH foot (3). They may, however, be more efficient than other feet at higher speeds. Geriatric amputees benefit from the light weight of these feet (Figure 7.8B).

TF PROSTHETICS

Traditional Socket Designs

TF sockets are often fitted in slight (5°) flexion and adduction to stretch the hip extensors and abductors to provide a mechanical advantage including knee stability at heel contact. The socket should allow stabilizing pressures on the skeletal structures while allowing for neurovascular integrity. Forces should be distributed over the largest area.

Quadrilateral Design – This ischial–gluteal weight-bearing, *narrow anteroposterior* design has four sides and four corners, which allow weight bearing through the ischium and gluteal muscles. It is easy to make and fit and most successful for long, firm residual limbs but less stable for shorter residual limbs and less comfortable in a seated position (Figure 7.9A).

Ischial Containment Design – A "bony lock" incorporates the ischial tuberosity, pubic ramus, and greater trochanter. The posterior rim provides weight bearing through the medial ischium and ischial ramus and is contoured for the ischial tuberosity and gluteal muscles. These features improve stability, particularly for shorter and fleshy residual limbs. The *narrow mediolateral* design also provides a more efficient energy cost of ambulation than the narrow anteroposterior design at high speeds (Figure 7.9B).

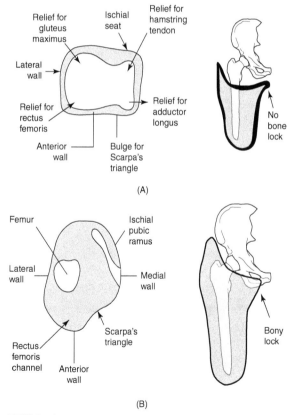

(A)

(B)

FIGURE 7.9 TF prosthetics. (A) Quadrilateral design. (B) Ischial containment design. TF, transfemoral.

Selected TF Suspension Options

Suction – Utilizes a one-way valve and liner with concentric rings to maintain prosthetic attachment during swing phase. It is lightweight, providing appropriate suspension and proprioceptive feedback, and indicated in active amputees with good balance and well-shaped and unfluctuating residual limbs. This can be provided using a silicone seal-in liner or via a skin suction suspension, pulling the residual limb into the socket with a pull sock or a donning sleeve through a hole in the bottom of the socket.

Silicone Seal-in liner With Pin-Locking or Lanyard Strap – Offers a secure suspension using a gel liner rolled onto the residual limb with either a pin or cord attached to the bottom as the interface between the residual limb and socket.

Lanyard Strap – The lanyard is attached to the distal end of the insert (generally silicone) and fed through the bottom of the socket.

Silesian Belt or Bandage – A belt that attaches from the socket at the greater trochanter and wraps around the opposite iliac crest (Figure 7.10A). It aids in rotational control and is adjustable; however, skin breakdown and chafing may be seen in obese patients.

Total Elastic Suspension (Belt) – Wraps around the proximal prosthesis and waist, enhancing rotational control. It retains body heat and has limited durability but is more comfortable than a Silesian belt (Figure 7.10B).

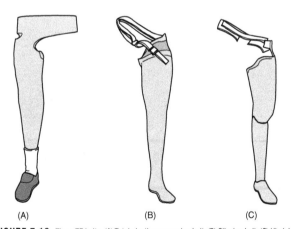

(A)   (B)   (C)

FIGURE 7.10 Three TF belts. (A) Total elastic suspension belt. (B) Silesian belt. (C) Hip joint with pelvic band.
TF, transfemoral.
Source: Adapted from Ref. (5).

Pelvic Band-and-Belt Suspension – A rigid belt is connected to a metal hip joint on the lateral side of the socket. It is indicated for improving rotational and mediolateral pelvic stability in obese patients with especially weak abductors and short or poorly shaped residual limbs. It is heavy and bulky and tends to interfere with sitting (Figure 7.10C).

Selected Knee Components: Key Features

Single-Axis Manual Locking Knee – This design provides the ultimate stability but the gait is awkward and energy consuming, as the knee remains locked for standing and ambulation and unlocked while seated. It is a durable and inexpensive knee with a fixed cadence to avoid an asymmetric swing phase. It is indicated for level surface ambulation and commonly used in geriatric and debilitated patients with poor hip control (Figure 7.11).

Stance Phase Control Knee – Provides KF control during weight bearing and constant friction during swing phase, which provides increased stability and allows for ambulation on uneven surfaces and prevents buckling. A delayed swing phase is noted, as full unloading is needed to flex the knee. The constant friction during swing phase is set for one general walking speed or fixed cadence.

Polycentric – This typically has a four-bar linkage design, and a shifting center of rotation provides a moment of force into extension at heel

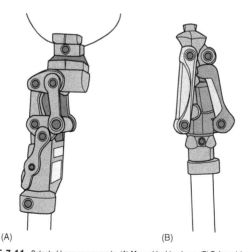

(A)   (B)

FIGURE 7.11 Selected knee components. (A) Manual locking knee. (B) Polycentric knee.
Source: Adapted from Ref. (5).

strike. The center of rotation moves proximally and posteriorly to the anatomic knees and provides increased stability during stance phase. Cosmesis is excellent, especially during sitting, but polycentrics are heavy and costly but quite durable. It is indicated for knee disarticulations and long TF amputees (Figure 7.11B).

Swing and Stance Phase Control Hydraulic Knee Unit (Oil or Pneumatic) – This design uses a piston in a fluid-filled cylinder, which provides variable resistance during swing phase, so the patient is able to vary the cadence. It provides a smooth and natural gait, but is heavy, costly, and requires higher maintenance. Available in single-axis and polycentric models.

Microprocessor-Controlled Hydraulic Knee Joint – Microprocessors gather information on the gait cycle (i.e., position, ankle movement, angular velocity of knee) and electronically adjust the resistance of the knee. There is a high level of resistance in stance phase, permitting weight bearing on the prosthesis during flexion, yielding low-energy expenditure and improved gait symmetry on stairs, inclines, and uneven terrain; it is thus appropriate for K3 or K4 amputees. Disadvantages include having to recharge the battery every night, increased cost, and high maintenance.

Functional Levels

In order to create an individualized prescription to include the appropriate components for a lower limb prosthesis, the provider must assess a patient's current and potential functional abilities as well as intended use of the prosthesis. Components of the prescription include socket, interface, suspension, pylon, and foot/ankle type.

Functional Level 0 (K0) – The patient lacks the ability to transfer or ambulate safely. The use of a prosthesis would not enhance mobility or quality of life. No prosthesis is provided.

Functional Level 1 (K1) – The patient is able/capable of transferring and ambulating on level surfaces at a fixed cadence—a *household ambulator*. Recommended: single-axis, constant friction knee and single-axis or SACH foot.

Functional Level 2 (K2) – The patient is able/capable of ambulating community distances and traverse small environmental barriers (uneven surfaces, curbs, stairs)—a *community ambulator*. Prosthesis components should be alignable and foot can be multiaxial or flexible.

Functional Level 3 (K3) – The patient is able/capable of ambulating community distances with variable cadence and traversing most environmental barriers and uneven terrain—an *unlimited community ambulator*. Prosthesis will include consideration of fluid and pneumatic control knees with an energy-storing or dynamic response foot.

Functional Level 4 (K4) – The patient's capabilities exceed everyday requirements for basic ambulation including *high level of impact, stress, and energy*—includes athletes, active adults, and children. A hydraulic knee and specialized feet (running, waterproof, adjustable heel height) may be considered as well as a backup suspension.

Selected Postamputation Complications

Pain – In one national survey, approximately 95% of amputees reported one or more types of pain related to amputation: 80% phantom pain, 68% residual limb pain, and 62% back pain (9). Poorly controlled pre- and postoperative pain may increase the risk of chronic amputation pain.

Phantom Pain – Phantom limb sensation, phantom limb pain, and generalized limb pain are maintained by afferent, central, and efferent dysfunction (4). Phantom limb pain can be sharp, burning, stabbing, tingling, shooting, electric, or cramping (10). Treatment options include desensitization (e.g., massaging and tapping), neuropathic pain agents, topical anesthetics, modalities (e.g., TENS units, mirror therapy), and injections into neuromas.

Choke Syndrome – Distal limb edema and painful *verrucous hyperplasia* may develop due to proximal limb pressure and a lack of total contact with the prosthesis. An underlying vascular disorder is usually present. Treatment involves adding a distal pad to the socket, correcting the suspension, removing proximal pressure, and/or refitting the socket.

PROSTHETIC GAIT ANALYSIS

Relationship between amputation level(s) and energy cost and speed is shown in Figure 7.12.

Causes of Stance Phase Problems

Excessive Trunk Extension/Lumbar Lordosis During Stance Phase – A poorly shaped posterior wall may cause patients to forward rotate their pelvis for pressure relief, with compensatory trunk extension. Other causes include insufficient initial socket flexion, HF contracture, and weak hip extensors or abdominal muscles.

Foot Slap – Foot slap may be noted with a TF locked-knee prosthesis if the foot is posteriorly placed or if socket flexion is excessive.

Knee Buckling/Instability – Causes include knee axis too anterior, insufficient PF, failure to limit DF, weak hip extensors, hard heel, large HF contracture, and posteriorly placed foot. Stability is achieved with a plantar-flexed or anteriorly placed foot, or a soft heel (i.e., SACH).

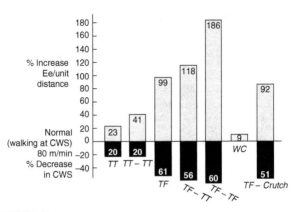

FIGURE 7.12 Graph showing relationship of amputation level(s) with energy cost and speed. CWS corresponds to the minimum energy cost per unit distance. Energy expenditure (Ee)/unit distance and CWS for amputees using prostheses are compared with able-bodied subjects at a CWS of 80 m/min (≈3 mi/h). The energy cost of ambulation at CWS for able-bodied subjects is 4.3 kcal/min.

TF, transfemoral; TT, transtibial; WC, wheelchair.
Source: Adapted from Ref. (7).

Lateral Bending – Generally occurs to the prosthetic side. Causes include a prosthesis that is too short, insufficient lateral wall, abducted socket, abduction contracture, and poor amputee balance.

Vaulting – Vaulting of the nonprosthetic limb may be due to a prosthesis that is too long, too much knee friction, or poor suspension.

Whip – A whip is an abrupt rotation of the heel occurring at the end of stance phase as the knee of a TF prosthesis is flexed to begin swing. If the heel moves medially during initial flexion, it is a medial whip; if laterally, a lateral whip. Causes include improper rotatory alignment of the knee axis, a knee axis not parallel to the floor, flabby muscles about the femur with the prosthesis rotating freely within the underlying soft tissue, or a socket that is too tight.

Causes of Swing Phase Problems

Abducted Gait – Causes include a prosthesis that is too long, an abduction contracture, or a medial socket wall encroaching the groin.

Circumducted Gait – Causes include a prosthesis that is too long, too much knee friction making it difficult to bend the knee during swing-through, or an abduction contracture.

Excessive Heel Rise – Causes include insufficient knee friction or excessive KF moment (i.e., posterior foot or insufficient PF at heel strike).

Foot Drag – Causes include inadequate suspension, a prosthesis that is too long, insufficient HF or KF, or weak PF of the nonprosthetic limb.

Terminal Swing Impact – Insufficient knee friction may cause the amputee to deliberately and forcibly extend the knee.

UPPER EXTREMITY AMPUTATION

Upper extremity amputations are most commonly due to traumatic injuries followed by malignancies and dysvascular disease (1). Additionally, approximately 58.5% of newborn congenital defects are upper limb deficiencies, most often left transverse terminal radial limb (6). The upper extremity orthosis must be able to perform gross and fine motor skills needed by the amputee. Unilateral amputees typically learn to perform most ADLs with their intact hand. Bilateral amputees often use their feet for many ADLs. Functional upper extremity prostheses should be prescribed for highly motivated patients with realistic expectations. Residual limb shaping with bandages may be required for 1 to 2 months before prosthetic fitting to ensure precise fit and appropriate alignment to protect bony prominences, avoid compression of peripheral nerves, and allow for sensory feedback for appropriate function. If fitting is not performed within a 3-to-6-month window after unilateral amputation, long-term prosthesis use is infrequently seen.

TR PROSTHETICS

A TR amputation allows for a high level of functional ability and can be performed at three levels: long (55%–90% residual limb), short (35%–55%), and very short (<35%). Longer residual limbs allow for improved cosmesis and functionally provide lever arm and more pronation/supination greater lever arm. Body-powered prostheses with hooks or hands are typically prescribed for manual laborers (the typical patient who is going to suffer a traumatic upper extremity amputation in the first place). Lifting up to 20 to 30 lb. can be expected. Myoelectric prostheses are typically more appropriate for relatively sedentary amputees (Figure 7.13).

TH PROSTHETICS

Longer residual limbs (up to 90% of original/expected length) are preferred. Function is usually much poorer than with a TR amputation. Key differences for TH prostheses include the need for an elbow unit and different harnessing and control systems. Lifting between 10 and 15 lb. can be expected (more with a shoulder saddle). Length estimates for bilateral TH amputees are 19% of patient height for the upper arm and 21% for the forearm component.

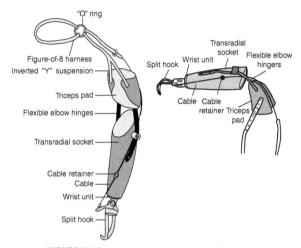

FIGURE 7.13 Commonly seen components in a TR prosthesis.
Source: Adapted from Ref. (5).

Functional Terminal Devices

Terminal devices (TDs) are the most important functional part of the upper extremity prosthesis. They are classified as active or passive. *Passive TDs* provide cosmesis and minimal function (e.g., ball handling or child mitt for crawling). *Active TDs* are broken into hooks and artificial hands. Hooks may have prehensors with thumb- and fingerlike components. The proximal limb/prosthesis essentially functions to position the TD in space. *Body-powered voluntary opening split hooks* are the most common and practical TDs. In these devices, the TD is closed at rest. Prehensile force is predetermined by the number of rubber bands in place (each rubber band requires 5 lb. of force to provide 1 lb. of pinch force). Up to 10 bands can be used (typical nonamputee male pinch force is 15 to 20 lb.; Figure 7.14A).

Voluntary closing TDs provide a better control of closing pressure, but active effort is required to maintain closure of the TD, or items may be dropped (Figure 7.14B).

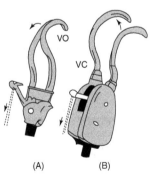

FIGURE 7.14 Functional terminal devices.
(A) Voluntary opening. (B) Voluntary closing.

Myoelectric hands offer spherical/palmar grasp with grip forces higher than body-powered TDs. They can have a lifelike appearance but are relatively fragile. Two-site two-function controllers use different muscles to open and close the TD, while one-site two-function controllers use weak versus strong contractions of the same muscle to operate the TD (Table 7.1).

Other Upper Limb Prosthesis Components

The **prosthetic wrist unit**, held in place by a friction or mechanical lock, provides orientation of the TD in space. The most common is the *friction wrist*, which allows passive pronation/supination, but it rotates and can slip when holding heavy objects. Bilateral amputees require at least one mechanical spring-assisted *flexion wrist* for access to the body midline.

The **elbow unit** is selected based on the level of amputation and residual function; pronation and supination decrease as the

TABLE 7.1 Upper Extremity Essential Components

	Control		Shape	
	Body powered	Myoelectric	Hook	Hand
Function				
Fine tip prehension	—	—	√	—
Cylindrical grip (large diameter)	—	—	—	√
Cylindrical grip (small diameter)	—	—	√	—
High grip force	—	—	—	—
Delicate grip force	—	√	—	—
Hook and pull	—	—	√	—
Pushing/holding down	—	—	—	√
Ruggedness	√	—	√	—
Comfort	—	—	—	—
Low weight	√	—	√	—
Harness comfort	—	√	—	—
Low effort	—	√	—	—
Reliability/convenience	√	—	√	—
Cosmesis	—	—	—	√
Low cost	√	—	—	—

Source: Adapted from Ref. (8).

amputation site becomes more proximal. Most TH prosthetic elbows have an *alternator lock*, which alternately locks and unlocks with the same movement. With the elbow unlocked, body movements will flex or extend the elbow using a cable; when locked, the same cable operates the TD.

The traditional **suspension** employs straps and cables, with a double-walled **socket** for optimal fit. The outer wall is rigid and connects to other components; the inner wall must fit precisely with the residual limb, or else the prosthesis may fail. The *suction socket* provides self-suspension without straps and is preferred for the TH amputee. The *Munster supracondylar socket* provides self-suspension for a very short TR or elbow disarticulation by encasing the humeral condyles and can be used for externally powered prostheses. Proper fit of the Munster socket limits full elbow extension.

The **body harness** uses cables to allow body motion and effort to operate prosthetic components. The *figure-of-8*, generally for a short TR or more proximal amputation, holds the socket firmly in place, usually with an elbow hinge and half-arm cuff or triceps pad. The *figure-of-9*, generally for a long TR or wrist disarticulation, requires a self-suspending socket but is more comfortable than the figure-of-8. The *shoulder saddle with chest strap* frees the opposite shoulder and relieves the pressure caused by the axillary loop of the figure-of-8. Heavy loads are better tolerated, but donning is difficult and cosmesis is inferior.

Body-Powered Prosthesis Control

Glenohumeral (GH) Forward Flexion (TR, TH) – This natural movement provides substantial power and reach, allowing for activation of the TD or flexion of an elbow joint (Figure 7.15A).

Biscapular Abduction (forequarter, shoulder disarticulation, TH, TR) – This movement permits activation of a TD, but it must stay relatively stationary. The forces generated are relatively weak and sufficient for fine motor activities located at the midline (Figure 7.15B).

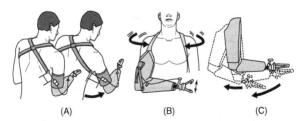

(A)   (B)   (C)

FIGURE 7.15 Body-powered prosthesis control. (A) GH. (B) Biscapular abduction. (C) GH depression, extension, abduction.
GH, glenohumeral.

GH Depression, Extension, Abduction (TH) – This movement locks or unlocks an elbow, but may be unnatural for some users and difficult to master (Figure 7.15C).

Scapular Elevation – This locks or unlocks the elbow and is easy to master. It requires a waist belt.

Chest Expansion/Scapular Adduction – This locks or unlocks the elbow. It is an awkward motion, but does not interfere with TD operations.

REFERENCES

1. Ziegler-Graham K, MacKenzie EJ, Ephraim PL, et al. Estimating the prevalence of limb loss in the United States: 2005 to 2050. *Arch Phys Med Rehabil.* 2008;89(3):422–429.

2. Dillingham TR, Pezzin LE, MacKenzie EJ. Limb amputation and limb deficiency: epidemiology and recent trends in the United States. *South Med J.* 2002;95(8):875–883.

3. Vemulapalli S, Greiner MA, Jones WS, et al. Peripheral arterial testing before lower extremity amputation among Medicare beneficiaries, 2000 to 2010. *Circ Cardiovasc Qual Outcomes.* 2014;7(1):142–150.

4. Higgins TF, Klatt JB, Beals TC. Lower Extremity Assessment Project (LEAP)—the best available evidence on limb-threatening lower extremity trauma. *Orthop Clin North Am.* 2010;41(2):233–239.

5. Cifu DX. *Braddom's Physical Medicine and Rehabilitation.* 5th ed. Philadelphia, PA: Elsevier; 2016.

6. Ephraim PL, Wegener ST, MacKenzie EJ, et al. Phantom pain, residual limb pain, and back pain in amputees: Results of a national survey. *Arch Phys Med Rehabil.* 2005;86(10):1910–1919.

7. Gonzalez EG, ed. *Downey and Darling's The Physiological Basis of Rehabilitation Medicine.* 3rd ed. Boston, MA: Butterworth Heinemann; 2001

8. Dillingham T (specialist ed.). *Rehabilitation of the Injured Combatant Part IV.* Office of the Surgeon General, Department of the Army; 1998.

9. Goktepe AS, Cakir B, Yilmaz B, Yazicioglu K. Energy expenditure of walking with prostheses: comparison of three amputation levels. *Prosthet Orthot Int.* 2010;34(1):31–36.

10. Potter BK et al. *Atlas of Amputations and Limb Prosthetics: Surgical, Prosthetic and Rehabilitation Principles.* Rosemont, IL; 2016.

SUGGESTED READING

Casale R, Alaa L, Mallick M, Ring H. Phantom limb related phenomena and their rehabilitation after lower limb amputation. *Eur J Phys Rehabil Med.* 2009;45(4):559–566.

Delussu AS, Paradisi F, Brunelli S, et al. Comparison between SACH foot and a new multiaxial prosthetic foot during walking in hypomobile transtibial amputees: Physiological responses and functional assessment. *Eur J Phys Rehabil Med.* 2016;52(3):304–309.

Eftekhari N. Amputation rehabilitation. In: O'Young BJ, ed. *Physical Medicine & Rehabilitation Secrets.* 2nd ed. Philadelphia, PA: Hanley & Belfus; 2002:553.

Foell J, Bekrater-Bodmann R, Flor H, Cole J. Phantom limb pain after lower limb trauma: origins and treatments. *Int J Low Extrem Wounds*. 2011;10(4): 224–235.

Garrison SJ. *Handbook of Physical Medicine and Rehabilitation Basics*. Philadelphia, PA: Lippincott Williams & Wilkins Handbook Series; 2003.

Hanley MA, Jensen MP, Smith DG, et al. Preamputation pain and acute pain predict chronic pain after lower extremity amputation. *J Pain*. 2007;8(2):102.

Kelly BM. Orthotic and prosthetic prescription for today and tomorrow. *Phys Med Rehabil Clin N Am*. 2007;18(4):785–858.

CHAPTER 8

PEDIATRICS: CEREBRAL PALSY

Definition – A group of disorders of the development of movement and posture, causing activity limitations that are attributed to a nonprogressive disturbance that has occurred in the developing fetal or infant brain (1).

Cerebral palsy (CP) affects approximately 3 per 1,000 school-aged children. Live birth incidence is about 2/1,000 for term infants. The highest incidence of 82/1,000 live births occurs in preterm infants <28 weeks gestation and decreases to 6.8/1,000 live births for those of 32 to 36 weeks of gestation. **Risk factors** include prenatal, perinatal, and postnatal infection, stroke, toxins, neonatal encephalopathy, complications of prematurity (small for gestational age [SGA], birth weight [BW] <800 g, intraventricular hemorrhage [IVH]), intrauterine growth restriction, maternal chorioamnionitis, fever during labor, coagulopathy or bleeding, placental infarction, thyroid disease, hyperbilirubinemia, multiple births, and trauma. The greatest risk factor is prematurity; neonatal encephalopathy is the best predictor of CP in term infants.

CP can be classified by movement type—spastic (70%–85%), dyskinetic, hypotonic, ataxic, and mixed or by anatomic distribution—hemiparesis, diparesis, and quadriparesis.

Mobility function based on age using the Gross Motor Function Classification System:

Level 1. Walks without limitations

Level 2. Walks with limitations

Level 3. Walks using a handheld mobility device

Level 4. May walk short distances with assistive device but may rely on power mobility

Level 5. Self-mobility severely limited

Diagnosis of CP is based on a careful history and examination. A few key items to look for based on developmental milestones include persistence of primitive reflexes after 6 months, asymmetry or obligatory response, early handedness/failure to use the involved hand or early rolling (from tone). Greater than 80% have abnormal neuroimaging, most often periventricular leukomalacia (PVL) following IVH in premature infants, focal cortical infarcts secondary to middle cerebral artery (MCA) stroke in hemiparesis, basal ganglia and thalamic lesions in dystonic CP, brain malformations, and generalized encephalomalacia in spastic quadriparesis. MRI is more likely to show an abnormality, compared with CT (2).

Associated disorders include the following: sensory impairments, especially in hemiparesis; hearing, visual, cognitive, psychological, oromotor, nutritional, genitourinary, respiratory, bone mineral density, and dental impairments in 10% to 50%; pain in 50% to 75%; gastrointestinal (GI) disorders in 90% with abdominal pain, constipation, gastroesophageal reflux disease (GERD), and swallowing disorders being most common; and seizures in 15% to 55% (3). Musculoskeletal disorders include hip dysplasia, dislocation, scoliosis, low bone mineral density, spasticity, and contractures. Gait impairments can include scissoring, intoeing, crouch gait, stiff knee, toe gait.

Treatment of CP includes therapy and medical management of spasticity. Spasticity treatment includes oral medications, chemical neurolysis, and intrathecal baclofen. In regard to therapy, no clear evidence in support of a particular approach exists. Neurodevelopmental treatment (NDT) and sensory integration therapy (SIT), however, are not recommended approaches. Therapy may include stretching, strengthening, tone management, and functional training. Surgical management of spasticity includes selective dorsal rhizotomy, which involves sectioning of a portion of abnormal L2 to S1 sensory nerve rootlets to reduce excitatory input. This procedure is favorable in patients aged 3 to 8 years who have selective motor control and functional strength with lack of significant contractures. Negative effects can include hypotonia and bladder dysfunction, which are usually transient, weakness, and spinal deformity including spondylolysis/listhesis and hip dislocation. Other orthopedic interventions such as serial casting, muscle–tendon lengthening and transfers, and osteotomy can be used as part of the treatment plan.

Outcomes may vary, but generally, there is good prognosis for ambulation if there is independent sitting by age 2 years, reciprocal crawl at 1½ to 2½ years, and supine to prone by 18 months (4–6). A poor prognosis for ambulation can generally be expected if there is presence of three or more primitive reflexes at 18 to 24 months. Life expectancy is reduced with immobility and inability to self-feed (7).

CONGENITAL BRACHIAL PLEXUS PALSY

Congenital brachial plexus palsy (CBPP) occurs in 1 to 2/1,000 live births in the United States. *Risk factors* include a multiparous mother, increased birth weight, and shoulder dystocia, which is the only established risk factor (8). Most cases are unilateral in presentation and clinical features depend on the affected level. Erb's palsy (C5, C6, C7) accounts for most cases and presents with shoulder internal rotation and adduction, elbow extension and pronation, and wrist flexion.

Main features in a C8, T1 lesion, which rarely occurs exclusively, include Horner's syndrome and isolated hand paralysis. This is more often seen in complete brachial plexus palsy C5–T1.

Spontaneous recovery is seen in 50% to 90% of cases. Associated injuries include facial palsy, cephalohematoma, clavicle or humerus fracture, torticollis, cervical spine injury, diaphragmatic injury, and Horner's syndrome (with lower plexus injury).

Diagnosis is often made at birth with weakness noted in the affected arm. Physical exam should include a detailed neurologic examination with focus on the stimulated motor and sensory responses a well as reflexes, noting any deficits. ROM should also be assessed both actively and passively. Neuroimaging such as MRI should be conducted to rule out fractures and neuromas. Ultrasound (US) needs to be studied further to determine its diagnostic utility in congenital brachial plexus injury. According to one review, electrodiagnostic studies should be conducted within 48 hours after birth and then repeated at approximately 1 week to aid outcome prediction (9). However, the role of electrodiagnostics as a reliable prognosticator has yet to be established.

Goals of treatment are to normalize limb function, optimize nerve regeneration, and allow elbow flexion and shoulder stabilization. Limb positioning is important to increase awareness, ROM, splinting, and developmental training. Surgery is indicated if antigravity strength is not present at the elbow at 6 months (10). Other literature cites early surgical intervention between age 3 and 9 months. Orthopedically, tendon releases/transfers may be used as well as early pinning to avoid shoulder stretch and gentle ROM to consider pain due to traumatic neuritis. Neurosurgical options include neurolysis of scar and fibrotic tissue, end-to-end anastomosis, nerve transfer of the sural or great auricular nerves, and end-to-side neurorrhaphy. Recovery by 3 months is a good prognosticator for normal function (11). Limited elbow flexion at 6 months may be predictive of poor prognosis.

Complications may include muscle atrophy, contracture, developmental concerns, glenoid dysplasia with posterior subluxation, issues of cosmesis, and pain, which may be indicated by biting the limb (possibly more in children who have had surgery).

SPECIAL CONSIDERATIONS IN PEDIATRIC SCI

Approximately 3% to 5% of all spinal cord injuries (SCIs) occur in children under the age of 15 years and 20% of all SCIs occur in those under 20 years of age (12). In children under 9 years of age, boys are four times more likely to be affected, compared with girls. Racial differences exist in those over 15 years, with overall increased risk for African Americans and Hispanic Americans.

The most common causes (in order) of pediatric SCI are motor vehicle accidents MVAs, falls (under 10 years), and sports (15 to 16 years). C5–C8 level injuries are most common. Pediatric patients are prone to higher cervical injuries due to their relatively large head size compared to adults and because the developing spine is more mobile, favoring stretch injury to ligaments without bony fracture. Fifty percent age <10 years had occiput-C1 injury, and 50% were neurologically intact SCI without radiographic abnormality (SCIWORA).

Management is an area of difference from the adult population. Deep vein thrombosis prophylaxis is not clear in children (13,14). Younger children with high lumbar or thoracic levels may be ambulatory with bracing but become more wheelchair dependent at adolescence (more energy efficient).

Children with SCI are at risk for orthopedic conditions not seen in skeletally mature adults with SCI, including scoliosis and hip subluxation or dislocation. Scoliosis occurs in almost all cases of pediatric SCI that have not reached skeletal maturity, with two thirds requiring surgical management. Although compliance rate is low, thoracolumbosacral orthoses (TLSOs) have been shown to decrease the curvature progression rate in children, thus delaying the need for surgery.

SPINA BIFIDA

Spina bifida is a type of neural tube defect (NTD) where there is failure of neural tube closure. Neural tube closure begins mid-cervical and proceeds caudally and rostrally by day 27. The risk of having a child with NTD is 0.1% to 0.2%, with the recurrence being 2% to 5% if one child has NTD. Recurrence rate further increases to 10% to 15% if two or more children have NTD. Rates are highest amongst the Hispanic population (15). Risk factors can be environmental—hyperthermia within the first 28 days from maternal fever, hot tubs, or sauna use; occupational—solvent exposure, health care workers, and agriculture; maternal—obesity, diabetes, medication use (valproic acid, antiretrovirals, isotretinoin, and methotrexate); and/or nutritional with folate deficiency being the most common. The American Academy of Pediatrics guidelines for folate supplementation is as follows (16): folate 0.4 mg/day for women of childbearing years and 0.4 mg/day prior to conception and through the first trimester in cases of a previous child with spina bifida or a high-risk pregnancy.

Diagnosis is often suspected based on prenatal screening. Elevation of α-fetoprotein, splaying of pedicles and lemon and banana sign on high-resolution US, and amniocentesis are some of the routine screenings where defects will be first noticed. Subcategories of NTDs are listed in the following text along with their common features.

A. Spina bifida occulta
   • Bony defect without herniation of neural elements
   • Incidental in 5% to 36% of adults
   • May have hair patch, dimple, sinus, or nevus
   • May be associated with tethered cord and bowel/bladder

B. Meningocele
   • Bony defect with herniation of meninges but not neural tissue
   • <10% of cases
   • Examination normal

C. Meningomyelocele
  • Herniation of meninges and neural elements
  • Associated with Chiari type 2 malformation in 90% of cases
  • Hydrocephalus in 80% to 90% of cases
  • 75% lumbosacral

D. Caudal regression
  • Absence of sacrum and parts of lumbar spine
  • Risk factor—maternal diabetes
  • Syrinx, anorectal stenosis, renal, cardiac, and external genitalia

Depending on the spinal level involved, there will be different sensory and motor deficits that may be present. These deficits are often asymmetric. At the thoracic level, the upper extremities are spared except when T1 is involved. Kyphoscoliosis from weak trunk occurs in 80% to 100% of the cases and lower extremity contractures may develop from position and wheelchair mobility. With L1 to L3 involvement, hip flexor and abductor tone is present, which predisposes to early hip dislocation and scoliosis. A child with this level of involvement may ambulate with bracing (hip knee ankle foot orthosis [HKAFO] and reciprocating gait orthosis [RGO]) and assistive device (AD) but stop due to high energy cost (17). An L4 to L5 lesion typically results in late hip dislocation. L4 lesions predispose to a calcaneovarus foot, while L5 predisposes to a calcaneus foot.

   Management can include closure in the first 24 to 48 hours of life; however, in utero repair has been reported. Rehabilitative management including the use of bracing depending on the level of the deficit, wheelchair fitting, seating, and standers are important as part of developmental training, mobility, and deformity prevention. Other issues and potential complications to address as they arise include obesity; latex allergy and potential cross-reactivity to kiwi, banana, avocado, and chestnuts; cognitive function and learning problems especially in higher level lesions (>T12) with hydrocephalus having more severe structural brain anomalies (18); shunt malfunction leading to headaches, vomiting, personality changes, concentration difficulty, or other neurological findings; tethered cord with possible findings of spasticity, decreased strength, scoliosis, deterioration in neurological status, bowel/bladder changes, contractures, gait deviations and back pain (found in only 20% but can improve after surgery (19)); diastematomyelia—sagittal cleavage of the spinal cord; syringomyelia in up to 40% of cases and is most often cervical and can present as scoliosis or decreased function above the lesion level; neurogenic bowel leading to episodes of fecal incontinence and constipation; and neurogenic bladder.

   In regard to management of the urinary tract, bladder studies including baseline US, urodynamics, and voiding cysto-urethrogram (VCUG) should be completed as a newborn. US should be repeated every 3 months during the first year, twice in the second year, and then yearly in subsequent years. Urodynamic studies and VCUG should be repeated at 3 months, at 1 year, once at 2 or 3 years of age, and then every 2 years following or sooner if there is a change in status of bladder function.

Determining bladder capacity—first year of life: weight in kg × 7 to 10 mL; age 1 to 12 years: (age + 2) × 30 mL; teen/adult: 400 mL.

Neurogenic bladder can be treated with intermittent catheterization (IC), with self-catheterization by age 5 years if adequate hand use and cognition are present. Additional treatments for neurogenic bladder include oral medication, botulinum toxin injections, vesicostomy, and surgical bladder augmentation.

PEDIATRIC NEUROMUSCULAR DISORDERS

Neuromuscular disorders can be caused by an abnormality of any component of the lower motor neuron (anterior horn cell, peripheral nerve, neuromuscular junction [NMJ] or muscle). They are frequently associated with systemic effects, as some of the pathologic changes may affect skeletal, smooth, and cardiac muscles, the brain, and mitochondria in multiple organs. The most common etiology is genetic but it may be progressive, acquired, or hereditary. It is crucial to obtain a detailed family history and if possible, to obtain diagnostic evaluation of the affected relatives. Diagnostic evaluation of a child with suspected neuromuscular disorder should include the following: comprehensive past medical history and surgical history, detailed family history, and meticulous physical examination. Request for additional laboratory and genetic data that may be costly and not readily available must be considered following ascertainment of developmentally appropriate assessment and history.

The most common cause of referral for possible neuromuscular disorder is when the infant appears floppy. See Table 8.1 on muscular dystrophy.

TABLE 8.1 Comparison of Duchenne Muscular Dystrophy With Becker Muscular Dystrophy

	Duchenne muscular dystrophy	Becker muscular dystrophy
U.S. prevalence (est.)	15,000	2,200
Incidence rate	1/3,500 male births	Unknown
Inheritance	X-linked	X-linked
Gene location	Xp21 (reading frame shifted)	Xp21 (reading frame maintained)
Protein	Dystrophin	Dystrophin
Onset	2–6 years	4–12 years (severe BMD) Late teenage to adulthood (mild BMD)

(continued)

TABLE 8.1 Comparison of Duchenne Muscular Dystrophy With Becker Muscular Dystrophy (*continued*)

	Duchenne muscular dystrophy	Becker muscular dystrophy
Severity and course	Relentlessly progressive Reduced motor function by 2–3 years Steady decline in strength Life span <35 years	Slowly progressive Severity and onset correlate with muscle dystrophin levels
Ambulation status	Loss of ambulation: 7–13 years (no corticosteroids) Loss of ambulation: 9–15 years (corticosteroids)	Loss of ambulation >16 years
Weakness	Proximal > distal Symmetric legs and arms	Proximal > distal Symmetric legs and arms
Cardiac	Dilated cardiomyopathy first to second decade Onset of signs second decade	Cardiomyopathy (may occur before weakness); third to fourth decade frequent
Respiratory	Profoundly reduced vital capacity in second decade Ventilatory dependency in second decade	Respiratory involvement in subset of patients Ventilatory dependency in severe patients
Muscle size	Calf hypertrophy	Calf hypertrophy
Musculoskeletal	Contractures: ankles, hips, and knees Scoliosis: onset after loss of ambulation	Contractures: ankles and others in adulthood
CNS	Reduced cognitive ability (reduced verbal ability)	Some patients have reduced cognitive ability
Muscle pathology	Endomysial fibrosis and fatty infiltration Variable fiber size and myopathic grouping Fiber degeneration/regeneration Dystrophin: absent Sarcoglycans: secondary reduction	Variable fiber size Endomysial connective tissue and fatty infiltration Fiber degeneration Fiber regeneration Dystrophin: reduced (usually 10%–60% of normal)
Blood chemistry and hematology	CK: Very high (10,000–50,000) High AST and ALT (normal GGT) High aldolase	CK: 5,000–20,000 Lower levels with increasing age

ALT, alanine transaminase; AST, aspartate transaminase; BMD, Becker muscular dystrophy; CK, creatine kinase; CNS, central nervous system; GGT, gamma-glutamyl transferase.

ANTERIOR HORN DISORDERS IN CHILDREN

Spinal Muscular Atrophy (SMA)

SMA comprises a group of autosomal recessive disorders caused by the degeneration of anterior horn cells of brain stem motor nuclei and is characterized by muscle weakness. There are four subtypes:

SMA type I (acute infantile or Werdnig-Hoffmann): Onset is from birth to 6 months.

SMA type II (chronic infantile): Onset is between 6 and 18 months.

SMA type III (chronic juvenile): Onset of subtype IIIa <3 years and IIIb >3 years.

SMA type IV (adult onset): Onset is in adulthood (mean onset, mid-30s).

SMA TYPE I (acute infantile or Werdnig-Hoffmann) is the most severe form and presents before 6 months of age—95% of patients have signs and symptoms by 3 months. Reports of impaired fetal movements are frequently observed in utero, and prolonged cyanosis may be noted at delivery. Severe, progressive muscle weakness and flaccid or reduced muscle tone are characteristic features. Children with this type do not attain sitting without support. Other clinical signs include severe limb and axial weakness with hypotonia, frog leg posture, weak cry, tongue fasciculations, diaphragmatic breathing, bell-shaped chest, internal rotation of arms and legs, feeding difficulty, no evidence of cerebral involvement, severe nonprogressive weakness, and proneness to respiratory infections.

Diagnostic workup includes a creatine kinase (CK) level, which is normal, nerve conduction study (NCS)/EMG, which shows decreased amplitude and possibly decreased velocity in motor conduction studies, a normal sensory conduction study, and a mild increase in amplitude and duration of motor unit potential and fibrillation potential. On muscle biopsy, early stages may be inconclusive. Large group atrophy and clusters of large fibers (type I) are noted at later (6–8 weeks) stages. Treatment is supportive and prognosis is poor, with death occurring in the vast majority within the first 3 years of life.

SMA TYPE II (chronic infantile) is an intermediate form characterized by developmental motor delay between 6 and 18 months. A unique feature of the disease is tremor affecting the fingers, attributed to fasciculations in the skeletal muscles. Tongue fasciculations may also be present. Sitting is usually attained, but independent ambulation is not. Children affected have hypotonia with slowly progressing symmetric muscle weakness (proximal > distal) and develop progressive kyphoscoliosis; restrictive lung disease and hip dislocations are common. They have normal to advanced intellect.

Diagnostic workup will show a CK that is normal to elevated. NCS/EMG will show decreased amplitude and possibly decreased velocity in motor conduction studies, a normal sensory conduction study, and a mild increase in amplitude and duration of motor unit potential and fibrillation potential. On muscle biopsy, large group atrophy will be present as well as clusters of large fibers (type I). The life spans of patients with SMA type II vary from 2 years to the third decade of life.

SMA TYPE III (chronic juvenile or Kugelberg-Welander syndrome) is a mild form with onset after age 18 months. There is slowly progressive proximal weakness, with the pelvic girdle more affected than the shoulder girdle. Children affected can stand and walk but may have trouble with motor skills such as going up and down the stairs.

Diagnostic workup will show a normal to elevated CK. NCS/EMG will show decreased amplitude and possibly decreased velocity in motor conduction studies, a normal sensory conduction study, and a mild increase in amplitude and duration of motor unit potential and fibrillation potential. On muscle biopsy, large group atrophy as well as clusters of large fibers will be seen. Also, focal small group atrophy may be seen.

SMA TYPE IV (adult) is a mild form with onset after the age of 20 years characterized by slowly progressive proximal weakness and normal life expectancy. There are other forms of anterior horn disorders that have been described in the medical literature. These disorders are rare and beyond the scope of this manual.

Peripheral Nerve Disorders

Acute inflammatory demyelinating polyradiculoneuropathy also known as Guillain–Barré syndrome (GBS) is a primarily demyelinating neuropathy and is the most common cause of acute motor paralysis in children. It is an autoimmune-mediated disease with environmental triggers and a number of different variants characterized by an acute monophasic, afebrile, postinfectious illness manifesting as an ascending weakness with areflexia. Pain and dysesthesias may also be present. Triggers of GBS include Epstein–Barr virus (EBV), cytomegalovirus (CMV), enteroviruses, hepatitis A and B, varicella, *Mycoplasma pneumoniae*, and *Campylobacter jejuni*. A variant of GBS, Miller Fisher syndrome, which is characterized by the triad of ophthalmoplegia, ataxia, and areflexia, is also linked to preceding infection with *C. jejuni*. Most of these patients have antibodies against the GQlb ganglioside. Recovery outcomes are more favorable in children than in adults and recurrence rate (5%–12%) is relatively uncommon in children.

In regard to treatment in children, the most effective form of therapy is generally considered to be intravenous immunoglobulin (IVIG). Plasmapheresis may decrease the severity and shorten the duration of GBS. Results of plasmapheresis and IVIG are similar, with possibly fewer side effects seen with IVIG. Care should be taken to monitor respiratory and cardiac function, especially in the acute, progressive stage of the disease. Respiratory compromise is the most concerning and life-threatening aspect of GBS in childhood.

Differential Diagnosis of GBS in Children

1. **Botulism** – In infants, botulism should be considered. Botulism is characterized not only by (descending) weakness but also by involvement of the extraocular muscles (ophthalmoplegia), miosis of the pupil, and constipation
2. **Myasthenia Gravis** – Can be present with primarily proximal weakness in childhood. A good history, testing for acetylcholine receptor antibodies, and electrophysiologic studies with NCSs and EMG, including repetitive stimulation, can help to distinguish myasthenia gravis from GBS
3. **Infectious Processes** – GBS-like syndromes can occur in certain infections, such as Lyme disease or HIV
4. **Peripheral Neuropathies** – Vincristine, glue sniffing, heavy metals, organophosphate pesticides, HIV, diphtheria, Lyme disease, inborn errors of metabolism, Leigh disease, Tangier disease, porphyria, and critical illness polyneuropathy
5. **NJ Disorders** – Tick paralysis, myasthenia gravis, botulism, and hypercalcemia

HEREDITARY MOTOR SENSORY NEUROPATHY

Hereditary motor sensory neuropathy (HMSN) is an inherited disorder of both motor and sensory peripheral nerves characterized by progressive neuromuscular impairments. Motor signs tend to develop before sensory signs. Other clinical features include weakness and atrophy first in the intrinsic foot muscles followed by ankle and toe dorsiflexors; and mismatch between strength in the affected peroneal-innervated muscles and the less affected tibial-innervated muscles results in the development of typical high-arched feet, hammertoes, and difficulty with heel walking seen early in physical examination. The onset is usually in the first or second decade of life and there are seven subtypes as follows:

- HMSN types 1A and IB (dominantly inherited hypertrophic demyelinating neuropathies): Charcot-Marie-Tooth (CMT) types 1A, 1B
- HMSN type 2 (dominantly inherited neuronal neuropathies): CMT type 2
- HMSN type 3 (hypertrophic neuropathy of infancy): Déjerine-Sottas disease
- HMSN type 4 (hypertrophic neuropathy associated with phytanic acid excess): Refsum disease

- HMSN type 5 (associated with spastic paraplegia)
- HMSN type 6 (with optic atrophy)
- HMSN type 7 (with retinitis pigmentosa)

The most common form of CMT1, known as CMT1A, is associated with a duplication within chromosome 17pll.2. The second most common form of CMT1 (CMT1B) and some cases of Déjerine-Sottas disease were found to be associated with mutations in the myelin protein zero (MPZ) gene in chromosome 1. Mutations of each of these genes have been associated with multiple, overlapping phenotypes. For example, MPZ mutations are associated with CMT1B, Déjerine-Sottas disease, and the axonal CMT2 phenotype. Inheritance patterns of HMSN disorders vary. CMT1 and CMT2 are both inherited dominantly as predominantly the demyelinating and axonal forms, respectively. Déjerine-Sottas is a severe form with onset in infancy. CMT4 includes the various demyelinating autosomal recessive forms of CMT disease.

The common foot deformities of CMT can lead to discomfort, impaired ambulation, and disability. Ankle weakness and instability can be treated with orthoses or shoe modifications. Moderate activity is recommended. Overexertion should be avoided.

NEUROMUSCULAR JUNCTION DISORDERS

Transient neonatal myasthenia occurs in 10% to 30% of neonates born to mothers with myasthenia gravis. It may occur any time during the first hours to first week of life. Signs are most commonly apparent by the third day of life. Infants should be monitored closely for any signs of respiratory distress. If treated and monitored, it is a self-limiting condition in vast majority of the cases. The major cause is transplacental transfer of circulating acetylcholine (ACh) antibodies from mother to fetus.

Congenital or infantile myasthenia occurs in infants of non-myasthenic mothers and may have an autosomal recessive inheritance. Antibodies to ACh receptor are usually absent.

Juvenile myasthenia gravis has a similar pathophysiologic origin as adult myasthenia gravis, but there are important differences, mostly relating to epidemiology, presentation, and therapeutic decision making.

Several considerations should be emphasized, such as postponement of corticosteroid therapy from an early age, which is associated with growth retardation, and avoidance of thymectomy due to the risks of induced immunodeficiency.

It particularly affects adolescent girls and is severe and labile in presentation. It presents clinically with weakness of other muscles including facial and mastication. It can affect swallowing, speech, respiration, as well as the neck, trunk, and limb muscles.

MYOPATHIES

Facioscapulohumeral muscular dystrophy (FSHD) is a slowly progressive dystrophic myopathy with predominant asymmetric involvement of facial and shoulder girdle musculature.

It has an autosomal dominant inheritance pattern with 10% to 30% caused by sporadic mutation. Presentation is usually before age 20 years and diagnosis is confirmed in over 90% by molecular genetic testing. Serum CK levels are normal or slightly elevated in the majority of patients. Clinical features include facial weakness and an expressionless appearance; difficulty with eye closure; involvement of scapular stabilizers, shoulder abductors, and external rotators, but deltoids are spared; mild, nonprogressive scoliosis; mild restrictive lung disease in 50% of patients. Contractures are uncommon. Coates syndrome, a rapidly progressive form of early onset of FSHD, is characterized by sensorineural hearing deficit and progressive exudative telangiectasia of the retina.

Emery-Dreifuss muscular dystrophy (EMD) is characterized by weakness, contractures, and cardiac conduction abnormalities. There are two subtypes: EMD-1 and EMD-2. **EMD-1** is an X-linked recessive progressive dystrophic myopathy. It typically presents in the second decade of life, but age of presentation may vary. Elbow flexion contractures are the hallmark of this form. Contractures in general are more limiting than weakness. There are functional limitations with ambulation and stair negotiation. However, due to slow progression, loss of ambulation is rare.

Progressive cardiac disease is almost invariably present with onset in the early second decade to the fourth decade. Arrhythmia may lead to emboli or sudden death; cardiomyopathy leads to progressive left ventricular myocardial dysfunction.

EMD-2 is caused by an abnormality due to lamin A/C protein linked to chromosome 1q21.2. Inheritance may be autosomal dominant, recessive, or missense. Missense mutation leads to childhood onset. The most prominent clinical feature is scapuloperoneal and facial distribution of weakness. Contractures are rare in this form of EMD.

Congenital myopathies are a group of heterogeneous disorders usually presenting with infantile hypotonia due to genetic defects, causing primary myopathies with the absence of any structural abnormality of the central nervous system or peripheral nerves.

JUVENILE IDIOPATHIC ARTHRITIS

Juvenile idiopathic arthritis (JIA) is the most common rheumatic disease of childhood. It affects the bone and joints and can lead to overgrowth, undergrowth, or aberrant growth. Possible anomalies related to JIA include micrognathia, leg length discrepancy, and hip dysplasia. Diagnosis should fulfill the following criteria: occur before age 16 years, persist for at least 6 weeks, and be a diagnosis of exclusion. Indicators of poor outcomes include but are not limited to greater severity and extension at disease onset, symmetrical disease, early wrist and hip involvement, serologic evidence of rheumatoid factor (RF), persistent active disease, and early radiographic changes. The seven subtypes of JIA are systemic arthritis, oligoarthritis, RF- negative polyarthritis, RF-positive arthritis, psoriatic arthritis, enthesitis-related arthritis, and undifferentiated arthritis. A few subtypes are highlighted in Table 8.2.

TABLE 8.2 Selected JIA Subtypes

Subtype and Key Diagnostic Features	Other Pertinent Features
Systemic arthritis • Diagnosis requires presence of both arthritis and arthritis preceded by fever with periodic spikes to 102°F or at least 2 weeks of fever • One or more of the following signs: evanescent salmon-colored rash, lymphadenopathy, hepatomegaly, splenomegaly, and/or serositis	• A small subset of children can develop macrophage activation syndrome, a life-threatening complication • Half of the patients with systemic JIA follow a relapsing–remitting course with good long-term prognosis • Another half have unremitting course with poor clinical and functional prognosis leading to joint destruction

Oligoarthritis
• Two subtypes:
  1. Persistent (four joints affected)
  2. Extended (more than four joints after first 6 months)
	• Early onset before 6 years of age, asymmetric predominately in females, and good outcome
	• Presence of ANA is a risk factor for the development of iridocyclitis
	• Silent uveitis can develop within 4 years of the onset of the disorder

Polyarthritis • Affects five or more joints	• RF positive: affects adolescent girls, symmetric joint involvement • RF negative: variable outcome in the subset of ANA-positive patients; development of chronic uveitis is possible
Psoriatic arthritis • Presence of arthritis and psoriatic rash	• If rash is absent, a positive history of psoriasis in a first-degree relative, dactylitis, and nail pitting
Enthesitis-related arthritis • Affects HLA B27–positive males after 6 years of age	**Enthesitis locations** • Calcaneal insertion of the Achilles tendon • Plantar fascia • Tarsal area • Hip involvement (common) The disease may progress to ankylosing spondylitis.*

Note: *Juvenile ankylosing spondylitis is not part of the JIA subclassfication but does have an arthritic component. It affects adolescent boys and is associated with HLA-B27. It is characterized by oligoarthritis that is episodic and asymmetric with sacroiliac (SI) joint involvement and "bamboo" spine.

ANA, antinuclear antibody; JIA, juvenile idiopathic arthritis; HLA, human leuko-cyte antigen; RF, rheumatoid factor.

The main goals of rehabilitation of children with JIA are to prevent joint damage, achieve normal growth and development, and maintain and improve function. **Treatment** includes resting the joint, splinting in functional position, ROM, modalities, and adaptive equipment. US is contraindicated in children with open growth plates. First-line treatments include NSAIDs and intra-articular steroid joint injections. Second-line treatments include tumor necrosis factor (TNF) inhibitors (etanercept and adalimumab) and T-cell blockers (abatacept) for TNF inhibitor nonresponders. Up to 75% of children may achieve remission with NSAIDs and methotrexate.

Special considerations, which need to be taken into account with JIA, are that the cervical spine is more often involved than in adults; TMJ is commonly affected and can lead to mandibular and facial growth disturbance (polyarticular form); wrist involvement is common and requires splinting, ROM and modalities; shoulder joint involved in polyarticular and psoriatic arthritis; hip flexion contractures with internal rotation and adduction unlike adults; knee is the most commonly involved joint and quadriceps weakness due to early contracture may not resolve (active quad strengthening is recommended); and leg length discrepancy due to bony overgrowth can lead to pelvic asymmetry and scoliosis.

REFERENCES

1. Bax M, Goldstein M, Rosenbaum P, et al. Proposed definition and classification of cerebral palsy. *Dev Med Child Neurol.* 2005;47(8):571–576.

2. Ashwal S, Russman BS, Blasco PA, et al. Practice parameters: diagnostic assessment of the child with cerebral palsy: report of the Quality Standards Subcommittee of the American Academy of Neurology and the Practice Committee of the Child Neurology Society. *Neurology.* 2004;62(6):851–863.

3. Molnar GE, Gordon SU. Cerebral palsy: predictive value of selected clinical sign of early prognostication of motor function. *Arch Phys Med Rehabil.* 1976;57:153.

4. Badell A. Cerebral palsy: postural locomotor prognosis in spastic diplegia. *Arch Phys Med Rehabil.* 1985;66:614–619.

5. Fedrizzi E, Facchin P, Marzaroli M, et al. Predictors of independent walking in children with spastic diplegia. *J Child Neurol.* 2000;15:228–234.

6. Bleck EE. Locomotor prognosis in cerebral palsy. *Dev Med Child Neurol.* 1975;17:18.

7. Strauss D, Brooks J, Rosenbloom R, Shavelle R. Life expectancy in cerebral palsy: An update. *Dev Med Child Neurol.* 2008;50(7):487–493.

8. Executive summary: Neonatal brachial plexus palsy. Report of the American College of Obstetricians and Gynecologists' Task Force on Neonatal Brachial Plexus Palsy. *Obstet Gynecol.* 2014;123(4):902–904.

9. Pitt M, Vredeveld JW. The role of electromyography in the management of the brachial palsy of the newborn. *Clin Neurophysiol.* 2005;116:1756–1761.

10. O'Brien DF, Park TS, Noetzel MJ, et al. Management of birth brachial plexus palsy. *Childs New Syst.* 2006;22:103–112.

11. Noetzel MJ, Park TS, Robinson S, et al. Prospective study of recovery following neonatal brachial plexus injury. *J Child Neurol*. 2001;16:488–492.

12. National Spinal Cord Injury Statistical Center. Spinal cord injury: Facts and figures at a glance. Birmingham, AL: University of Alabama; 2008.

13. Levy ML, Granville RC, Hart D, Meltzer H. Deep venous thrombosis in children and adolescents. *J Neurosurg Pediatr*. 2004;101(2):32–37.

14. Truitt AK, Sorrells DL, Halvorson E, et al. Pulmonary embolism: which pediatric trauma patients are at risk? *J Pediatr Surg*. 2005;40:124–127.

15. Centers for Disease Control and Prevention (CDC). Racial/ethnic differences in the birth prevalence of spina bifida–United States, 1995–2005. *MMWR Morb Mortal Wkly Rep*. 2009;57(53):1409.

16. Diamond M, Armento M. Children with disabilities. In: DeLisa JA, Gans BM, Walsh NE, et al, eds. *Physical Medicine and Rehabilitation: Principles and Practice*. 4th ed. Philadelphia, PA: Lippincott Williams & Wilkins; 2005.

17. Williams EN, Broughton NS, Menelaus MB. Age related walking in children with spina bifida. *Dev Med Child Neurol*. 1999;41(7):446–449.

18. Fletcher JM, Copeland K, Frederick JA, et al. Spinal lesion level in spina bifida; a source of neural and cognitive heterogeneity. *J Neurosurg*. 2005;102(3):268–279.

19. Schoenmakers MA, Goosekens RH, Gulmans VA, et al. Long-term outcome of neurosurgical untethering on neurosegmental motor and ambulation levels. *Dev Med Child Neurol*. 2003;45(8):551–555.

SUGGESTED READING

Alexander MA, Matthews DJ eds. *Pediatric Rehabilitation: Principles and Practice*. 5th ed. New York, NY: Demos Medical Publishing, LLC; 2015.

Butler C, Darrah J. Effects of neurodevelopmental treatment (NDT) for cerebral palsy: an AACPDM evidence report. *Dev Med Child Neurol*. 2001; 43:778.

Davis PJC, Mc Donagh JE. Principles of management of musculoskeletal conditions in children and young people. *Best Pract Res Clin Rheumatol*. 2006;20(2):263–278.

Hofer M. Spondyloarthropathies in children–are they different from those in adults? *Best Pract Res Clin Rheumatol*. 2006;20(2):315–328.

Krach LE, Gormley, ME, Jr., Ward M. Traumatic brain injury. In: Alexander M, Matthews D. *Pediatric Rehabilitation: Principles and Practice*. 4th ed. New York, NY: Demos Medical Publishing; 2010:231–260.

Massagli TL. Medical and rehabilitation issues in the care of children with spinal cord injury. *Phys Med Rehabil Clin N Am*. 2000;11(1):169–182.

Novak I, Hines M, Goldsmith S, Barclay R. Clinical prognostic messages from a systematic review on cerebral palsy. *Pediatrics*. 2012;130:e1285.

Powell A, Davidson L. Pediatric spinal cord injury: A review by organ system. *Phys Med Rehabil Clin N Am*. 2015;26:109–132.

Veugelers R, Benninga MA, Calis EA, et al. Prevalence and clinical presentation of constipation in children with severe generalized cerebral palsy. *Dev Med Child Neurol*. 2010; 52:e216.

Wallace SJ. Epilepsy in cerebral palsy. *Dev Med Child Neurol*. 2001;43(10):713–717.

CHAPTER 9

CONCUSSION

DEFINITION AND PATHOPHYSIOLOGY

In the most recent Consensus Statement on Concussion in Sport held in 2016, it was noted that the terms *mild traumatic brain injury* and *concussion* are often being used interchangeably. Concussion is a subset of traumatic brain injury (TBI) and is defined as a complex pathophysiological process affecting the brain, induced by biomechanical forces (1).

A concussion may be caused by a direct or indirect force transmitted to the brain resulting in rapid-onset and short-lived neurological impairments, which may evolve over hours. Loss of consciousness (LOC) does not always occur. A constellation of symptoms may develop and resolution of these symptoms typically follows a sequential course, but some cases may be prolonged. Neuropathological changes are usually due to a functional rather than a structural injury (1).

A concussion leads to complex cellular dysfunction primarily caused by neurotransmitters released after the injury. The ensuing responses cause a cascade of events, each further exacerbating the other:

Glutamate release → efflux of potassium, influx of calcium → hyperglycolysis → release of free radicals and enzymes (proteases, lipases, NO) → damage to cytoskeletons → inflammatory damage, glucose utilization, energy crisis (increased adenosine triphosphate [ATP] use) → mitochondrial failure → lactate production → increased membrane permeability → apoptosis, necrosis

As a result of the energy crisis, symptoms develop and may worsen when physical or cognitive activities are performed. Concussion symptoms can be somatic (headache, nausea, vomiting, light and noise sensitivity, dizziness, poor balance, tinnitus, blurry vision), cognitive (fogginess, difficulty concentrating or remembering), sleep-related (disturbances of, fatigue), and/or emotional (sadness, irritability). Headache is the most common symptom. LOC occurs in less than 10% of concussions, whereas confusion and amnesia (retrograde and/or anterograde) are more common (2).

ASSESSMENT

For on-field assessment of a sport-related concussion, one must recognize the symptoms and signs of a concussion. Athletes should be medically evaluated on-site by a health care provider and removed from the game. After serious medical conditions have been ruled out, sideline evaluation with the Sport Concussion Assessment Tool 5th edition (SCAT5) assessment tool should be performed. Serial monitoring for deterioration should be performed over the initial few hours, and a player with a diagnosed concussion should not be allowed to return to play the same day. A health care professional knowledgeable in the management and treatment of concussion should be consulted.

Assessment of a concussion requires a thorough history and physical exam, which includes

- Injury details (how it occurred, immediate symptoms and evolution, presence of LOC or amnesia)
- Current symptom description, guided by the 22-item Post-Concussion Symptom Scale (Table 9.1). *Do not use concussion grading scales*
  - Determine how the symptoms manifest (what makes them better or worse)
  - Discuss how they may interfere with physical activities, work, school, computer/cell phone use, and so forth
  - Identify how the symptoms are interrelated with each other (insomnia may cause fatigue, headaches, irritability, etc.)

TABLE 9.1 Post-Concussion Symptom Scale

	None	Mild		Moderate		Severe	
Headache	0	1	2	3	4	5	6
Nausea	0	1	2	3	4	5	6
Vomiting	0	1	2	3	4	5	6
Dizziness	0	1	2	3	4	5	6
Balance problems	0	1	2	3	4	5	6
Trouble falling asleep	0	1	2	3	4	5	6
Sleeping more than usual	0	1	2	3	4	5	6
Drowsiness	0	1	2	3	4	5	6
Sensitivity to light	0	1	2	3	4	5	6
Sensitivity to noise	0	1	2	3	4	5	6
More emotional than usual	0	1	2	3	4	5	6
Irritability	0	1	2	3	4	5	6
Sadness	0	1	2	3	4	5	6
Nervousness	0	1	2	3	4	5	6
Numbness or tingling	0	1	2	3	4	5	6
Feeling slowed down	0	1	2	3	4	5	6
Feeling like in a "fog"	0	1	2	3	4	5	6
Difficulty with concentrating	0	1	2	3	4	5	6
Difficulty with remembering	0	1	2	3	4	5	6

- ○ Symptoms can be affected by the patient's age, motivation, or gender, or by a learning disability
- Physical exam
  - ○ Neurological exam
  - ○ Balance assessment using the Balance Error Scoring System (BESS). The BESS tests balance with eyes closed, on firm and soft surfaces, in three stances—feet together, tandem, and on only the nondominant foot
  - ○ Visuomotor exam (nystagmus, saccades, convergence, vestibular–ocular reflex)
  - ○ If needed, brief neurocognitive testing with SCAT5 (Child SCAT5 for those aged 5–12 years). Computerized testing not recommended. Often, cognitive complaints are secondary to the somatic and emotional symptoms experienced and should be addressed first
- A head CT and MRI are usually negative and their use is limited to high suspicion for structural intracerebral injury, including intracranial hemorrhage, prolonged LOC, post-traumatic amnesia, persistently altered mental status (Glasgow Coma Scale [GCS] < 15), focal neurologic deficit, evidence of skull fracture on examination, or signs of clinical deterioration (3)

MANAGEMENT AND TREATMENT

In sports, no athlete should be allowed to return to play until assessed for the presence of concussion. When in doubt, sit them out. Risk of reinjury is high, given the symptoms described. Reinjury can lead to worsened symptoms and a prolonged recovery. The term *second impact syndrome* (SIS) should NOT be used. This is when one who has sustained an initial head injury sustains a second head injury before symptoms associated with the first have fully cleared. After further investigation, SIS was based upon 17 case reports of which none fulfilled the criteria of SIS; additional cases have not been reported since, nor have such cases been reported outside of the United States. Furthermore, if it were a true syndrome, the prevalence would be significant in boxers.

Concussion management is individualized. However, protocols have been established to assist in guiding management and treatment. Goal of recovery should focus on return to play, sports, work, and daily life activities.

The first step in the management of a concussion is to educate and provide reassurance about recovery. Education also involves providing information on how to ensure symptoms improve in a timely fashion. This includes being active, as tolerated by the symptoms. Previous guidelines recommended complete rest; however, this led to prolonged symptoms and unnecessary anxiety. Children and young adults should be allowed to use computers and video games to test their reactions, and use should be limited if it causes exacerbation, as not all concussions respond similarly. In addition, allowing such activities can provide the clinician guidance in ongoing management.

Physical activities should be limited to those that are contact in nature. If the patient is an athlete, he or she should be allowed to return to some form of physical activity, as tolerated by the symptoms. For example, recommend slow or brisk walks and if symptoms develop, modify the activity to where the patient does not develop or exacerbate symptoms. Goal is to allow some form of activity because complete rest is not beneficial to improving return to previous level of activity.

Cognitive activity should be limited to activities as tolerated by the symptoms. Students should not be removed from school unless there are significant symptoms. Trial of school with rest breaks and modifications is recommended. This should be the treatment management for return to work as well.

The process for returning athletes to sports can be guided by the Graduated Return to Play Protocol (Table 9.2). The athlete is progressed through each of the six stages of activity, where each stage lasts at least 24 hours. The athlete should only progress to the next stage if asymptomatic. If symptoms develop at any stage, the athlete is returned to the previous stage and reattempts progression the following day. Return to play should not occur on the same day, and adequate time, at least 1 week, is recommended to ensure that recovery has occurred.

Pharmacological use in concussion management should be limited to those with ongoing symptoms beyond the usual course.

TABLE 9.2 Graduated Return to Play Protocol

Rehabilitation Stage	Functional Exercise	Objective
1. Symptom-limited activity	Daily activities that do not provoke symptoms	Gradual reintroduction of work/school activities
2. Light aerobic exercise	Walking or stationary cycling at slow to medium pace No resistance training	Increased HR
3. Sport-specific exercise	Running or skating drills No head impact activities	Add movement
4. Noncontact training drills	Harder training drills, e.g., passing drills May start progressive resistance training	Exercise, coordination, and increased thinking
5. Full contact practice	Following medical clearance, participate in normal training activities	Restore confidence and assessment of functional skills by coaching staff
6. RTP	Normal game play	—

HR, heart rate; MPHR, maximum predicted heart rate; RTP, return to play.
Source: Adapted from Ref. (1).

However, treatment of sleep with melatonin is recommended in the initial weeks to ensure adequate rest is achieved. Headache medications should be limited to acetaminophen or ibuprofen as needed and ice or heat to sear areas.

If dizziness or balance disturbances exist with the presence of oculomotor dysfunction, vestibular therapy should be recommended. Physical therapy can also be used to aid in reintegration into sports if no athletic trainer/coach available. Cognitive therapy with speech or occupational therapy should not be utilized, unless there is objective data indicating deficits after neurocognitive assessment by a neuropsychologist (via pen-and-paper testing).

Symptoms normally improve over the course of days to weeks, and it is essential to provide reassurance to both athletic and non-athletic populations. The Berlin expert consensus denotes the term *persistent symptoms* as a reflection of the failure of normal clinical recovery—that is, symptoms that persist beyond expected time frames (i.e., >10–14 days in adults and >4 weeks in children; 1). When concussion symptoms last >2 months, further evaluation into underlying causes must be sought, as it most likely related to other confounding factors. Common risk factors related to prolonged symptoms are presence of migrainous symptoms, fogginess, or amnesia; being younger in age, female, or prone to overexertion; or having a history of multiple concussions, psychiatric disturbances, or learning disability (4). In addition, a higher PCSS score can also lead to a delay in recovery. Postconcussion syndrome is a nonspecific wastebasket psychiatric diagnosis often used by clinicians for symptoms lasting >3 months after a concussion. *This term should never be used* as it can describe many diagnoses related to psychological distress or cognitive inefficiencies related to distress.

For optimal management of concussion, especially when faced with complex cases, it is important to have a multidisciplinary team approach. This team should consist of a physiatrist, vestibular therapist, and neuropsychologist. Neurology, neurosurgery, neuro-ophthalmologists, and neuro-optometrists can be consulted when specialty care is needed.

REFERENCES

1. McCrory P, Meeuwisse W, Dvorak J, et al. Consensus statement on concussion in sport-the 5th international conference on concussion in sport held in Berlin, October 2016. *Br J Sports Med.* 2017.
2. Lovell M, Collins M, Bradley J. Return to play following sports-related concussion. *Clin Sports Med.* 2004;23(3):421–441, ix.
3. Giza CC, Kutcher JS, Ashwal S, et al. Summary of evidence-based guideline update: evaluation and management of concussion in sports: report of the Guideline Development Subcommittee of the American Academy of Neurology. *Neurology.* 2013;80(24):2250–2257.
4. Sabini RC, Nutini DN, Nutini M. Return-to-play guidelines in concussion: revisiting the literature. *Phys Sportsmed.* 2014;42(3):10–19.

CHAPTER 10

PAIN MEDICINE

TERMINOLOGY

Pain

A subjective unpleasant sensory or emotional experience due to actual or potential tissue damage (1). It is often described in terms of a penetrating or tissue-destructive process such as stabbing, squeezing, tearing, burning, or twisting. It may also be characterized using emotionally descriptive words such as *sickening* or *nauseating* and is often associated with anxiety when moderate or severe. When pain is acute, it renders a behavioral arousal or stress response typically manifested as increased blood pressure, tachycardia, increased pupil size, and increased plasma cortisol levels.

Nociceptor

A receptor preferentially sensitive to a noxious stimulus or to a stimulus that would become noxious if prolonged.

Allodynia

Pain due to a stimulus that does not normally provoke pain.

Dysesthesia

An unpleasant abnormal sensation, whether spontaneous or evoked.

Hyperalgesia

An increased response to a stimulus that is normally painful. For pain evoked by stimuli that usually are not painful, the term *allodynia* is preferred, whereas the term *hyperalgesia* is more appropriately used for cases with an increased response at a normal threshold or at an increased threshold, for example, in patients with neuropathy.

Hyperesthesia

Increased sensitivity to stimulation.

Hyperpathia

A painful syndrome characterized by an abnormally painful reaction to a stimulus, especially a repetitive stimulus, as well as an increased threshold.

Hypoalgesia

Diminished pain in response to a <u>normally painful</u> stimulus.

Hypoesthesia

Decreased sensitivity to stimulation, excluding the special senses.

Neuralgia

Pain in the distribution of a nerve or nerves.

Neuropathic Pain

Pain initiated or caused by a primary lesion or dysfunction in the nervous system.

Neuropathy

A disturbance of function or pathologic change in a nerve: in one nerve, mononeuropathy; in several nerves, mononeuropathy multiplex; if diffuse and bilateral, polyneuropathy.

Paresthesia

An abnormal sensation, whether spontaneous or evoked.

Somatic Pain

Can be superficial or deep. Superficial somatic pain is from nociceptive input from skin or subcutaneous tissues. It may be characterized as localized and sharp, throbbing, or burning.

Deep somatic pain arises from joints, muscles, tendons, or bones. It usually is dull, aching, and less localized (2).

Visceral Pain

Due to pathology involving an internal organ or parietal pleura, pericardium, or peritoneum. Often described as dull and diffuse. It is frequently associated with abnormal sympathetic or parasympathetic activity resulting in sweating, changes in blood pressure and heart rate, and nausea and vomiting (2).

Chronic Pain

Pain that persists beyond the typical course of an acute insult or after healing. Chronic pain may be nociceptive, neuropathic, or both. Psychological mechanisms or environmental factors frequently play a role.

The most common causes of chronic pain are derived from musculoskeletal disorders, visceral disorders, peripheral nerve disorders, or the dorsal root ganglia. Additional causes are injuries to the central nervous system (CNS; cerebrovascular accident [CVA], spinal cord injury [SCI], and multiple sclerosis [MS]) and/or cancer pain. Most musculoskeletal pain is nociceptive, whereas neurological pain from the CNS or peripheral nervous system (PNS) is typically neuropathic. The pain associated with other disorders such as cancer pain or chronic lower back pain is often mixed (2).

PATHOPHYSIOLOGY

The sensation of pain travels via three primary neuronal pathways that transmit noxious stimuli from the periphery to the brain. Primary afferent neurons contain cell bodies in the dorsal root ganglia, which are located in the vertebral foramina at each spinal cord level.

Each of these primary afferent neurons contains a single axon that bifurcates to the periphery and to the dorsal horn of the spinal cord.

In the dorsal horn, the primary afferent neuron synapses with a second-order neuron whose axon crosses midline and ascends through the contralateral spinothalamic tract to the thalamus. These neurons then synapse in the thalamic nuclei with third-order neurons, which then transmit the signal to the internal capsule and corona radiata, and then to the postcentral gyrus of the brain cortex (2).

EXAMINATION

A comprehensive history and physical examination is fundamental to the diagnosis and treatment of patients with pain. Pain assessments and diagrams help the physician in stratifying a patient's pain, especially the recognition of red flags that warrant emergent treatment (e.g., progressive numbness, weakness, bowel/bladder incontinence, and saddle anesthesia).

ANATOMY

As neck and low back pain are often encountered by physiatrists in myriad settings, it is important to understand spinal anatomy when evaluating a patient and forming a differential diagnosis. Cervical and lumbar vertebral bodies are complex structures, with multiple possible pain generators present (Figure 10.1).

The spinal cord gives off spinal nerves in pairs: 8 cervical, 12 thoracic, 5 lumbar, 5 sacral, and 1 coccygeal. The spinal cord and nerves are surrounded by a sac called the *dura mater*, which contains the cerebrospinal fluid (CSF).

Knowing and understanding the dermatomal distributions of each nerve root is also important and this aids in obtaining history and during examination and treatment. As will be discussed, different types of spine pathology and radicular irritation/dysfunction can be treated differently. As a rule of thumb, in the cervical spine, a nerve root comes out *above* its corresponding vertebral body, meaning that at C6/C7, the C7 nerve root exits. *At C7/T1, the C8 nerve root exits.* The

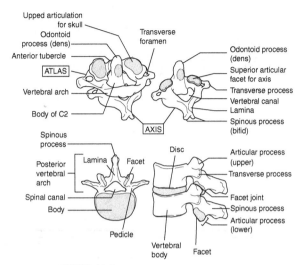

FIGURE 10.1 Cervical and lumbar vertebral anatomy.

presence of C8 translates to *the thoracic and lumbar nerve roots exiting below their corresponding vertebral body* (Figure 10.2).

Similarly, the direction of the disc herniation can determine which nerve root is impacted. Posterolateral disc herniations typically spare the root that exits at that level and affect the root exiting at the level below. The majority of disc herniations are posterolateral, given the additional support provided by the posterior longitudinal ligament (Figure 10.3). Far lateral disc herniations can affect the nerve root at that level as it exits via the lateral recesses (Figure 10.4).

IMAGING

Imaging of the spine plays a large role in the workup/evaluation of low back pain. X-rays are often the first-line imaging obtained. It is important to know how the normal anatomy appears in x-ray/CT/MRI to better appreciate spinal pathology when present (Figure 10.5).

X-rays can demonstrate multiple pathologies including

- Spondylitic changes
- Instability (best seen with flexion/extension films)
- Compression fractures
- Intervertebral disc degeneration
- Lytic/blastic lesions
- Pathologic findings in spine diseases (e.g., ankylosing spondylosis)

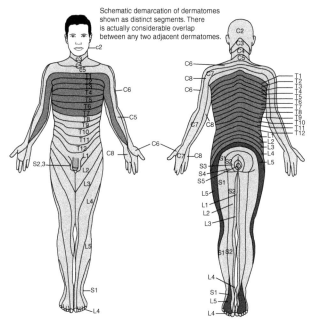

Schematic demarcation of dermatomes shown as distinct segments. There is actually considerable overlap between any two adjacent dermatomes.

Levels of principal dermatomes

C5 Clavicles
C5,6,7 Lateral parts of upper limbs
C8,T1 Medial sides of upper limbs
C6 Thumb
C6,7,8 Hand
C8 Ring and little fingers
T4 Level of nipples

T10 Level of umbilicus
T12 Inguinal or groin regions
L1,2,3,4 Anterior and inner surfaces of lower limbs
L4,5,S1 Foot
L4 Medial side of great toe
S1,2,L5 Posterior and outer surfaces of lower limbs
S1 Lateral margin of foot and little toe
S2,3,4 Perineum

FIGURE 10.2 Dermatomal distribution of spinal nerve roots.

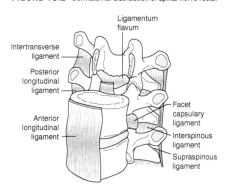

FIGURE 10.3 Support structures of the lumbar spine.

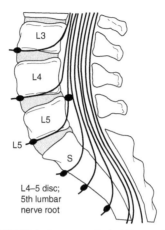

FIGURE 10.4 Disk herniation in relation to level affected.

CT and MRI are usually the next modalities ordered if further radiographic evaluation is warranted (Figures 10.6 and 10.7). Unless contraindicated, MRI is often ordered to evaluate for soft tissue pathology (i.e., disc disease) and to better evaluate bony pathology (e.g., assessing acuity of fracture).

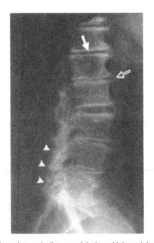

FIGURE 10.5 X-ray demonstrating spondylosis and intervertebral disk degeneration.

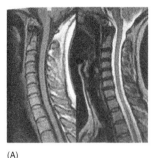 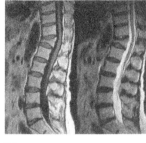

(A)   (B)

FIGURE 10.6 T1 (left) versus T2 (right) MRI of cervical spine (A) and lumbar spine (B).

The main MRI types are T1, T2, sagittal short T1 inversion recovery (STIR), and T1 with fat suppression. Different tissues appear differently on different types, however.

Water and pathology: white on T2, dark on T1

Fat: white on T1 and T2

Bone cortex, stones, and ligaments: dark on every type. Contusions are white.

Among the most common complaints in the physiatrist's office are neck and low back pain. Due to the interplay of multiple musculoskeletal and neurologic structures, pain is often multifactorial in origin. Nachemson reported that after approximately 1 month of symptoms, only 15% of patients have definable disease or injury (3). *Radiculopathic* (nerve root) pain typically follows a dermatomal/myotomal distribution and can stem from irritation from disc fragments, bone, and others. In the cervical spine, the most common roots involved are C6 and C7. The most commonly involved levels in the lumbar spine are L5 and S1. A thorough physical exam with tests for root irritation (cervical loading/distraction and straight leg raising) aids in accurate diagnosis.

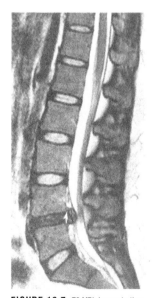

FIGURE 10.7 T2 MRI demonstrating disk herniation at L4/L5.

COMPLEX REGIONAL PAIN SYNDROME I/II

CRPS I

- A relatively common disabling disorder with 50,000 new cases diagnosed each year in the United States (4)
- Unknown pathophysiology
- Underlying mechanisms may include changes in the peripheral and central somatosensory, autonomic, and motor processing systems and a pathologic interaction of sympathetic and afferent systems, neurogenic inflammation, and autoimmunity (4)

Clinical Picture of CRPS

- Disproportionate extremity pain
- Swelling
- Autonomic (sympathetic) and motor symptoms

The condition can affect the upper or lower extremities, but it is slightly more common in the upper extremities.

CRPS I (previously known as reflex sympathetic dystrophy [RSD]) is the definition given in the setting of known trauma to an area without specific nerve injury. CRPS II (previously known as causalgia) is defined by a known injury to a nerve.

Causes may include trauma, underlying neurologic pathology, musculoskeletal disorders, and malignancy.

CRPS is subdivided into the following three phases:

- Acute stage: Usually warm phase of 2 to 3 months
- Dystrophic phase: Vasomotor instability for several months
- Atrophic phase: Usually cold extremity with atrophic changes

DIAGNOSIS/WORKUP

- No single diagnostic test has proven sensitive and specific enough to diagnose CRPS
- Radiographic findings
  - X-ray imaging may show osteoporosis
  - The *triple-phase bone scan* has also been useful in diagnosis. According to Kozin et al., scintigraphic abnormalities were reported in up to 60% of CRPS patients and may be useful in arriving at the diagnosis of CRPS. The most suggestive and sensitive findings on bone scan include diffuse increased activity in the *delayed (third) phase*, including juxta-articular accentuation (5)
  - Skin thermography: can reveal temperature disparities between limbs
  - Quantitative Sudomotor Axon Reflex Testing (QSART; 6)
  - Electrodiagnostic studies: nerve conduction velocity (NCV)/EMG is usually normal
  - Laser Doppler imaging

Budapest Criteria: Currently, the most widely used diagnostic criteria for CRPS. In 1994, the International Association for the Study of Pain (IASP) published consensus-based diagnostic criteria for CRPS with the objective of becoming the internationally accepted standard. Ongoing research studies elucidated issues with validation and low specificity leading to potential overdiagnosis. This prompted an international task force to develop and validate CRPS diagnostic criteria with high sensitivity and improved specificity. In 2012, the Budapest Criteria became the official IASP diagnostic criteria for CRPS (3).

1. Continuing pain, which is disproportionate to any inciting event
2. Must report at least one symptom in *three of the four* following categories:
   - *Sensory:* reports of hyperesthesia and/or allodynia
   - *Vasomotor:* reports of temperature asymmetry and/or skin color changes and/or skin color asymmetry
   - *Sudomotor/edema:* reports of edema and/or sweating changes and/or sweating asymmetry
   - *Motor/trophic:* reports of decreased range of motion and/or motor dysfunction (weakness, tremor, dystonia) and/or trophic changes (hair, nail, skin)
3. Must display at least one sign at the time of evaluation in *two or more* of the following categories:
   - *Sensory:* evidence of hyperalgesia (to pinprick) and/or allodynia (to light touch and/or deep somatic pressure and/or joint movement)
   - *Vasomotor:* evidence of temperature asymmetry and/or skin color changes and/or asymmetry
   - *Sudomotor/edema:* evidence of edema and/or sweating changes and/or sweating asymmetry
   - *Motor/trophic:* evidence of decreased range of motion and/or motor dysfunction (weakness, tremor, dystonia) and/or trophic changes (hair, nail, skin)
4. There is no other diagnosis that better explains the signs and symptoms

TREATMENT/MEDICATIONS

The mainstay of treatment for CRPS involves early restoration of function.

Initiation of physical therapy (PT)/occupational therapy (OT) program with focus on the affected limb.

Oral steroids early in the course can help quell symptoms.

Sympathetic Blocks – Diagnostic and therapeutic

- Stellate ganglion block: good for upper extremity CRPS
- Lumbar sympathetic block: good for lower extremity CRPS

Sympathectomy – Can be performed interventionally (radiofrequency [RF] and cryoablation) or surgically

Dorsal Column Stimulation – Can be a tremendous help with upper extremity/lower extremity CRPS. Appropriate diagnosis (good response to sympathetic block) and patient screening help to improve outcomes of neuromodulation

NECK/LOW BACK PAIN

Spinal Stenosis – Pain typically has a more insidious onset, with the patient complaining of pain that is worse after arising in the morning as well as after ambulating a certain distance. The former is said to be due to the additive compression by engorged epidural veins overnight. The latter is called *neurogenic claudication* (or pseudoclaudication—pain worsening when walking down a hill versus up the hill, which is vascular claudication). As with radicular pain, signs and symptoms may have a dermatomal distribution but are typically more diffuse. Further, spinal stenosis and degenerative disc disease are not mutually exclusive. More often than not, stenosis results from disc herniation/bulges coupled with spondylitic changes such as facet joint and ligamentous hypertrophy.

Sacroiliac Joint Pain – The sacrum supports the axial spine and articulates with the iliac wings to form the left and right sacroiliac (SI) joints. Several ligamentous and muscle attachments contribute to the stability of this joint. Imbalance or dysfunction in the SI joint can result from repeated lifting and bending, causing a shift on the anteroposterior axis. Additionally, repeated forces can cause stress on the myofascial attachments and irritation of the joint articulations. The SI joint is innervated by L3 to S1 root levels and may cause radicular-type symptoms when irritated, making diagnosis difficult or delayed. Common areas of pain in SI joint pathologies include the ipsilateral hip and greater trochanter regions (7). While evaluating the SI joint as a pain source, one must obtain appropriate history, radiography, and tests for pathologic causes of sacroiliitis (i.e., ankylosing spondylosis). A variety of provocation maneuvers exist (i.e., Faber and Gaenslen tests) to evaluate for SI joint dysfunction, although their sensitivity and specificity vary.

Treatment

Treatment typically begins with a short period of rest and initiation of PT (i.e., "Back School" and McKenzie treatment programs) along with initiation of medications including NSAIDs and cyclo-oxygenase-2 (COX-2) inhibitors. Over the past few years, multiple topical formulations for NSAID delivery have augmented the tools available to the physician. A tapering dose of oral steroids may also be given concomitantly, depending on the severity of clinical presentation.

SPINAL INTERVENTIONS

Cervical/Lumbar Epidural Nerve Blocks

Epidural injections involve the introduction of local anesthetics, opioids, or steroids that have utility in the management of pain of various etiologies. They are mainly performed in an interlaminar technique with loss-of-resistance or a transforaminal (described in the following text) approach. The interlaminar technique involves traversing the supraspinous ligament, interspinous ligament, and then the ligamentum flavum, after which a "sudden loss of resistance" indicates entry to the epidural space.

Indications:
- Cervical/lumbar radiculopathy
- Pain from cervical/lumbar spondylosis (8)
- Post-laminectomy syndrome
- Pain from vertebral compression fractures (9)
- Diabetic polyneuropathy
- Phantom limb pain
- Chemotherapy-related neuropathy/plexopathy
- Cancer pain
- As a diagnostic procedure to help identify the pain source (i.e., pelvic, back, groin, genital, and lower extremity pain)

Contraindications:
- Local infection
- Patient on anticoagulants
- Coagulopathy
- Sepsis (10)

Complications:
- Dural puncture – Incidence ranges from 0.16% to 1.3% in experienced hands and may result in CSF loss or introduction of air (pneumocephalus), responsible for significant postprocedure headaches (11)
- Intravenous needle placement, given the preponderance of epidural veins/arteries
- Epidural hematoma – Usually self-limiting. In the setting of anticoagulation, it may cause cord compression, cauda equina syndrome paralysis, apnea, and death
- Infection – High chance of spread, given epidural vascularity
- Urinary retention and incontinence (12)
- Direct trauma to spinal cord/nerve roots

Caudal Epidural Nerve Block

Though currently used relatively infrequently, this injection preceded its lumbar counterpart by nearly 20 years (1901).

Proper technique for the caudal epidural steroid injection (ESI) involves the patient positioned in a lateral or prone position. The caudal space is approached through the *sacrococcygeal ligament* that covers the sacral hiatus. The needle is placed over the sacrococcygeal membrane at an angle of about 60° to the coronal plane and perpendicular to the other planes. There is usually a loss of resistance as the membrane is pierced. General indications/contraindications mimic those of the lumbar/cervical approaches where anatomically relevant. There are, however, several key indications where the caudal injection may be preferred:

- Prior lumbar surgery – Can distort anatomy, making lumbar approach difficult (i.e., fusion and hardware in place)
- Patients on anticoagulation or coagulopathic therapy (since epidural venous plexus usually ends at S4)

Contraindications include infection, sepsis, pilonidal cysts, and congenital anomalies of dural sac and contents.

Complications include dural puncture, needle misplacement, hematoma/ecchymosis, infection, and urinary retention/incontinence.

Facet Joint Injection/Medial Branch Block

The cervical and lumbar facet (zygapophyseal) joints are common and significant sources of chronic neck and low back pain (13). The facet joints are diarthrodial, made up of the inferior articular process and the superior articular process of the vertebra one level below. They are dually innervated, receiving inputs from the medial branch nerves of each level comprising the joint. For example, the L4/L5 facet joint is innervated by the medial branches of L4 and L5. Facet blocks are performed by first properly identifying anatomic landmarks, utilizing oblique images at 10° to 40° from midline for optimal needle visualization with rotation by another 5° to 10° for joint visualization. Using proper imaging and feel, a mixture of dye, local anesthetic, and steroid is injected.

Indications:
- When making the decision to inject the facet joint or perform a medial branch block, one must identify those with facet syndrome and the levels causing the pain. Classically, symptoms are characterized by dull, aching pain with tenderness to palpation over the facet joints with occasional overlying muscle spasm. Pain may be unilateral or bilateral with occasional radiation. Definitive diagnosis can be made with pain relief following injection of local anesthetic into the facet joint.

Contraindications:
- Like other injections, these should be avoided in patients with medication allergies, systemic or local infection, or coagulopathies.

Complications:
- The most common complication is a transient increase in pain. Other complications include dural penetration, spinal anesthesia, capsule rupture, infection, and vertebral artery puncture (cervical facets).

Selective Nerve Root Blocks/Transforaminal ESI

Nerve root blocks/transforaminal steroid injections are useful tools in the workup and treatment of back pain, but they are used in a patient subset that differs from one where facet joint blocks are used. Nerve root blocks attempt to anesthetize the painful nerve for both diagnostic and therapeutic purposes. Steroids are used in an attempt to provide long-term relief, primarily in patients with radicular symptoms. Transforaminal ESIs can be utilized when physical exam and radiologic findings suggest a specific nerve root as the cause for pain. Pressure on such a nerve may result in an autoimmune response that can further elicit pain and facilitate inflammation. Because venous drainage occurs outside of the nerve, pressure on a nerve may increases the venous pressure. Further, extrinsic forces on the nerve can lead to ischemia and pain at the nerve root, manifested as pain being referred down a particular dermatome. Similar to other injections, the selective nerve root block (SNRB) or transforaminal ESI involves placing a mixture of local anesthetic and steroid in the superior region of the neural foramen where the postganglionic nerve root exits.

There exist two main approaches for transforaminal ESIs. The most common approach utilizes the "safe triangle" and approaches the affected nerve root in a subpedicular fashion. In this method, the injection needle is progressed toward the safe triangle under the inferior surface of the pedicle to locate the superolateral spinal nerve related to the patient's symptoms (Figure 10.8). This approach is common and favored because medication can be injected into the anterior extradural space and the risk of damaging dura is decreased (14). However, Murthy et al. reported that the Adamkiewicz artery (AKA artery) runs through this "safe triangle" and injection at this site runs the risk of damage to the vessel wall or injection into the artery itself (15).

The second approach is the utilization of Kambin's triangle. In 1972, Kambin introduced endoscopic intervertebral discectomy by posterolateral approach, defining Kambin's triangle as the best approach to the intervertebral disc (16). Kambin's triangle is defined as a right-angled triangle over the dorsolateral disc, with the hypotenuse as the exiting nerve root, the base (width) as the superior border of the caudal vertebra, and the height as the traversing nerve root (16; Figure 10.9). It is believed that this approach can protect epidural and neurological structures and prevent chronic nerve edema, epidural bleeding, and scarring (14).

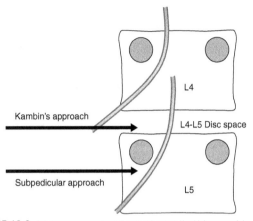

FIGURE 10.8 Safe triangle (subpedicular) approach versus Kambin's approach to transforaminal ESIs.

ESI, epidural steroid injection.
Source: Adapted from Ref. (14).

Indications:
- After discectomy in patients who have recurrent radiculopathy but no recurrent disc herniation, symptoms are often caused when scar tissue tethers the nerve. Many patients can be treated successfully by using SNRB/TFESI.

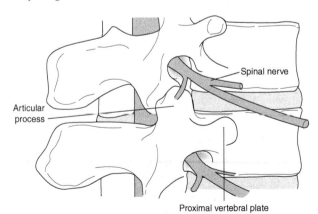

FIGURE 10.9 Schematic depiction of Kambin's triangle.
Source: Adapted from Ref. (14).

- In patients with disc herniations, nerve root blocks are helpful. Since the body naturally resolves 90% of disc herniations when given enough time, early pain relief is important to try to avoid surgery. The pain is believed to result from an inflammation of the nerve root more than from direct compression. As a result, potent anti-inflammatories such as steroids work well in mitigating the process.
  - The injections are also efficacious when facet joint hypertrophy or cysts cause an irritation of the nerve root, though not so much as with discogenic disease.

Contraindications:

- Include a history of allergy to local anesthetics or steroids, systemic or overlying infection, coagulopathy, or, in the case of facet joint injections, severe foraminal stenosis (which can become worse if an injection is made into the joint itself). Severe foraminal stenosis is a relative contraindication to intra-articular facet joint injections. Injections into the facet joints can cause joint swelling, worsening a preexisting foraminal stenosis.

Complications:

- Rare, but can include bleeding, infection, and allergic reactions.
- Intravascular injection may be harmless, but it results in a suboptimal or false-negative result. Furthermore, intravascular injection can be dangerous if the agent is injected into the vertebral artery or radicular branches that enter the neural foramina at various levels.
- Spinal cord infarcts have occurred from both cervical and lumbar SNRBs.
- Direct trauma to the nerve root can occur via the spinal needle, causing increased pain and occasional root avulsion.
- Spinal anesthesia may occur if local anesthetic is inadvertently injected into the nerve root sleeve.
- During cervical procedures, doing so can lead to respiratory arrest. Some patients experience adverse effects from the steroids.
- Consider the total steroid dose when performing injections at multiple levels.

SI Joint Injection

- Indicated for sacroiliitis or chronic SI joint arthropathy. Serves both diagnostic and therapeutic purposes. Under fluoroscopic guidance, the joint space is visualized. A spinal needle is then introduced at the junction of the posterior one third of the joint line with the middle one third of the joint. The posterior iliac spine obstructs the superior portion of the joint, making the lower portion of the joint easier to inject. Once the joint space is entered, a small amount of contrast is injected to confirm needle placement. Once the arthrogram is satisfactory, the medication, which is usually a mixture of anesthetic and steroid, is injected.

Other Procedures

Radiofrequency Ablation

Involves using a needle (electrode) to deliver a current in either a constant (hot) or a pulsatile (cold) fashion to cause neurolysis of the nerves in the vicinity of the lesion created by the electrode. General indications include failed conservative treatments, transient relief from repeated medial branch blocks, or no indication for surgical intervention. Again, contraindications include coagulopathy, platelet dysfunction, and severe cardiopulmonary disease for procedures involving cervical and thoracic regions (16). Complications include local post-procedure soreness, sensorimotor deficits from improper needle placement, vascular trauma (cervical region), pneumothorax (thoracic), entry into subarachnoid space via neural foramen (dorsal root ganglion RF), diaphragmatic paralysis and hoarseness (from cervical sympathectomy RF), puncture of abdominal viscera (lumbar sympathectomy RF), or direct disk, cord, and nerve root trauma.

Vertebroplasty/Kyphoplasty

A minimally invasive procedure aimed at treating the pain and spinal instability surrounding acute vertebral compression fractures from the age of 2 weeks to 1 year. Anecdotally, many practitioners use a 6-month age limit for compression fractures. Further indications for vertebroplasty include refractory pain from the fracture. Absolute contraindications include discitis, sepsis, and osteomyelitis. Relative contraindications include significant spinal canal compromise secondary to bone fragments, fractures older than 2 years, >75% collapse of vertebral body, fractures above T5, and traumatic compression fractures or disruption of posterior vertebral body wall. Vertebroplasty focuses on treating pain, while kyphoplasty focuses on restoring stability and vertebral height. Vertebroplasty involves tunneling a large gauge needle into the vertebral body and injecting 3 to 5 mL of methyl methacrylate cement into the vertebral body. Similarly, in kyphoplasty, two balloons are introduced via catheter into the vertebral body. The inflated balloon restores height and then allows for filling with the cement.

Spinal Cord Stimulators

Stimulate dorsal column of the spinal cord to treat patients with chronic intractable pain. Though the exact mechanism is unknown, several theories exist including the "gate" theory and direct inhibition of pain pathways in the spinothalamic tract. The spinal cord stimulator (SCS) can either be totally implantable or have an external transmitter. SCS placement first involves a trial stage where the lead is placed and managed externally. The latter is internalized pending satisfactory results. Indications for SCS include failed neck/back surgery, peripheral neuropathy, post-herpetic neuralgia, CRPS I/II, epidural fibrosis/

arachnoiditis causing chronic pain, radiculopathy, phantom limb pain, and ischemic pain from peripheral vascular disease (17).

Most patients have had chronic pain for greater than 12 months that is refractive to other conservative therapies. Contraindications include coagulopathy, platelet dysfunction, local or systemic infection, and patients with psychological issues (i.e., drug seeking). The most common complications are scar formation, lead migration, and infection.

Neuromodulation has more recently begun to be used for peripheral stimulation in subcutaneous tissue with promising results. It has been used successfully for occipital neuralgia (18) and recalcitrant trigeminal neuralgia, among others (19).

Intrathecal Pumps

Intrathecal pumps have a place in the management of chronic pain as well as spasticity. A catheter is inserted intrathecally and connected to a pump. Initially, during the trial, the pump is external. If a satisfactory result is achieved, a permanent catheter is placed intrathecally and is tunneled through the subcutaneous tissue to an internal pump that usually sits in a pocket in the anterior abdomen. The pump can then be adjusted to deliver different amounts of medication. Intrathecal infusion bypasses the blood–brain barrier and hence allows a more directed effect on brain and spinal neuroreceptors with less medication. Several medications are used in these pumps, with the two most common ones being preservative-free morphine and baclofen for spasticity management.

REFERENCES

1. Rathmell JP, Fields HL. Pain: Pathophysiology and management. In: Longo DL, Fauci AS, Kasper DL, et al., eds. *Harrison's Principles of Internal Medicine, 18e.* New York, NY: McGraw-Hill; 2012.

2. Rosenquist RW, Vrooman BM. Chronic pain management. In: Butterworth JF, IV, Mackey DC, Wasnick JD. eds. *Morgan.* Appleton & Lange; 2013.

3. Harden RN, Bruehl S, Perez RS, et al. Validation of proposed diagnostic criteria (the 'Budapest Criteria') for complex regional pain syndrome. *Pain.* 2010;150(2):268–274.

4. Tajerian M, Clark JD. New concepts in complex regional pain syndrome. *Hand Clin.* 2016;32(1):41–49.

5. Kozin F, Soin JS, Ryan LM, et al. Bone scintigraphy in the reflex sympathetic dystrophy syndrome. *Radiology.* 1981;138(2):437–444.

6. Chelimsky TC, Low PA, Naessens JM, et al. Value of autonomic testing in reflex sympathetic dystrophy. *Mayo Clin Proc.* 1995;70(11):1029–1040.

7. Fortin JD, Aprill CN, Ponthieux B, et al. Sacroiliac joint: pain referral maps upon applying a new injection/arthrography technique. Part I. *Spine.* 1994;19:1475–1482.

8. Pages E. Anestesia metamerica. *Rev Sanid Mil Madr.* 1921;11:351–385.

9. Bromage PR. Identification of the epidural space. In: Bromage PR, ed. *Epidural Analgesia.* Philadelphia, PA: WB Saunders; 1978:178.

10. Cousins MJ, Bromage PR. Epidural neural blockade. In: Cousins MJ, Bridenbaugh DO, eds. *Neural Blockade*. Philadelphia, PA: JB Lippincott; 1988:340-341.

11. Ghaleb A, Arjang K, &Devanand M. Post-dural puncture headache. *Int J Gen Med*. 2012;5:45–51.

12. Armitage EN. Lumbar and thoracic epidural. In: Wildsmith JAW, Armitage EN, eds. *Principles and Practice of Regional Anesthesia*. New York, NY: Churchill Livingstone; 1987:109.

13. Bogduk N, Aprill C. On the nature of neck pain, discography, and cervical zygapophyseal joint blocks. *Pain*. 1993;54:213–217.

14. Park JW, Nam HS, Cho SK, et al. Kambin's triangle approach of lumbar transforaminal epidural injection with spinal stenosis. *Ann Rehabil Med*. 2011;35(6):833–843.

15. Murthy NS, Maus TP, Behrns CL. Intraforaminal location of the great anterior radiculomedullary artery (artery of Adamkiewicz): a retrospective review. *Pain Med*. 2010;11:1756–1764.

16. Kambin P, Savitz MH. Arthroscopic microdiscectomy: an alternative to open disc surgery. *Mt Sinai J Med*. 2000;67:283–287.

17. Carter ML. Spinal cord stimulation in chronic pain: a review of the evidence. *Anaesth Intensive Care*. 2004;32:11–21.

18. Weiner RL, Reed KL. Peripheral neurostimulation for control of intractable occipital neuralgia. *Neuromodulation*. 1999;2:217–221.

19. Slavin KV, Burchiel KJ. Peripheral nerve stimulation for painful nerve injuries. *Contemp Neurosurg*. 1999;21(19):1–6.

SUGGESTED READING

Falco FJE, Kim D, Zhu J, et al. Interventional pain management procedures. In: Braddom R, ed. *Physical Medicine and Rehabilitation*. 3rd ed. Philadelphia, PA: WB Saunders; 2006.

Nachemson A, ed. *Neck and Back Pain: The Scientific Evidence of Causes, Diagnosis, and Treatment*. Philadelphia, PA: Lippincott Williams & Wilkins; 2000.

CHAPTER 11

MUSCULOSKELETAL/ SPORTS/ORTHOPEDICS

LIMB JOINT PRIMARY MOVERS

Motion (ROM in degrees)	Muscles	Nerves	Roots
Shoulder flexion (180)	Anterior deltoid Coracobrachialis	Axillary Musculocutaneous	C5, C6 C6, C7
Shoulder extension (45)	Latissimus dorsi Teres major Posterior deltoid	Thoracodorsal Inferior subscapular Axillary	C6, C7, C8 C5, C6, C7 C5, C6
Shoulder abduction (180)	Middle deltoid Supraspinatus	Axillary Suprascapular	C5, C6 C5, C6
Shoulder adduction (40)	Pectoralis major Latissimus dorsi	Med + lat pectoral Thoracodorsal	C5-T1 C6, C7, C8
Shoulder external rotation (90)*	Infraspinatus Teres minor	Suprascapular Axillary	C5, C6 C5, C6
Shoulder internal rotation (80)*	Subscapularis Pectoralis major Latissimus dorsi Teres major	Sup + inf subscapular Med + lat pectoral Thoracodorsal Inferior subscapular	C5, C6 C5-T1 C6, C7, C8 C5, C6, C7
Shoulder shrug	Trapezius Levator scapulae	Spinal accessory (CN XI) C3, C4 ± dorsal scapular (C5)	
Elbow flexion (150)	Biceps brachii Brachialis Brachioradialis	Musculocutaneous Musculocutaneous Radial	C5, C6 C5, C6 C5, C6
Elbow extension	Triceps brachii	Radial	C6, C7, C8
Forearm supination (80)	Supinator Biceps brachii	Posterior interosseous Musculocutaneous	C5, C6, C7 C5, C6

(continued)

(*continued*)

Motion (ROM in degrees)	Muscles	Nerves	Roots
Forearm pronation (80)	Pronator teres Pronator quadratus	Median Anterior interosseous	C6, C7 C8, Tl
Wrist flexion (80)	Flexor carpi radialis Flexor carpi ulnaris	Median Ulnar	C6, C7, C8 C7, C8, Tl
Wrist extension (70)	Ext carpi rad longus Ext carpi rad brevis Ext carpi ulnaris	Radial Radial Posterior interosseous	C6, C7 C6, C7 C7, C8
MCP flexion (90)	Lumbricals Dorsal + palmar interossei	Median, ulnar Ulnar	C8, Tl C8, Tl
PIP flexion (100)	Flexor digitorum superficialis Flexor digitorum profundus	Median Median, ulnar	C7-T1 C7, C8, Tl
DIP flexion (90)	Flexor digitorum profundus	Median, ulnar	C7, C8, Tl
MCP, finger extension	Extensor digitorum Extensor indicis Extensor digiti minimi	Posterior interosseous Posterior interosseous Posterior interosseous	C7, C8 C7, C8 C7, C8
Finger abduction (20)	Dorsal interossei Abductor digiti minimi	Ulnar Ulnar	C8, Tl C8, Tl
Finger adduction	Palmar interossei	Ulnar	C8, Tl
Thumb flexion	Flexor pollicis brevis Flexor pollicis longus	Median, ulnar Anterior interosseus	C8, Tl C7, C8, Tl
Thumb extension	EPB Extensor pollicis longus	Posterior interosseous Posterior interosseous	C7, C8 C7, C8
Thumb abduction	Abductor pollicis longus Abductor pollicis brevis	Posterior interosseous Median	C7, C8 C8, Tl

(*continued*)

(*continued*)

Motion (ROM in degrees)	Muscles	Nerves	Roots
Thumb adduction	Adductor pollicis	Ulnar	C8, T1
Hip flexion (120)	Iliopsoas	Femoral	L2, L3, L4
Hip extension (30)	Gluteus maximus	Inferior gluteal	L5, S1, S2
Hip abduction (40)	Gluteus medius Gluteus minimus	Superior gluteal Superior gluteal	L4, L5, S1 L4, L5, S1
Hip adduction (20)	Adductor longus Adductor magnus	Obturator Obturator, sciatic	L2, L3, L4 L2, L3, L4, L5, S1
Hip external rotation (45)	Obturator int + ext	n. obt int, obturator	L3-S2
	Quadratus femoris	n. quadratus femoris	L2, L3, L4
	Piriformis	n. piriformis	S1, S2
	Sup + inf gemelli	n. obt int, n. quad fem	L4-S2
	Gluteus maximus (postfibers)	Inferior gluteal	L5, S1, S2
Hip internal rotation (45)	Gluteus minimus	Superior gluteal	L4, L5, S1
	Gluteus medius	Superior gluteal	L4, L5, S1
	Tensor fasciae latae	Superior gluteal	L4, L5, S1
Knee flexion (135)	Semitendinosus	Tibial div. of sciatic	L5, S1, S2
	Semimembranosus	Tibial div. of sciatic	L4, L5-S2
	Biceps femoris	Tib + per div. sciatic	L5, S1, S2
Knee extension	Quadriceps femoris	Femoral	L2, L3, L4
Ankle dorsiflexion (20)	Tibialis anterior	Deep peroneal	L4, L5, S1
Ankle plantar flexion (45)	Gastrocnemius	Tibial	L5, S1, S2
	Soleus	Tibial	L5, S1, S2
Ankle inversion (35)	Tibialis posterior	Tibial	L4, L5, S1
Ankle eversion (25)	Peroneus longus	Superficial peroneal	L4, L5, S1
	Peroneus brevis	Superficial peroneal	L4, L5, S1

(*continued*)

(continued)

Motion (ROM in degrees)	Muscles	Nerves	Roots
Toe extension	Extensor hallucis longus	Deep peroneal	L4, L5, S1
	Extensor digitorum brevis	Deep peroneal	L5, S1

*Shoulder internal rotation/external rotation varies with elevation of the arm.
CN, cranial nerve; div, division; EPB, extensor pollicis brevis; ext, extensor; inf, inferior; int, internal; lat, lateral; med, medial; MCP, metacarpophalangeal; obt, obturator; PIP, proximal interphalangeal; rad, radial; sup, superior.
For ROM, 0° is anatomic position. Please note that there is no absolute consensus regarding which muscles are the primary movers of joints or that for the root innervations of muscles.

TREATMENT OF SELECTED MUSCULOSKELETAL CONDITIONS

Upper Limb

Acromioclavicular (AC) Sprains/Tears – AC injuries often occur with falls on an adducted shoulder. AC joint injuries are classified according to the Rockwood criteria. A type I (Rockwood classification) injury is a nondisplaced sprain of the AC ligament, manifested by local tenderness without anatomic deformity. A type II injury (see Figure 11.1) involves an AC tear and coracoclavicular (CC) ligament sprain, but the CC interspace is intact. Treatment for type I or II injuries are nonoperative and includes an arm sling, ice, analgesics, and progressive ROM exercises. An unstable type II injury may require arm sling use for 2 to 4 weeks. Sports activities can be resumed when full painless ROM is achieved and deltoid is near baseline. Type III to VI lesions involve rupture of the AC *and* CC ligaments with varying displacements of the clavicle. These require orthopedic consultation for potential open reduction internal fixation (ORIF), although many separations may be followed conservatively with several weeks of sling-and-swathe immobilization, followed by long-term therapy.

AC Joint Osteoarthritis (ACJ OA) – OA is a very common cause of ACJ pain, especially in the elderly. The presence of ACJ tenderness and pain with cross-body adduction suggests ACJ OA. Radiologic studies such as x-rays and ultrasound (US) evaluation can help confirm the diagnosis. Treatment includes topical or oral analgesics, physical therapy (PT), injections, and surgery if refractory to conservative care. Traditional injection techniques have

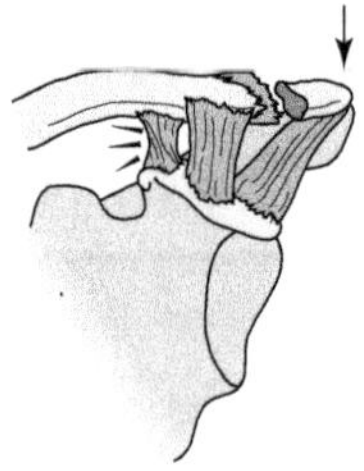

FIGURE 11.1 Type II injury.
Source: Adapted from Ref. (1).

proven to be inaccurate; therefore, fluoroscopic or US-guided injections are preferred (2).

Rotator Cuff Tendinopathy/Shoulder Impingement Syndrome – As a common cause of rotator cuff pathology, shoulder impingement syndrome can lead to rotator cuff tendinitis, subacromial bursitis, rotator cuff tendinosis, and rotator cuff tears. Most common tendon affected is the supraspinatus tendon. Impingement of the shoulder can be caused by many factors, including predisposing acromion shape, repetitive overhead activities (i.e., throwing, racquet sports, and swimming), and age, just to name a few of the most known. Pain is often worse at night and may be aggravated by overhead activities. Shoulder flexion and abduction may be limited.

Exam maneuvers to assess for shoulder impingement include Hawkin's and Neer's. Other common maneuvers to assess rotator cuff pathology include painful arc, drop arm test, and empty can maneuver, all described in the following text.

In Neer's test (Figure 11.2), the examiner passively flexes the patient's shoulder forward to 180° while the arm is internally rotated. A positive test is pain in the subacromial area. The Hawkin's test is performed by flexing the elbow and abducting the shoulder passively to 90° in the scapular plane and internally rotating the glenohumeral joint. A positive test is pain in subacromial region.

A *painful arc* (Figure 11.3) may be present at about 70° to 110° on active arm abduction. In the *drop arm test*, the arm is passively elevated to 90° in abduction and the patient is asked to hold the arm in position and then slowly lower the arm to the side. The inability to slowly lower the arm or having severe pain when attempting to do so may be indicative of a severe or complete tear of the rotator cuff. The *empty can test* is assessed with arm at 90° of abduction and the shoulder is internally rotated and angled in the scapular pain (approximately 30° of abduction) with thumb pointing to the floor. The examiner applies downward pressure on the distal forearm against resistance. Pain and/or weakness in the shoulder is considered positive of rotator cuff pathology.

Treatment for rotator cuff pathology. The painful shoulder should initially be *rested* until pain and swelling subside. *Ice* and *NSAIDs* may be helpful. Overhead activities should be avoided. *PT* can institute gentle stretching to preserve ROM and isometric strengthening. Exercises should progress until strength and ROM are restored. If these conservative measures fail, imaging should be ordered,

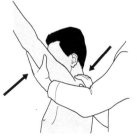

FIGURE 11.2 Neer's test.

including diagnostic US and/or MRI of the shoulder depending on imaging availability and type of injury. A *steroid injection* into the subacromial space may relieve pain and improve motion if these measures fail.

US-guided steroid injection can be performed; however, there is conflicting evidence to suggest the benefit of US-guided injection versus blind steroid injection into the subacromial space. Evolving medical practice does include the use of US guidance for shoulder injections to ensure accurate medication placement, especially

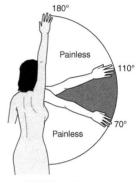

FIGURE 11.3 Painful arc.

after failure of initial blind shoulder injection for additional diagnostic and therapeutic purposes (3,4). *Surgery* is an option if there is a failure of conservative treatment/steroid injections, prolonged duration of symptoms, large rotator cuff tear, history of trauma, and limitations of ADLs (5). Surgery involves repairing the rotator cuff, and it may also include an acromioplasty, which involves acromial shaving to increase the space around the inflamed tendon if shoulder impingement is suspect. The tendon may also be debrided. Recovery averages 4 to 6 months to regain full strength after surgery.

Anterior Shoulder Dislocation – Anterior dislocations are more common than posterior dislocations. Complications include axillary nerve injury, recurrent dislocations, and rotator cuff tears (especially in older patients). A *Bankart lesion* (Figure 11.4) is an avulsion of the anteroinferior glenoid labrum and capsule from the glenoid rim and is felt to be a primary etiologic factor in recurrent dislocations. A *Hill-Sachs lesion* is a compression fracture of the humeral head when the posterolateral aspect of the humeral head compresses against the anterior glenoid rim. Various techniques exist for acute reduction, including the modified *Stimson technique*, where the patient lies prone with a wrist weight (i.e., 5–10 lb.) on the affected arm as it hangs over the side of the table. Reduction is achieved over 15 to 20 minutes as the shoulder muscles relax.

There is no strong evidence to show that immobilization or the duration of immobilization has an effect on outcome. One option includes bracing in external rotation (ER), which may reduce the rate of recurrence, though

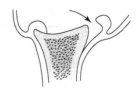

FIGURE 11.4 Bankart lesion.

this should be initiated 24 to 48 hours following injury. Early rehabilitation may include icing and sling immobilization for 1 to 3 weeks to allow healing of the capsule. Maintenance of elbow, wrist, and hand ROM is important. Isometric exercises and gentle pendular exercises with the arm in the sling are encouraged, but passive abduction for hygiene is limited to 45° and ER is avoided. The duration of sling use may be shortened in older patients due to the higher risk of frozen shoulder. Once the capsule has healed, shoulder ROM and strengthening are progressed. There is debate regarding the optimal type and timing of surgery after shoulder dislocation and in shoulder instability.

Adhesive Capsulitis – A syndrome characterized by a progressive painful loss of passive and active glenohumeral ROM that occurs more commonly in females and is frequently seen in individuals between the ages of 40 and 60 years (6). All ROM is affected. This condition may be the end result of other conditions that result in prolonged immobility (i.e., bursitis and rotator cuff tendinitis) and has also been associated with other medical conditions (i.e., DM, thyroid dysfunction, and autoimmune diseases). Treatment consists of aggressive ROM, NSAIDs, and heat modalities to improve tolerance. Other techniques include intra-articular steroid injections, brisement (hydrodilation of the capsule), manipulation under anesthesia, and suprascapular nerve blocks. Of these additional options, intra-articular steroid injection has been well studied and appears to improve short-term outcomes. Recovery may take several months to beyond a year (7).

Bicipital Tendinitis – This overuse injury can be associated with overhead activities or sports and often coexists with shoulder impingement syndrome, rotator cuff tears, or labral pathology (i.e., superior labral tear from anterior to posterior [SLAP] lesions). Examination often reveals a tender bicipital groove. While palpating this structure, assess for instability/subluxation of the bicipital tendon by internally and externally rotating the shoulder. If unstable, the tendon may sublux medially over the lesser tuberosity and a clunk or snap may be appreciated. *Speed's test* (Figure 11.5) is performed by elevating the subject's arm to 90° with the elbow extended and palm upward, then having the patient attempt forward flexion of the arm against resistance. Pain in the bicipital groove is indicative of a positive test. Treatment includes NSAIDs, activity modification, and progressive exercise program, which may include the use of modalities such as heat and postactivity icing. Local corticosteroid injection may be

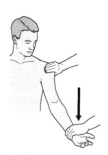

FIGURE 11.5 Speed's test.

used in refractory cases, and US guidance may help increase the accuracy of
performing injections into the tendon
sheath (8).

Scapular Winging – Medial scapular
winging (Figure 11.6) is caused by
weakness of the serratus anterior (long
thoracic nerve). It is elicited by having the patient push against a wall
and using resisted forward flexion or
resisted scapular protraction.

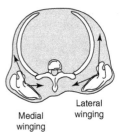

FIGURE 11.6 Scapular winging.

Lateral winging is caused by weakness of the trapezius muscle (CN XI)
and is elicited by shoulder abduction. Most cases of medial or lateral
winging resolve with a full rehabilitation and strengthening program,
although traumatic and refractory cases can be surgically corrected.

Golfer's Elbow (Medial Epicondylitis) – An overuse syndrome of the
tendinous origin of the flexor–pronator mass and medial collateral
ligament (MCL) of the elbow. The initial treatment is *rest, ice, compression, and elevation (RICE)* and *NSAIDs*. Stretching the elbow during
the painful period is important. Once pain and inflammation subside, strengthening exercises are started (important groups include
the wrist flexors/extensors, wrist radial deviators, forearm pronator/
supinators, and elbow flexor/extensors). A *tennis elbow counterforce
strap* may be helpful. *Injection of local steroids* into the area of maximum tenderness can also be considered, with care taken not to injure
the ulnar nerve.

Tennis Elbow (Lateral Epicondylitis) – An extensor tendinopathy affecting
the extensor carpi radialis brevis (ECRB), but some studies suggest the
problem arises from the common extensor tendon shared by the ECRB
and extensor carpi radialis longus (ECRL). Provocative testing using
Cozen's Test can elicit pain over the lateral epicondyle. To perform this
test, the examiner stabilizes the patient's elbow while palpating the
lateral epicondyle. The patient then pronates the forearm as well as
radially deviates and extends the wrist against resistance applied by
the examiner. A positive test would be the reproduction of pain near
the lateral epicondyle. Initial treatment is *relative rest, NSAIDs,* and *heat*
or *cold* modalities. Wrist extensor *stretching and strengthening* should be
initiated when tolerated. Conservative measures are usually effective,
but recurrences are common. A tennis elbow strap worn circumferen-
tially around the forearm just distal to the elbow may be helpful and
a wrist splint may be considered to rest the common wrist extensor
tendons. Modifications to the racquet include a *larger racquet grip and
head* and *lesser string tension*. A *corticosteroid injection* into the area of
maximum tenderness may be indicated if conservative treatment fails.
Treatment with platelet-rich plasma (PRP) or autologous whole blood

has been shown to be more effective than corticosteroids in those patients who have failed conservative treatment (9,10). No more than three injections should be given at intervals of 5 days to 1 week. Surgical fasciotomy or fixing the conjoined tendon may be considered if these measures fail.

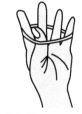

FIGURE 11.7 Strengthening.

De Quervain's Disease – A tenosynovitis of the first dorsal compartment of the hand, which is made up of the abductor pollicis longus (APL) and extensor pollicis brevis (EPB) tendons. *Finkelstein's test* is positive when pain is elicited in the radial wrist while the wrist is forced into ulnar deviation with the thumb enclosed in a fist. Treatment includes *activity modification* and *NSAIDs* followed by a *stretching* and *strengthening* program (Figure 11.7). A *thumb spica splint* with the wrist in neutral position and the first metacarpophalangeal (MCP) immobilized (interphalangeal [IP] joint is free) is helpful in resting the tendons. *Local corticosteroid injections* into the compartment reduce acute pain and inflammation. US-guided injections have been described and may improve accuracy while decreasing the risk of intratendinous injections (11). *Surgical decompression* may be curative in severe, refractory cases.

Scaphoid Fracture (Most Common Carpal Bone Fracture) – Often due to a fall on an outstretched hand. Snuffbox tenderness may be noted. If initial plain films (approximately three to four views) are negative, the wrist should be immobilized (short arm cast or splint with thumb spica) and films repeated in approximately 2 weeks (some fractures may not be visible until bone has resorbed around the fracture line). If repeat films are negative and clinical suspicion persists, CT or MRI can be considered. Because the main blood supply (Figure 11.8) enters from the distal pole, there is a high incidence of nonunion and avascular necrosis (AVN) in waist and proximal pole fractures. For nondisplaced fractures, a *long arm thumb spica cast* should be used. Isometric muscle contractions can be performed in the cast to counter atrophy. Displaced fractures or nondisplaced fractures with persistent nonunion should be referred for surgical evaluation.

Trigger Finger (Digital Stenosing Tenosynovitis) – Digital tendon sheath inflammation may result in a tendinous knot that gets stuck in the finger pulley system as the finger extends. Patients with DM or rheumatoid arthritis are

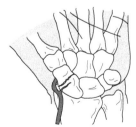

FIGURE 11.8 Blood supply of the scaphoid.

particularly at risk for developing trigger finger. *NSAIDs* and *steroid injections* help to reduce inflammation and pain. Use of a *volar static hand splint* that immobilizes the MCP but allows full IP flexion rests the flexor tendons and helps break the vicious cycle of inflammation and catching. In some cases, surgery may be necessary to release tendons in fingers that are locked in flexion.

Lower Limb

Greater Trochanteric Pain Syndrome – Classically described as trochanteric bursitis, but improved visualization of the hip via MRI and arthroscopy has proven that other etiologies of lateral hip pain exist (such as gluteus medius or minimus tendinosis or tears, and snapping hip syndrome; 12). Pain is noted with walking, running, climbing stairs, sitting, and especially when lying on the side of the involved hip. Physical examination often reveals point tenderness over greater trochanter and pain-limited hip abductor strength, and lateral hip pain with Patrick's Flexion ABduction External Rotation (FABER) test is noted. Conservative treatment includes *NSAIDs*, an iliotibial band (ITB) *stretching* program, and hip abductor/extensor strengthening. If refractory to these measures, a *steroid injection* into the bursas, as noted on imaging (Figure 11.9), can relieve symptoms in many patients. Various etiologies may be responsible for greater trochanteric region pain; therefore, musculoskeletal US may become a valuable tool for both diagnostic and therapeutic reasons (13,14). For instance, true trochanteric bursitis can be blindly injected, but other bursas including, but that are not limited to, subgluteus medius bursa, will require US image guidance to reach target.

ITB Syndrome – Potential causes include overtraining or running on uneven surfaces. Lateral knee pain is noted as the ITB slides over the lateral femoral condyle, especially between 20° and 30° of flexion. Predisposing factors include genu varum, tibial varum, varus hindfoot, and foot pronation. Tenderness over the lateral knee and Gerdy's tubercle may be noted on examination. *Ober's test* may be positive. Rehabilitation should be aimed at *stretching* the ITB, hip flexors, and gluteus maximus. Adductors may be strengthened to counteract the tight ITB, and hip abductor strengthening may also be performed to improve dynamic hip stability (Figure 11.10). Helpful *modalities* include ice, US, and phonophoresis. Foot pronation should be corrected; running only on even surfaces may help. A *steroid injection* into the area of the lateral femoral condyle may relieve pain. Symptoms can generally take 2 to 6 months to improve.

Figure 11.11 illustrates the Ober test for ITB/tensor fasciae latae (TFL) contraction. The

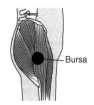

FIGURE 11.9 Bursa.

patient lies on the side with the involved side uppermost. The hip is flexed and then abducted as far as possible while stabilizing the pelvis. Next, the hip is brought into extension and the limb is released. The limb will remain abducted if there is tightness at the ITB or TFL when compared to the contralateral side.

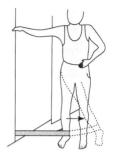

FIGURE 11.10 Hip adduction strengthening with TheraBand.

Sacroiliac Joint (SIJ) Pain – SIJ pain is a common but underestimated cause of chronic low back pain. SIJ pain is usually localized to the buttocks but can also be referred to the upper or lower lumbar region, groin, abdomen, lower limb, or the foot (15,16). Due to the myriad of presenting symptoms, no single physical examination or historical feature can reliably elucidate SIJ or iliolumbar pain, often necessitating multiple provocative physical exam maneuvers or diagnostic nerve blocks to confirm diagnosis (17). There are many physical exam maneuvers with varying sensitivities and specificities. Figure 11.12 illustrates Patrick's test (also known as FABER test). This test is commonly used to elicit SIJ pain. Many therapeutic approaches focus on interventional options, but conservative management with PT and NSAIDs may provide a viable option with fewer risks in the early course of treatment (17). Referral for diagnostic or therapeutic interventions should be considered after conservative management has failed or for refractory pain.

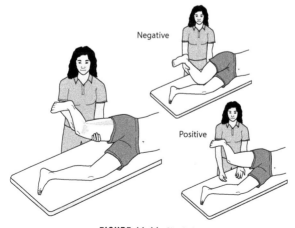

Negative

Positive

FIGURE 11.11 Ober test.

Pes Anserine Bursitis (Bursa Under Sartorius, Gracillis, SemiTendinosis; Mnemonic: "Say Grace Before Tea") – Pain and tenderness at the insertion of the medial hamstrings at the medial proximal tibia may be noted. The treatment should emphasize *stretching* of the medial hamstrings and improving knee biomechanics. Athletes may wear *protective knee padding. Steroid injections* may be very effective, but US guidance should be considered since unguided injections rarely infiltrate the pes anserine bursa (18).

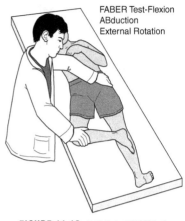

FABER Test-Flexion
ABduction
External Rotation

FIGURE 11.12 Patrick's test (FABER test).

Anterior Cruciate Ligament – The ACL proceeds superiorly and posteriorly from its anterior medial tibial attachment to attach to the medial aspect of the lateral femoral condyle (Figure. 11.13). It prevents excessive anterior translation of the tibia and abnormal ER of the tibia on the femur and knee hyperextension. A primary function in the athlete is maintaining joint stability during deceleration. The most common mechanism of injury is ER of the femur on fixed tibia with a valgus load. Injuries may be due to excessive *pivoting or cutting*, as well as hyperextension, hyperflexion, or lateral trauma to the knee. A "pop" is often heard or felt at the time of injury. Immediate swelling due to hemarthrosis and a sense of instability usually follow. Commonly injured with the ACL is the MCL and medial meniscus, known as the terrible triad or O'Donoghue's triad.

The *Lachman test* (Figure 11.14) is performed at 20° to 30° of knee flexion and particularly assesses the posterolateral fibers. Some laxity may be normal, so comparison with the contralateral leg is recommended. Sensitivity is higher than the anterior drawer test (99% vs. 54%) (19). The *pivot shift (Macintosh) test* is performed in the lateral decubitus position with the

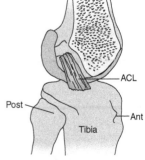

ACL

Post

Ant

Tibia

FIGURE 11.13 Anterior cruciate ligament.

affected knee extended and the tibia internally rotated. Valgus stress is applied to the knee as it is flexed. A "clunk" felt at 30° of knee flexion is indicative of ACL injury. An *MRI* confirms the diagnosis and may identify other concomitant injuries.

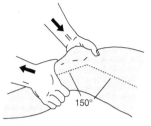

FIGURE 11.14 The Lachman test.

Nonoperative rehabilitation of ACL injury should concentrate on proprioceptive training and strengthening of the hamstrings (i.e., TheraBand; see Figure 11.15) to prevent anterior subluxation of the tibia. Bracing should limit terminal extension and rotation. Activity modification (e.g., avoiding cutting and pivoting sports) is extremely important if nonoperative management is given a trial to avoid injury to other intra-articular structures, such as the menisci.

The need for *operative treatment* depends on the amount of damage and degree of laxity and is patient specific as well. A younger, more active patient is more likely to require surgical repair versus the older, sedentary patient. Post-op rehab can last up to 6 to 9 months, although the trend is to shorten this time. Patients are typically weight bearing as tolerated (WBAT) with an extension brace immediately after surgery. As with nonoperative rehab, the emphasis is on strengthening the hamstrings and proprioceptive training. During the first 6 weeks, it is important to regain ROM (can be assisted by continuous passive motion [CPM]) and enhance patellar mobility. Intensity and resistance should progressively increase between weeks 6 and 10. By week 10, there should be essentially no limitation in strengthening.

Prevention of these injuries is of utmost importance as well and has been a recent focus of sports medicine research. Young female athletes, especially those who play soccer and basketball, are at a much higher risk of ACL injury than their male peers. ACL injury prevention programs that incorporate proprioceptive and neuromuscular control training may reduce the risk of ACL injuries and, therefore, should be considered in high-risk athletes (21).

Posterior Cruciate Ligament – The PCL (Figure 11.16) arises from the posterior intercondylar tibia and extends anteriorly, superiorly, and medially to attach to the medial femoral condyle. It prevents abnormal internal rotation (IR) and posterior

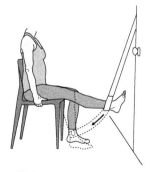

FIGURE 11.15 Strengthening with TheraBand

translation of the tibia on the femur, which aids knee flexion. Injury of the PCL classically occurs secondary to a motor vehicle accident (MVA) when the tibia strikes the dashboard, forcing the tibia posteriorly. Injury also occurs with high valgus stress or when falling on a flexed knee. Swelling is uncommon. Tenderness in popliteal region is a common finding after injury. Integrity of the PCL can be tested by the *posterior drawer test* and the *sag test*, where the examiner tries to observe a posterior displacement of the tibial tuberosity (or tibial joint line in relation to the femur) while the patient is supine and the knees are flexed to 90° to allow the quadriceps to relax. After a sag sign is assessed for, the *posterior drawer test* can

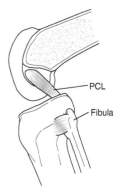

FIGURE 11.16 The posterior cruciate ligament.
Source: Adapted from Ref. (20).

be used to further test the integrity of the PCL. In addition, a *varus stress* can be applied to an extended knee to assess for concomitant injuries to the PCL and posterolateral corner of the relaxed knee. MRI is the preferred imaging although less sensitive for PCL pathology compared to ACL pathology; arthroscopy is more accurate in making the diagnosis. Treatment of a mild PCL sprain usually involves quadriceps strengthening without need for bracing. Severe PCL injuries will often need to be repaired arthroscopically.

Meniscal Injury – The menisci (Figure 11.17) are fibrocartilaginous structures of the intra-articular knee that increase the contact area between the femur and tibia and can act as "shock absorbers" for the knee.

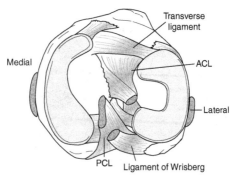

FIGURE 11.17 The menisci.
Source: Adapted from Ref. (20).

Mechanisms of injury include excessive rotational stresses, typically the result of twisting a flexed knee. The medial meniscus is more often injured than the lateral. Knee locking, popping, and/or clicking are characteristic complaints. On examination, an effusion, joint line tenderness, and loss of full knee flexion or extension may be noted. *McMurray's test* is performed with the patient supine and hip and knee maximally flexed. A valgus–tibial ER force is applied while the knee is extended; a pop or snap suggests a medial meniscus tear. Varus–tibial IR forces are used to evaluate the lateral meniscus. McMurray's test may be poorly tolerated due to pain, and some consider it to be relatively unreliable (22). Apley's grind test may be positive, but it is avoided by some clinicians for fear of aggravating the injury. The *Thessaly test* has recently been described and validated. It is performed in single leg stance with 20° of knee flexion with assistance from the examiner, who holds the hands while the subject rotates the knee internally and externally (23). *MRI* may help confirm the clinical diagnosis and identify other injuries. *Arthroscopy* is the gold standard for diagnosis of a tear.

Treatment is dependent on the severity of injury. For the nonsurgical candidate, early management consists of RICE, NSAIDs, hamstring and ITB stretching, and a progressive resistive exercise program for quadriceps/hamstring/hip strengthening. A joint aspiration is sometimes useful to reduce effusion and relieve pain. *Aquatic exercises* and the use of *canes* can unload the affected meniscus. The intensity can be gradually increased with avoidance of activities involving compressive rotational loading. It may be reasonable to gradually resume sports activities once strength in the affected limb approaches 70% to 80% of that of the unaffected limb. Orthopedic referral for possible *arthroscopic surgery* is indicated if the patient is experiencing mechanical symptoms including locking, buckling, or recurrent swelling with pain and has not responded to conservative treatment. Surgical treatment has been evolving. Total meniscectomy is no longer considered acceptable; efforts are now aimed at preserving as much cartilage as possible in order to prevent degenerative changes. The outer thirds of the menisci are vascular and may be repaired; the inner two thirds are avascular and may need to be debrided. Following partial meniscectomy, full weight bearing (WB) may occur once the patient is pain-free. Following meniscal repair, full WB may be delayed for up to 6 weeks. ROM exercise, stretching, and progressive strengthening of the lower limbs are the mainstays of post-op therapy. Deep squatting is discouraged.

Patellofemoral Pain Syndrome – The etiology is postulated to be a combination of overuse, muscular imbalance (i.e., hip abductor and external rotator weakness; 24), and/or biomechanical problems (i.e., pes planus or pes cavus, increased Q angle [Figure 11.18]). Anterior knee pain may occur with activity and worsen with prolonged sitting or descending stairs. Acute management involves *relative rest, ice,* and

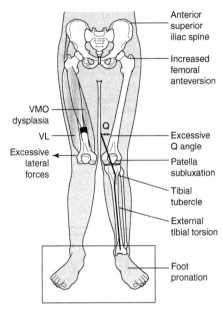

FIGURE 11.18 Sequelae of an increased Q angle. Normally, the male Q is 13°; the female is 18°.

VL, vastus lateralis; VMO, vastus medialis obliquus.

Source: Adapted from Ref. (20).

NSAIDs. Prolonged sitting should be avoided. The mainstay of rehabilitation is to address the biomechanical deficits through a combination of *quadriceps strengthening exercises* with *stretching* of the quadriceps, hamstrings, ITB, and gastroc-soleus complex. Classically, short arc terminal knee extension (0°–30°) exercises were utilized, with the belief that they selectively strengthened the vastus medialis oblique (VMO). Currently, the idea of VMO selectivity is controversial. In general, *short arc (0°–45°) closed kinetic chain leg press* exercises are recommended to strengthen all four heads of the quads, which are thought to be weakened in aggregate. Full arc and open kinetic chain exercises should be avoided to reduce symptom aggravation.

Taping the patella so that it tracks properly (*McConnell technique*) may improve pain symptoms during exercise. *Orthotics* to correct pes planus or foot pronation and soft braces with patellar cutouts may provide modest symptomatic relief in appropriate cases. Occasionally, *electrical stimulation* and *biofeedback* are useful. Prolonged PT with modalities such as US is generally not helpful or cost-effective. *Surgery* is rarely necessary and is reserved for recalcitrant instability or symptomatic malalignment.

Exercise-Induced Leg Pain – Shin splint, a nonspecific term, refers to exercise-induced tibial pain, without evidence of fracture on x-ray. It is believed to represent periostitis, usually of the posteromedial tibial border (*medial tibial stress syndrome*). Runners, gymnasts, and dancers are at risk, with causes including an increase in exercise intensity, inadequate footwear, hard surface training, or poor biomechanics. Local pain and tenderness are noted along the distal one third of the tibia. Pain is often quickly relieved by rest and not aggravated by passive stretch. Bone scan may be positive in severe cases. Treatment includes rest, NSAIDs, US, preactivity icing, and correction of aggravating factors.

Causes of tibial stress fractures (TSFs) are similar to those of tibial stress syndrome. Stress fractures are also common in the fibula and the metatarsals, especially the second metatarsal. Pain is initially exercise induced only, but it progresses to pain with WB or even at rest. There is often exquisite point tenderness along the distal or middle third of the tibia. X-rays may be negative initially, but may show a clear fracture after several weeks (i.e., a positive "dreaded black line" on oblique radiograph, representing an anterior TSF). Bone scans are more sensitive. TSFs can be treated with *relative rest* (i.e., crutches). Medial TSFs can be treated with relative rest for 4 to 6 weeks, NSAIDs, and TENS. Anterior TSFs may require several months of rest from sports activities and ongoing conservative treatment. Recalcitrant cases may eventually require a bone graft.

In *chronic compartment syndrome of the leg,* pain is felt after a specific period of exercise and can be associated with paresthesias, numbness, and weakness in the distribution of the nerve within the compartment. Electrodiagnostics studies are usually normal. Resting and postexercise compartment pressures should be obtained. Resting pressures >30 mmHg, 15-second postexercise pressures >60 mmHg, or 2-minute postexercise pressures >20mm Hg are all suggestive of chronic compartment syndrome. An initial conservative approach should include NSAIDs, proper footwear selection, and correction of training errors. If symptoms persist 1 to 2 months after a trial of conservative treatment, referral for surgical fasciotomy may be warranted.

Achilles Tendinitis – Overuse, overpronation, heel varus deformity, and poor flexibility of the Achilles tendon/gastroc-soleus/hamstrings may be contributing factors. Basketball players may be particularly susceptible because of the frequent jumping. It is also noted in runners who increase their mileage or hill training. Symptoms include pain and swelling in the tendon during and after activities. On examination, there may be swelling, pain on palpation, a palpable nodule, and inability to stand on tiptoe. Chronic tendinosis may result in tendon weakness, potentially leading to rupture.

There is no consensus on the optimal mode of treatment, but most rehabilitation will likely begin with the PRICE (Protection Rest Ice Compression Elevation) principle. Modalities, especially *US*, may be helpful. Plantar flexor strengthening is important. *Downhill exercises* should be emphasized; uphill running should be discouraged, especially early in rehab. Heel lifts may provide early relief but may lead to heel cord shortening with prolonged use. A properly fitted shoe, often with a stiff heel counter, is important. Steroid injections into the Achilles tendon is not recommended by many sources due to the risk of tendon rupture, as the Achilles tendon does not have a true synovial sheath. For severe or chronic cases, recovery to near-normal strength may take up to 24 months, even with good circulation. For this reason, novel treatments (i.e., PRP) are currently being studied, but results are inconclusive (25,26). Young, active persons with ruptured tendons are usually operated on; casting is an option for older, sedentary persons.

Ankle Sprains – Lateral ankle sprains are usually due to inversion of a plantar flexed foot. The anterior talofibular ligament (ATFL) is typically the first structure to be involved. With increasing severity of injury, the calcaneofibular ligament (CFL) may be involved next, followed by the posterior talofibular ligament (PTFL). The anterior drawer test checks ankle ligament stability, primarily the ATFL (displacement ≥5 mm is considered positive). The talar tilt test (Figure 11.19) checks the CFL; it is performed by providing an inversion stress on the talus (a positive test is a marked difference, i.e., >10°, in the inversion of the affected vs. the unaffected side). X-rays to check the tibiofibular syndesmosis may be necessary in the event of severe sprains; these require surgical consultation.

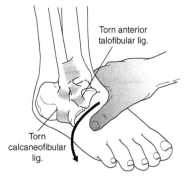

FIGURE 11.19 Talar tilt test.
Source: Adapted from Ref. (20).

Injuries of the medial (deltoid) ankle ligament due to an eversion injury are less common; an associated proximal fibula fracture (Maisonneuve fracture) should be ruled out.

Rehabilitation of ankle sprains involves three phases: *Phase I* normally lasts 1 to 3 days, until the patient is able to bear weight comfortably. This phase involves the *RICE* principle: rest (i.e., crutches), ice 20 minutes 3 to 5x/day, compression with Ace wrap, and elevation of the foot above the heart. Hot showers, alcohol, methyl salicylate counterirritants (e.g., Bengay), and other treatments that may increase swelling should be avoided during the initial 24 hours. *Phase II* usually lasts days to weeks. The goals in this phase are to restore ROM, strengthen the ankle stabilizers, and stretch/strengthen the Achilles tendon. *Phase III* is initiated when motion is near normal and pain and swelling are almost absent. Reestablishing motor coordination via proprioceptive exercises and endurance training are emphasized, that is, balance board, running curves (*figure-of-8*), and zigzag running.

Return to play guidelines vary. Some recommendations may be as follows: Grade I (no laxity and minimal ligamentous tear): 0 to 5 days, Grade II (mild to moderate laxity and functional loss): 7 to 14 days, Grade III (complete ligamentous disruption and cannot bear weight): 21 to 35 days, and syndesmosis injury: 21 to 56 days. Recent literature has demonstrated that an early and accelerated rehabilitation program results in better short-term outcomes for grades I and II lateral ankle sprains (27).

Plantar Fasciitis – Commonly seen in athletes and in persons whose jobs require much standing or walking. Repetitive microtrauma to the plantar fascia can cause inflammation and pain in the acute phase. In chronic conditions, the fascia is less commonly inflamed; instead, it becomes degenerative and painful and is commonly termed plantar fasciopathy. Biomechanical issues (i.e., an overpronated foot with increased tension on the fascia) are often at fault. The classic symptoms are medial heel pain and pain across the entire area of plantar fascia, noted especially with the first few steps in the morning or pain that is worse at the beginning of an activity.

The key component of treatment is a home exercise program of *routine, daily stretching* of the plantar fascia (Figure 11.20) and Achilles tendon, which has proven to be superior to other treatment modalities (29,30). Patients should be on *relative rest* from walking, running, and jumping and consider switching

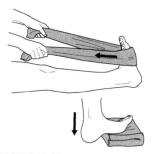

FIGURE 11.20 Stretching for plantar fasciitis.
Source: Adapted from Ref. (28).

to activities such as swimming or cycling to allow the fascia to heal. *Proper footwear* includes well-cushioned soles, possible use of an extra-deep heel pad/cup insert, and avoiding high heels. *Soft medial arch supports* are generally preferable to rigid orthotics, which can exacerbate symptoms. NSAIDs and ice may help decrease inflammation. For patients not responding to other measures, *splints* may be useful to supply a gentle constant stretch across the sole of the foot and gastrocnemius at night while sleeping. Once the pain resolves, patients should return to increased levels of activity only gradually, while continuing their stretching program.

The majority of cases will improve with conservative measures within 6 to 12 weeks, if faithfully followed. In the rare, persistent case, a *local corticosteroid injection* may be considered. A potential complication is necrosis of the fatty pad of the heel, which cannot be easily reversed or treated. Surgical intervention, which consists of a release of the involved fascia from its attachment to the calcaneus, can be considered if all other measures fail, but is necessary in only very rare cases.

SPORTS/EXERCISE PREPARTICIPATION EVALUATION (PPE)

General Guidelines

Questions about personal and family history of cardiovascular disease are the most important initial components of the history and physical examination (H&P). A thorough history of neurologic or musculoskeletal problems should also be emphasized. Physical examination should emphasize cardiac auscultation with provocative maneuvers to screen for hypertrophic cardiomyopathy (see the following text), which is the most common cause of sudden death in young male athletes. The use of ECG in the PPE screen remains controversial (31–33). For most young, asymptomatic persons, screening tests such as ECG, treadmill stress testing, and lab tests are not indicated in the absence of symptoms or a significant history of risk factors. For older asymptomatic persons without cardiopulmonary risk factors or known metabolic disease, the American College of Sports Medicine recommends exercise stress testing in men ≥45 years and women ≥55 years before starting a vigorous exercise program (≥60% of Vo$_2$max). Most older persons can begin a moderate aerobic and resistance training program without stress testing if they begin to slowly and gradually increase their level of activity (31–33).

Example of an Appropriate PPE

The following table is a guideline for a PPE.

Examination feature	Comments
Blood pressure	Must be assessed in the context of participant's age, height, and gender

(continued)

Examination feature	Comments
General	Measure for excessive height and observe for evidence of excessive long bone growth that suggests Marfan syndrome
Eyes	Important to detect vision defects that leave one of the eyes with worse than 20/40 corrected vision
Cardiovascular	Palpate the point of maximal impulse for increased intensity or displacement that suggests hypertrophy or failure, respectively Perform auscultation with the patient supine and again standing or straining during Valsalva maneuver (a loud systolic murmur that increases with upright posture or Valsalva and decreases with squatting suggests hypertrophic cardiomyopathy) Femoral pulse diminishment suggests aortic coarctation
Respiratory	Observe for accessory muscle use or prolonged expiration and auscultate for wheezing. Exercise-induced asthma will not produce manifestations on resting examination and requires exercise testing for diagnosis
Abdominal	Assess for hepatic or splenic enlargement
Genitourinary (males only)	Hernias/varicoceles do not usually preclude sports participation, but it may be appropriate to screen for testicular masses
Musculoskeletal	The "2 minute orthopedic examination" is a commonly used systematic screen (31) Consider supplemental shoulder, knee, and ankle examinations
Skin	Evidence of molluscum contagiosum, herpes simplex infection, impetigo, tinea corporis, or scabies would temporarily prohibit participation in sports in which direct skin-to-skin competitor contact occurs (i.e., wrestling and martial arts)

Contraindications to Sports Participation

The following conditions preclude participation: active myocarditis or pericarditis; hypertrophic cardiomyopathy; uncontrolled severe HTN (static resistance exercises are particularly contraindicated); suspected coronary artery disease (CAD) until fully evaluated; long QT interval syndrome; history of recent concussion and symptoms of post-concussion syndrome (no contact or collision sports); poorly controlled convulsive disorder (no archery, riflery, swimming, weight lifting, strength training, or sports involving heights); recurrent episodes of burning upper extremity pain or weakness or episodes of transient quadriplegia until stability of cervical spine can be assured (no contact or collision sports); sickle cell disease (no high exertion, contact, or collision sports); mononucleosis with unresolved splenomegaly; eating disorder where athlete is not compliant with treatment or follow-up or where there is evidence of diminished performance or potential injury because of eating disorder.

REHABILITATION AFTER HIP FRACTURE

The lifetime risk of hip fractures in industrialized countries is 18% for females and 6% for males (34). Osteoporosis and falls are the primary risk factors. Mortality and morbidity following hip fractures are high: 20% are not alive by 1 year after fracture and 33% by 2 years (35).

Nearly one of three survivors is in institutionalized care within a year after the fracture, and as many as two of three survivors never regain their preoperative activity status (36). Surgery is usually indicated for most hip fractures, unless medically contraindicated or in nonambulatory patients.

Femoral Neck Fracture – Screw fixations (Figure 11.21) are typical for stable, nondisplaced fractures. Ambulation with WBAT and an appropriate assistive device may be started during the first few days post-op. Bipolar endoprostheses (Figure 11.22) may be used for unstable, displaced fractures when satisfactory reduction cannot be achieved and the patient is >65 years of age or has preexisting articular pathology (e.g., OA). Patients are usually mobilized quickly and allowed WBAT within the first few days post-op. Abduction pillows and short-term ROM restrictions (no adduction past midline and no IR) may be ordered to reduce the risk of prosthetic displacement.

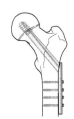

FIGURE 11.21
Screw fixation.

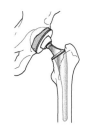

FIGURE 11.22
Bipolar endoprosthesis.

Intertrochanteric Fractures (Figure 11.23) – Sliding hip screw fixation allows for early WBAT for stable fractures (intact posteromedial cortex) and provides dynamic compression of the fracture during WB. Intramedullary hip screws are another surgical option. A period of limited WB may be necessary following fixation of unstable fractures. Surgical management for *subtrochanteric fractures* also includes the use of sliding screw fixation and intramedullary nails/rods, although initial WB may be more limited.

Complications seen during rehabilitation and convalescence after hip fracture include

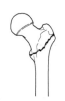

FIGURE 11.23
Intertrochanteric fracture.

atelectasis, pneumonia, anemia, fracture nonunion, AVN, surgical site infection, component loosening, leg length discrepancy, heterotopic ossification (HO), DVT, constipation, and skin breakdown.

REHABILITATION AFTER JOINT REPLACEMENT

Total Hip Arthroplasty

Indications for total hip arthroplasty (THA): unstable hip fractures, OA, osteonecrosis, inflammatory arthritis, post-traumatic arthritis, malignancy, hemoglobinopathies, hip dysplasia.

Various surgical approaches for THA have been described in literature. Two of the most commonly used approaches are the anterolateral and the posterior approaches. The anterolateral approach utilizes the plane between the tensor fascia latae and gluteus medius. To expose the acetabulum, the abductor mechanism must be neutralized via trochanteric ostomy or partial detachment of the anterior gluteus minimus and medius (37). The posterior approach splits the gluteus maximus and remains posterior to the gluteus medius and minimus. The hip capsule is divided and the external rotators such as piriformis, superior and inferior gemelli, and obturator internus are necessarily detached (37). Both approaches are routinely performed and debate continues as to the benefits and limitations of each.

Biologically fixed or *"cementless" implants* provide a more durable bioprosthetic interface, but require a longer period of protective WB (i.e., touchdown WB to partial WB [PWB] × ≥2 to 3 months) to allow for osseous integration into the porous prosthetic surface. *Cement-fixed implants* are cheaper and may offer immediate WBAT. The cement, however, can be prone to deterioration, which may result in component loosening and ultimately require revision.

Precautions following surgery using different approaches vary. For a posterior THA, patients may be out of bed to chair with assist on post-op day 1. A triangular hip abduction pillow in bed is highly recommended for the first 6 to 12 weeks. *Hip precautions* generally continue for up to 12 weeks post-op to allow for the formation of a pseudocapsule and minimize the chance of dislocation. Patients are allowed flexion up to 90°, passive abduction, and gentle (≤30°) IR while extended. There should be no adduction past midline and no IR while flexed. Active abduction, hyperextension and external rotation are allowed with a posterior approach (gluteus medius preserved) but avoided after an anterolateral approach (gluteus medius split open). Typical patient instructions are diagrammed in Figure 11.24.

Other key issues include DVT prophylaxis, monitoring for post-op anemia and infection, and pain control. Patients may often complain about perceived leg length discrepancies during the first several months post-op; PT to address muscle imbalances and tight capsules may be helpful. In general, prognosis following THA is excellent,

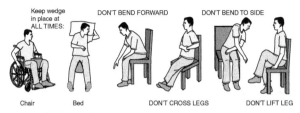

FIGURE 11.24 Rehabilitation after posterior total hip arthroplasty.

although being younger, male, obese, and highly active may adversely affect outcomes.

Total Knee Arthroplasty

Indications for total knee arthroplasty (TKA): OA, inflammatory arthritis.

Cemented fixation may allow immediate WBAT; cementless fixation may require several months of restricted WB for complete stability. Neither addresses the issue of polyethylene liner wear, which may be the key factor in eventual prosthetic failure. Microscopic wear debris can trigger an inflammatory response with ensuing osteolysis and component loosening.

Regaining *knee ROM* (i.e., 0°–90° before going home) is an important rehabilitation goal for all TKA patients. Pillows under the knee should be avoided. The use of CPM is controversial. Some have argued that it may decrease length of inpatient rehabilitation stay and improve ROM (by 10°) at 1 year post-op, but most studies have *not* demonstrated long-term benefits in ROM or functional outcome.

Regenerative Medicine in Orthopedics and Sports Medicine

Regenerative medicine is a rapidly growing field within musculoskeletal and sports medicine. Prolotherapy, PRP, and stem cells are still being investigated as facilitators and stimulators of healing, and evidence-based support for their use in clinical setting is still debated.

Prolotherapy is a technique that involves injecting an irritant, usually a hyperosmolar dextrose solution for the treatment of chronic painful musculoskeletal conditions. The most frequent indications are the treatment of low back pain, tendinopathies, and OA. Prolotherapy may be an option for the treatment of painful musculoskeletal conditions, particularly those refractory to other conservative, standard treatments (38). Its precise mechanisms of action and effectiveness are still being investigated.

PRP involves the injection of concentrated platelets derived from centrifugation of autologous blood. Platelets contain products that are believed to enhance healing, specifically in soft tissue. Such products include growth factors important for cell proliferation, differentiation, and neovascularization (39).

It has also been demonstrated that PRP contains cell adhesion molecules and chemotactic properties that aid in the recruitment of mesenchymal stem cells (MSCs) and fibroblasts (39). Therefore, PRP may employ the healing potential of concentrated platelets and may be considered as an adjunct treatment modality for various conditions when conservative treatments fail. Its efficacy continues to be investigated.

The use of MSCs and its increasing popularity originates from their pluripotent characteristics and their ability to differentiate into many adult cell types including bone, cartilage, and fat (39). Stem cells derived from bone marrow yield both hematopoietic and non-hematopoietic precursor cells, red and white blood cells, and platelets. When centrifuged and concentrated, the non-hematopoietic cells and platelets can be isolated. Depending on where the cells are obtained from, the isolate can contain varying levels of stem cells. It has been shown that harvest from bone marrow of the iliac crest provides the greatest number of bone-forming MSCs. The ability of these stem cells to differentiate into a particular adult cell and the degree to which they may release growth factors is of great interest to the field of regenerative medicine. This treatment has been employed in the treatment of OA, rotator cuff, and meniscal tears (39). Its efficacy continues to be investigated.

REFERENCES

1. Rockwood CA, ed. *Rockwood & Green's Fractures in Adults.* 3rd ed. Philadelphia, PA: JB Lippincott; 1988.
2. Bisbinas I, Belthur M, Said HG, et al. Accuracy of needle placement in ACJ injections. *Knee Surg Sports Traumatol Arthrosc.* 2006;14(8):762–765.
3. Naredo E, Cabero F, Beneyto P, et al. A randomized comparative study of short term response to blind injection versus sonographic-guided injection of local corticosteroids in patients with painful shoulder. *J Rheumatol.* 2004;31(2):308–314.
4. Panditaratne N, Wilkinson C, Groves C, Chandramohan M. Subacromial impingement syndrome: a prospective comparison of ultrasound-guided versus unguided injection techniques. *Ultrasound.* 2010;18(4):176–181.
5. Iannotti JP. Full-thickness rotator cuff tears: Factors affecting surgical outcome. *J Am Acad Orthop Surg.* 1994;2(2):87–95.
6. Connolly J. Unfreezing the frozen shoulder. *J Musculoskel Med.* 1998: 47–58.
7. Neviaser AS, Hannafin JA. Adhesive capsulitis: a review of current treatment. *Am J Sports Med.* 2010;38(ll):2346–2356.
8. Sofka CM, Collins AJ, Adler RS. Use of ultrasonographic guidance in interventional musculoskeletal procedures: a review from a single institution. *J Ultrasound Med.* 2001;20(l):21–26.
9. Mishra A, Collado H, Fredericson M. Platelet-rich plasma compared with corticosteroid injection for chronic lateral elbow tendinosis. *Phys Med Rehabil.* 2009;1(4):366–370.

10. Kazemi M, Azma K, Tavana B, et al. Autologous blood versus corticosteroid local injection in the short-term treatment of lateral elbow tendinopathy: A randomized clinical trial of efficacy. *Am J Phys Med Rehabil.* 2010;89(8):660–667.

11. Jeyapalan K, Choudhary S. Ultrasound-guided injection of triamcinolone and bupivacaine in the management of De Quervain's disease. *Skeletal Radiol.* 2009;38(11):1099–1103.

12. Strauss EJ, Nho SJ, Kelly BT. Greater trochanteric pain syndrome. *Sports Med Arthrosc.* 2010;18(2):113–119.

13. Fearon AM, Scarvell JM, Cook JL, Smith PN. Does ultrasound correlate with surgical or histologic findings in greater trochanteric pain syndrome? A pilot study. *Clin Orthop Relat Res.* 2010;468(7):1838–1844.

14. Labrosse JM, Cardinal E, Leduc BE, et al. Effectiveness of ultrasound-guided corticosteroid injection for the treatment of gluteus medius tendinopathy. *AJR Am J Roentgenol.* 2010;194(1):202–206.

15. Vanelderen P, Szadek K, Cohen S, et al. 13. Sacroiliac joint pain. *Pain Pract.* 2010;10(5):470–478.

16. Slipman C, Jackson H, Lipetz J, et al. Sacroiliac joint pain referral zones. *Arch Phys Med Rehabil.* 2000;81.

17. Cohen SP, Yian C, Neufeld, N. Sacroiliac joint pain: A comprehensive review of anatomy, diagnosis and treatment. *Expert Review of Neurotherapeutics.* 2013;13(1):99–116.

18. Finnoff JT, Nutz DJ, Henning PT, et al. Accuracy of ultra-sound-guided versus unguided pes anserinus bursa injections. *Phys Med Rehabil.* 2010;2(8):732–739.

19. Torg JS. Clinical diagnosis of ACL instability in the athlete. *Am J Sports Med.* 1976;4:84–93.

20. Fu F, Stone D. *Sports Injuries: Mechanisms, Prevention & Treatment.* Baltimore, MD: Williams & Wilkins; 1994.

21. Gilchrist J, Mandelbaum BR, Melancon H, et al. A randomized controlled trial to prevent noncontact anterior cruciate ligament injury in female collegiate soccer players. *Am J Sports Med.* 2008;36(8):1476–1483.

22. Karachalios T, Hantes M, Zibis AH, et al. Diagnostic accuracy of a new clinical test (the Thessaly test) for early detection of meniscal tears. *J Bone Joint Surg Am.* 2005;87(5):955–962.

23. Cichanowski HR, Schmitt JS, Johnson RJ, Niemuth PE. Hip strength in collegiate female athletes with patellofemoral pain. *Med Sci Sports Exerc.* 2007;39(8):1227–1232.

24. de Vos RJ, Weir A, van Schie HT, et al. Platelet-rich plasma injection for chronic Achilles tendinopathy: a randomized controlled trial. *JAMA.* 2010;303(2):144–149.

25. Gaweda K, Tarczynska M, Krzyzanowski W. Treatment of achilles tendinopathy with platelet-rich plasma. *Int J Sports Med.* 2010;31(8):577–583.

26. Bleakley CM, O'Connor SR, Tully MA, et al. Effect of accelerated rehabilitation on function after ankle sprain: randomised controlled trial. *BMJ.* 2010;340:c1964.

27. Rompe JD, Cacchio A, Weil L, et al. Plantar fascia-specific stretching versus radial shock-wave therapy as initial treatment of plantar fasciopathy. *J Bone Joint Surg Am.* 2010;92:2514–2522.

28. Rouzier P. *The Sports Medicine Patient Advisor.* Amherst, MA: SportsMed Press; 1999.

29. Corrado D, Basso C, Schiavon M, et al. Screening for hypertrophic cardiomyopathy in young athletes. *N Engl J Med.* 1998;339:364–369.

30. Baggish A, Hutter AM, Wang F, et al. Cardiovascular screening in college athletes with and without electrocardiography. *Ann Int Med.* 2010;152:269–275.

31. Kurowski K, Chandran S. The preparticipation athletic evaluation. *Am Fam Physician.* 2000;61:2683–2698.

32. ACSM. *Guidelines for Exercise Testing and Prescription.* 6th ed. Baltimore, MD: Lippincott Williams & Wilkins; 2000.

33. Neid RJ. Promoting and prescribing exercise for the elderly. *Am Fam Physician.* 2002;65:419–428.

34. Meunier PJ. Prevention of hip fxs. *Am J Med.* 1993;95(suppl):75–78.

35. Emerson S. 10yr survival after fxs of the proximal end of the femur. *Gerontology.* 1988;34:186–191.

36. Osteoporosis Prevention, Diagnosis, and Therapy. *NIH Consensus Statement* March 27–29. 2000;17:1–36.

37. Palan J, David JB, David WM, et al. Which approach for total hip arthroplasty: Anterolateral or posterior? *Clin Orthop Relat Res.* 2009;467(2):473–477.

38. Distel LM, Best TM. Prolotherapy: A clinical review of its role in treating chronic musculoskeletal pain. *PM R.* 2011;3(6):S78–S81.

39. Gobbi A, Fishman M. Platelet-rich plasma and bone marrow-derived mesenchymal stem cells in sports medicine. *Sports Med Arthrosc.* 2016;24(2):69–73.

SUGGESTED READING

Sayegh FE, Kenanidis EI, Papavasiliou KA, et al. Reduction of acute anterior dislocations: a prospective randomized study comparing a new technique with the Hippocratic and Kocher methods. *J Bone Joint Surg Am.* 2009;91:2775–2782.

CHAPTER 12

ULTRASOUND

INTRODUCTION

Ultrasound (US) is sound above the human audible limit of 20 kilo-hertz (KHz). Use of US as an imaging modality has become integral to the evaluation of musculoskeletal (MSK) and peripheral nervous system disorders. The advantages of US over conventional imaging techniques include point-of-service availability, lower costs, increased safety versus other modalities, and the ability to view, in real time, targeted anatomy and neighboring structures including vascular flow, internal organ movement, dynamically moving MSK structures, and the administration of injected medication. There are no true contraindications for its use in MSK imaging.

Limitations of MSK US include an inability to evaluate tissue types such as bone due to acoustic impedance. Imaging is not possible for structures located below or within bony encasements. Imaging can also be somewhat limited for patients with large body habitus. Finally, the quality of a study is highly operator dependent, with appropriate training required in the interpretation of US images, including the limitations and unique artifacts related to US.

Safety – US has an excellent safety record because it does not utilize radiation. US energy, however, has the potential to be harmful if used improperly. US images can raise tissue temperatures and produce cavitation in body fluids. The long-term effects are still unknown. Thus, the FDA recommends the As Low As Reasonably Achievable (ALARA) principles to be followed when utilizing US.

MACHINE BASICS

The US machine transmits and receives ultrasonic waves, typically 2 to 15 megahertz (MHz), to produce two-dimensional (2D) images. The main components of an US machine are the (a) central processing unit (CPU), (b) transducer, and (c) display. The CPU transmits an electrical current to the transducer probe, which contains piezoelectric crystals, causing them to vibrate. This produces acoustic waves that are transmitted through a water-based gel interface on the skin and internally into the tissues. The acoustic waves interact with tissue interfaces and are then reflected back to the transducer, causing an electrical current that the CPU converts into an image. The brightness mode (B mode) is a black-and-white 2D image mode typically used for MSK US.

Higher transducer frequencies increase the resolution and are optimal for visualization of more superficial structures. Lower frequencies will penetrate deeper structures but with less resolution. The basic types of transducer probes used in MSK medicine are curvilinear (or convex), with an average frequency range of 4 to 9 MHz (lower frequency); linear, with an average frequency range of 5 to 12 MHz; and compact linear, with an average frequency range of 7 to 15 MHz (higher frequency). Other important components of the sound wave include speed and the amplitude. The speed at which the acoustic wave returns to the transducer determines the placement, that is, depth of the image on the screen. The strength of the acoustic wave is the amplitude and is represented by the brightness of the image on screen.

The quality of an US image depends in large part on the amount of energy that is reflected back to the transducer. Acoustic impedance, scattering, refraction, and attenuation affect the sound wave signal returning to the transducer. *Reflection* occurs when the sound wave hits the interface of two adjacent structures or tissues. The larger the acoustic impedance (the amount of resistance a sound wave encounters as it passes through tissue) between the tissues, the more energy reflected back and the brighter the image. *Scattering* occurs when the energy originally transmitted hits a surface and the waves are retransmitted in different directions, with only a portion of the sound returning to the transducer. *Refraction* occurs when a sound wave deviates from its original direction due to acoustic impedance. *Attenuation* is the conversion of sound to heat, which is not reflected back to the transducer. The image will appear darker.

Knobology – The sonographer has access to various controls on an US machine to optimize the image.

Gain – This knob controls image brightness by altering the overall amplitude of the US signal returning to the probe. Increasing the gain increases the amplitude, producing a brighter image.

Depth – This knob adjusts the depth of the field view. The greater the depth, the less the resolution and vice versa.

Frequency – This knob alters the transducer probe frequency to balance depth and resolution needs. Lower frequencies penetrate deeper structures, but with less resolution.

Focus – If present, this knob allows focus of the US wave to an area of interest. Newer machines can have permanent focus, which is shown in the middle of the screen.

US NOMENCLATURE AND COMMON ARTIFACTS

Various terms are commonly used in MSK US for scanning orientation. The *longitudinal axis* (aka long axis) is a sagittal view. The *transverse axis* (aka short axis) is a cross-sectional view. *In-plane* (used with needle guidance) is a reference to the orientation of the needle relative to the probe. The needle enters the skin in long axis to the probe, traversing the plane of the transducer. The whole shaft and tip of needle can be seen within the tissue. A needle is *out-of-plane* when it is perpendicular to the transducer, appearing as a bright dot within the tissue, that is, it is a cross-sectional view of the needle.

Echogenicity refers to a structure's ability to produce echoes, that is, reflections of the acoustic waves transmitted by the transducer. *Anechoic* structures produce no echoes, appearing black on US. *Hypoechoic* structures produce weaker echoes, appearing darker than other structures. *Hyperechoic* structures produce stronger echoes, appearing brighter than other structures. *Homogeneous* structures have an echo pattern that is uniform in its composition. *Heterogeneous* structures show an uneven pattern of echoes of varying echodensities. *Isoechoic* describes a tissue that produces an echo of the same strength as another (e.g., surrounding) tissue.

Artifacts are common in MSK US and must be well understood to prevent misdiagnosis of pathology. Some examples of artifacts include:

Anisotropy – The property of a tissue that causes significant reflection changes. Slight changes in the direction of an acoustic wave can lead to drastic changes in the sound waves reflected in some tissue types and thus impact the image greatly.

Shadowing – The partial or total reflection or absorption of US waves as they hit or pass through an object, causing the structures deep to it to appear hypoechoic or anechoic.

Enhancement – The opposite of shadowing, it is an increase in brightness of structures deep to other structures that transmit sound easily. Generally, images are automatically processed to enhance (brighten) deeper structures to compensate for the loss of acoustic waves that naturally occurs at deeper versus more superficial levels. A structure such as a fluid-filled cyst, however, absorbs a minimal amount of acoustic energy, and the structures deep to the cyst will appear hyperechoic because the processor is expecting more attenuation of the signal at this level. This phenomenon is also referred to as posterior acoustic enhancement.

Reverberation is a phenomenon that occurs when a US wave hits highly reflective surfaces that lie parallel to each other and perpendicular to the US wave. The initial reflection is manifested as an anatomic structure (or needle) at its proper depth, but some of the signal gets caught between the surfaces before returning to the transducer in increments. The CPU assumes that waves return to the transducer after a single reflection, so these additional reflections (which take longer to return) are interpreted by the CPU to be separate structures that are deeper to the original structure, with depth corresponding to the time it takes for each reflection to come back. This phenomenon can be seen with a hollow bore needle in soft tissue when the long axis of the needle shaft is parallel to the transducer.

NORMAL TISSUE TYPES

Skin presents as a thin, uniform hyperechoic layer. *Fat* is hypoechoic with echogenic septa representing connective tissue. *Blood vessels* are anechoic, with a tubular structure. Veins collapse with pressure from the transducer, while arteries do not collapse as easily.

Synovium is generally hypoechoic. *Hyaline cartilage* is hypoechoic to anechoic over the hyperechoic bony cortex. *Ligaments* are hyperechoic, homogeneous bands. *Tendons*, in longitudinal view, have a dense, fibrillar hyperechoic appearance. In transverse view, their appearance is hypoechoic. Tendons are subject to a high degree of anisotropy. Artefactual hypoechoicity due to anisotropy may result in an inappropriate diagnosis of tendinosis or tendon tear. On the other hand, the anisotropy can be used productively to help distinguish tendon tissue from other surrounding hyperechoic tissues such as deep fat.

Muscle, in longitudinal view, appears as a hypoechoic, irregularly striated tissue with thin hyperechoic lines of fascia. In transverse view, muscle appears as a hypoechoic mass with hyperechoic speckles. Muscle tissue is subject to anisotropy.

Nerves have a fascicular "railroad track" pattern in longitudinal view, and a "honeycomb" appearance in transverse view, with hyperechoic epineurium and hyperechoic fascicles. Nerves are subject to anisotropy, albeit less than tendons are, and are also generally hypoechoic compared to tendons.

Bone appears as a bright echogenic line with no visible structures (acoustic shadowing) deep to the bone.

DIAGNOSTIC APPLICATIONS

In *bone and joint disorders*, US is sensitive in the detection of joint effusions that are anechoic and compressible. Heterogeneous-appearing fluid may be indicative of infection, for which aspiration may be indicated. Synovitis appears as noncompressible, echogenic tissue within a joint. Erosions and gouty tophi can also be seen on US. Inflamed bursae contain simple anechoic fluid or complex heterogeneous fluid.

With *nerve injury*, affected nerves can show regional swelling, hypoechogenicity, and loss of typical fascicular pattern.

In *tendon injury*, tendinosis appears as tendon enlargement, with hypoechogenicity. Partial-thickness tears present with regions of anechogenicity accompanied by loss of the normal fibrillar pattern of tendons. High-grade, partial-thickness tearing manifests as tendon thinning. Full-thickness tears manifest as gaps in the tendon. Tenosynovitis may appear either as anechoic with displaceable fluid surrounding the tendon or as heterogeneous fluid with mixed echogenicity.

In *muscle injury*, low-grade muscle strains exhibit subtle regions of hypoechogenicity with echotexture reduction, making the affected area look "washed out." High-grade injuries exhibit evidence of fiber disruption and heterogeneous fluid.

THERAPEUTIC APPLICATIONS

US as an imaging modality in MSK medicine is primarily employed to guide needle placement into joints for aspiration and/or injection. Acknowledging that there are multiple approaches and a high degree of variability in clinical practice, some basic approaches to a few joints that are commonly targeted are delineated below:

Glenohumeral (GH) Joint – The patient is typically seated or in the lateral decubitus position. The patient's hand is positioned resting on the opposite shoulder, and key landmarks including the humeral head, labrum, and joint capsule are identified. The GH joint is best accessed from the posterior approach. The needle is usually introduced lateral to medial in the axial plane, with the target between the posterior aspect of the humeral head and posterior labrum.

Elbow Joint – The patient can be positioned in a seated or supine position with elbow flexed and arm across the chest. The probe is positioned along the posterior elbow and oriented sagittally. The needle should be introduced superiorly, passing the triceps tendon and through the posterior fat pad to enter the joint space. Key landmarks are the olecranon fossa, posterior fat pad, and the olecranon.

Hip Joint – The patient is supine, and the joint is accessed anterolaterally. The probe should be aligned along the long axis of the femoral neck and the distinctive transition between femoral head and neck identified. The needle is introduced from an inferior approach, entering the joint capsule near the subcapital femur and lateral to the neurovascular bundle. In slimmer patients, the US probe may be oriented axially. With the femoral head and acetabular rim in view, the needle is introduced from an anterolateral approach.

Knee Joint – For knee joints with effusions, optimal access is typically with the patient supine and knee slightly flexed. The probe is held parallel to the quadriceps tendon and moved medially or laterally until the quadriceps fibers no longer appear. The needle is then directed into the bursa. For knee joints without effusions, the medial patellofemoral area is a potential target access point. The probe is initially oriented in the axial plane of the patella and medial femoral condyle, then turned 90° and oriented along the joint line. The needle is then introduced either inferiorly or superiorly to the probe.

Ankle Joint – With the patient lying supine, the anterior tibiotalar joint can be visualized in the sagittal plane. The examiner can plantarflex and dorsiflex the foot to identify the movement of the talus across the tibia. The dorsalis pedis artery and extensor tendons should be identified and avoided. The needle is then introduced into the joint in the sagittal plane via an inferior approach.

SUGGESTED READING

Abu-Zidan FM, Hefny AF, Corr P. Clinical ultrasound physics. *J Emerg Trauma Shock*. 2011;4(4):501–503.

Barys I, Boezaart AP. Ultrasound: Basic understanding and learning the language. *Int J Shoulder Surg*. 2010;4(3):55–62.

McNally EG. The development and clinical applications of musculoskeletal ultrasound. *Skeletal Radiol*. 2011;40:1223–1231.

CHAPTER 13

ELECTRODIAGNOSTIC STUDIES

Electrodiagnostic studies (also known as NCS/EMG or sometimes just EMG) include nerve conduction studies (NCSs or NCVs) and EMGs. Other less commonly performed electrodiagnostic tests include somatosensory evoked potentials, brain stem auditory evoked potentials or responses, single-fiber EMG (SFEMG), repetitive stimulation studies, and sympathetic skin response. This discussion is limited to the most commonly used studies, NCS and EMG. As they are usually performed together and reported as one comprehensive report, they will be referred to as a single test (NCS/EMG). This test provides physiologic information about nerves and muscles in real time. It gives information about muscle and nerve function, unlike most radiologic studies, which give a static picture of anatomy and do not directly assess function.

Indications for electrodiagnostic testing include numbness, tingling/paresthesias, pain, weakness, atrophy, depressed deep tendon reflexes, and/or fatigue. EMG/NCS can serve as an important part of a patient's clinical picture. Electrodiagnostic tests are used to (a) establish a correct diagnosis, (b) localize a lesion, (c) determine the treatment when a diagnosis is already known, and (d) provide information about the prognosis (1). NCS/EMG should be considered an extension of a good history and physical examination.

INITIAL SETTINGS FOR NCS

Sweep speed is the horizontal axis on the recording in units of time (milliseconds [ms]). *Gain* is the vertical axis on the graph in units of voltage (millivolts [mV] for motor studies or microvolts [µV] for sensory studies).

Motor settings: sweep—2 ms/division, gain—5 mV/division
Sensory settings: sweep—2 ms/division, gain—20 µV/division (1)

INITIAL SETTINGS FOR EMG

Sweep speed: 10 ms/division
Low-frequency filter: 10 to 30 Hz
High-frequency filter: 10,000 to 20,000 Hz
Amplifier sensitivity: 50 to 100 µV (1)

INTRODUCTION TO NCS

NCS is the recording of an electrical response of a nerve that is stimulated at one or more sites along its course. The nerve is stimulated electrically using a probe, and the response is recorded over the muscle (for motor studies) or dermatome (for sensory studies) that the nerve supplies. The action potential (AP) that is propagated is the summative response of many individual axons or muscle fibers. For motor nerves, this response is called a compound motor action potential (CMAP) and represents the summative response of motor units (MUs) that are firing. CMAPs are usually recorded in mV. For sensory nerves, the response is called a sensory nerve action potential (SNAP) and represents the summation of individual sensory nerve fibers. SNAPs are very small-amplitude potentials that are usually recorded in μV. Late responses (evoked potentials that record over a very long pathway) include F waves and H-reflexes. *Orthodromic* refers to conduction in the same direction as occurs physiologically (i.e., a sensory fiber conducts from the extremity toward the spine). *Antidromic* refers to conduction in the opposite direction to the physiological direction.

Components of the AP

Latency is the time it takes from stimulation to the beginning of the CMAP or SNAP (the distal speed of transmission). The latency of a sensory nerve is dependent on the conduction speed of the fastest fibers and the distance it travels. The latency of a motor nerve also includes the time it takes for the AP to synapse at the neuromuscular junction (NMJ) and the speed of conduction of the electrical potential through the muscle. Since there is no myoneural junction of sensory nerves, the latency of a sensory nerve is directly related to the conduction velocity (CV). Latency measurement requires standardized and accurately recorded distance or else the results are meaningless.

Conduction velocity reflects how fast the nerve AP is propagating. In sensory studies, the velocity is measured directly from the time it takes the AP to travel the measured distance (distance/latency). In a motor nerve, two different sites have to be stimulated to calculate the velocity (velocity = change in distance/change in time) and account for the myoneural junction. The presence of a myelin covering speeds up NCV via a process known as saltatory conduction. Myelinated nerves conduct impulses approximately 50 times faster than unmyelinated nerves. In myelinated nerves, the CV is primarily dependent on the integrity of the myelin covering. Slowing or latency prolongation usually implies demyelination.

Amplitude correlates with axonal integrity. Decreased amplitude could indicate an axonal lesion (if the amplitude is decreased both distally and proximally) or it can indicate a conduction block across the site of injury (if the amplitude is low distally and not proximally; 1,2).

TYPES OF NERVE INJURIES

Nerve injuries can be classified depending on whether there is injury to the axon, the myelin, or both. Often, especially with trauma, the affected structures do not always fit into one category. It is the job of the electromyographer to diagnose and communicate the type of injury that exists, the severity, and the location. Seddon proposed a classification of nerve injuries in 1943 that is still commonly used as it correlates well with electrophysiology:

1. **Neurapraxia** – Defined as conduction block. This type of nerve injury occurs in the peripheral nerve with minor contusion or compression. There is preservation of the axon; only the myelin is affected. In neurapraxia, there is an area of demyelination that is so severe that the AP cannot propagate (saltatory conduction cannot occur). The transmission of AP is interrupted for a brief period, but recovery is usually complete in days to weeks.

2. **Axonotmesis** – More significant injury: breakdown of axon with accompanying Wallerian degeneration distal to the lesion. There is preservation of some of the supporting connective tissue stroma (Schwann cells and endoneurial tubes). Regeneration of axons (through collateral sprouting or axonal growth) can occur with good functional recovery, depending on the amount of axonal loss and the distance from the injury to the muscle.

3. **Neurotmesis** – Severe injury with complete severance of the nerve and its supporting structures; extensive avulsing or crushing injury. The myelin, axon, perineurium, and epineurium are all disrupted. Spontaneous recovery is not expected.

Injury to the myelin can be focal (local), uniform (throughout the nerve), or segmental (affecting some parts of the nerve but not others):

1. *Uniform demyelination* – Slowing of CV along the entire nerve (e.g., Charcot-Marie-Tooth disease).

2. *Segmental demyelination* – Uneven degree of demyelination in different areas along the course of the nerve; may have variable slowing (temporal dispersion).

3. *Focal nerve slowing* – Localized area of demyelination causing nerve slowing; decreased CV is noted across the lesion.

4. *Conduction block* – Severe focal demyelination that prevents propagation of the AP through the area. There will be more than 20% amplitude decrement when the nerve is stimulated proximal to the lesion. The distal CMAP amplitude remains intact. Clinically, conduction block presents as weakness.

Axonal injuries will lead to Wallerian degeneration distal to the lesion. Low-amplitude CMAPs will be noted with both proximal and distal stimulation. On EMG, abnormal spontaneous potentials (fibrillations [fibs] and positive sharp waves [PSWs]) are seen. The MU recruitment will be decreased (increased firing frequency of existing MUs). With reinnervation, MUs may become polyphasic with high amplitude and long duration (1,3).

H-REFLEX

The *H-reflex* (Hoffmann reflex) is a true reflex and is the electrical equivalent of the monosynaptic or oligosynaptic stretch reflex. It is a sensitive but nonspecific tool for possible S1 radiculopathy, especially when clinical, radiologic, and electrophysiologic signs of motor root involvement are lacking. In some cases, it may be the only abnormal study. The H-reflex is usually elicited by submaximally stimulating the tibial nerve in the popliteal fossa. Such stimulation can be initiated by using slow (less than 1 pulse/s), long-duration (0.5–1 ms) stimuli with gradually increasing stimulation strength. The stimulus will travel along the most excitable 1a afferent nerve fibers, through the dorsal root ganglion (DRG). It then gets transmitted across the central synapse to the anterior horn cell, which then sends it down along the alpha motor axon to the muscle. Hence, the H-reflex is a measure of the time it takes for the orthodromic sensory response to get to the spinal cord proximally and the orthodromic motor response to reach the muscle distally (on which the recording electrode is placed). A generally acceptable result would be a motor response usually between 0.5 and 5 mV in amplitude and a latency of 28 to 30 ms. H-reflex studies are usually performed bilaterally because asymmetry of responses is an important criterion for abnormality. An abnormal latency greater than 0.5 to 1.0 ms (as compared with the other side) or H-reflex absence in patients under 60 years may suggest a lesion along the H-reflex pathway (afferent and/or efferent fibers). This may be due to an SI radiculopathy or any other source of slowing along this pathway. The standard formula for calculating the H-reflex is 9.14 + 0.46 (leg length in cm from the medial malleolus to the popliteal fossa) + 0.1 (age). For a patient older than 60 years, 1.8 ms will be added to the total calculated value.

In normal infants or adults with upper motor neuron (corticospinal tract) lesions, the H-reflex may be elicited in muscles other than the gastrocnemius/soleus muscles or flexor carpi radialis. It is often absent in patients older than 60 years. The reflex can be potentially inhibited by antagonist muscle contractions and initiated by agonist muscle contractions.

The H-reflex does have some limitations. It is unable to distinguish between acute and chronic lesions, may be normal with incomplete lesions, is diluted by focal lesions, and is nonspecific in terms of injury location. Once the H-reflex is found to be abnormal, it will usually remain so, even with resolution of symptoms.

F WAVES

F wave or F response is a small-amplitude, variable-latency late motor response that occurs following the activation of motor nerves. It derives its name from the word "foot" because it was first recorded from the intrinsic foot muscles. Unlike the H-reflex, the F wave does not represent a true reflex because there is no synapse from an afferent impulse to a motor nerve. Depolarizing peripheral nerves with external stimuli evokes potentials propagating both proximally and distally. Electrical stimulation of a peripheral nerve results in an orthodromic CMAP. In addition, the proximally (antidromically) propagating potential activates a small percentage of anterior horn motor neurons. In turn, this generates an orthodromic motor response (the F wave) along the same axon that activates a few muscle fibers picked up by the recording electrode (4).

F waves can be obtained from any muscle by a supramaximal stimulus. Because of their variability (as opposed to H-reflexes), multiple stimulations must be used to obtain the shortest latency. F waves may be useful in the evaluation of peripheral neuropathies with predominantly proximal involvement, such as Guillain-Barré syndrome and chronic inflammatory demyelinating polyneuropathies, in which distal conduction velocities may be normal early in the disease. However, the value of the F wave in evaluating focal nerve lesions, such as radiculopathy or peripheral nerve entrapment, is extremely limited largely due to the variability of F-wave responses. In addition, most muscles receive innervation from multiple roots, so the fastest (unaffected) fibers will be normal. In addition, the results are nonspecific. It is a pure motor response, and its long neural pathway dilutes focal lesions and hinders the specificity of injury location. F waves are also generally not seen in nerves where the CMAP amplitude is severely reduced, such as severe axonal loss, since the F-wave amplitude is only 1% to 5% of the amplitude of the CMAP.

Normal latency of F wave, upper limb: 28 ms; lower limb: 56 ms. Side-to-side difference: <2.0 ms for upper limbs; <4.0 ms for lower limbs.

BLINK REFLEX

The most complicated of the late responses is the blink reflex. It is the electrophysiologic correlate of the corneal reflex. The sensory afferent limb of the reflex is the supraorbital nerve, a branch of the ophthalmic division of the trigeminal nerve (CN V_1). Intervening synapses (pons and medulla) are stimulated. The motor efferent limb is the facial nerve (CN VII), which innervates the orbicularis oculi muscle. As with the corneal reflex, stimulation of one side of the supraorbital branch of the trigeminal nerve elicits a motor response (eye blink) bilaterally through the facial nerves. Abnormalities anywhere along the reflex arc (central or peripheral) can be detected.

There is an early response (R1) due to a disynaptic reflex arc from the ipsilateral sensory nucleus of V to the ipsilateral facial nerve. There is also a late response (R2) due to multiple interneurons connecting the ipsilateral sensory nucleus of V to the ipsilateral spinal motor nucleus of V and then to the bilateral facial nuclei.

Recording electrodes are placed below and slightly lateral to the pupils bilaterally. Reference electrodes are placed just lateral to the

TABLE 13.1 Basic Abnormal Patterns*

Lesion	Electrodiagnostic pattern if affected side stimulated	Electrodiagnostic pattern if unaffected side stimulated
Unilateral CN V	Delayed (partial injury) or absent (complete injury) R1 and bilateral R2	Normal R1 and bilateral R2
Unilateral CN VII	Delayed or absent R1 and ipsilateral R2	Delayed or absent contralateral R2
Unilateral midpontine	Delayed R1 and normal bilateral R2	Normal R1 and bilateral R2
Unilateral medullary	Delayed ipsilateral R2	Delayed contralateral R2
Demyelinating peripheral neuropathy	Possible delay or absence of R1 and bilateral R2	Possible delay or absence of R1 and bilateral R2

*Using the anatomy outlined here and these basic patterns, complex and bilateral lesions can be extrapolated.
CN, cranial nerve; R1, early response; R2, late response.
Source: Adapted from Ref. (4).

lateral canthus bilaterally. The ground can be placed on the chin. The stimulator is placed over the medial supraorbital ridge of the eyebrow. The sweep speed should be 5 or 10 ms with initial sensitivity of 100 or 200 μV.

Normal latency for R1 response is <13 ms. Normal latency for ipsilateral R2 is <41 ms. Normal latency for contralateral R2 is 44 ms. Acceptable normal bilateral variation for R1 is <1.2 ms, for ipsilateral R2 is <5 ms, and for contralateral R2 is <7 ms (Table 13.1).

EMG USING MONOPOLAR VERSUS CONCENTRIC NEEDLE

EMG testing involves evaluation of the electrical activity of skeletal or voluntary muscles. Muscles contract and produce movement through the orderly recruitment of MUs. An MU is defined as one anterior horn cell, its axon, the NMJ, and all the muscle fibers (ranging from five to hundreds), innervated by that motor neuron. An MU is the fundamental structure that is assessed in EMG testing. EMG requires a thorough knowledge of the anatomy of the muscle being tested in order to place the needle electrode in the appropriate muscle.

Monopolar needles are 22-G to 30-G Teflon-coated stainless steel needles with an exposed tip of 0.15 to 0.2 mm² (Figure 13.1A). They require a surface electrode or a second needle as a reference lead. Another surface electrode serves as a ground. A monopolar needle records the voltage changes between the tip of the electrode and the

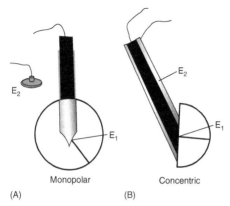

FIGURE 13.1 Needle electrodes. (A) Monopolar needle. (B) Concentric needle.

reference. Since it picks up from a full 360° field around the needle, it registers larger amplitude and has increased polyphasicity when compared with the concentric needle. The smaller diameter and the Teflon coat make the monopolar needle less uncomfortable. This, combined with its cost advantage over the concentric, has led to its preferential clinical use.

Concentric needles are 24-G to 26-G stainless steel needles (Figure 13.1B). The needle comprises a reference (cannula) electrode with a bare inner wire in the center of the shaft that is the recording electrode. The concentric needle can register the voltage changes between the wire and the shaft. The pointed tip of the needle has an oval (beveled) shape. Since the exposed active recording electrode is on the beveled portion of the cannula, the concentric needle picks up from a 180° field. Therefore, it registers smaller amplitude (since it has a smaller recording area). A separate surface electrode serves as the ground.

EFFECTS OF TEMPERATURE AND AGE ON NCS

Cooling is thought to prolong the opening of Na^+ channels (1,5). Decreasing the temperature of a limb affects SNAPs and CMAPs by prolonging latency, decreasing CV, and increasing amplitude and duration. CV decreases 2.4 m/s per 1°C decrease. Correction formulas exist but the best approach is to warm the limb prior to the NCS (32° in the upper limbs and 30° in the lower limbs).

As patients age, SNAP and CMAP amplitudes decrease and latencies increase. Motor NCSs for newborns are 50% of adult values since myelination is incomplete. Normal adult values are attained by age 5 years. After age 60 years, there is a progressive decline of 1 to 2 m/s per decade in the NCS of the fastest motor fibers.

THE NEEDLE EMG EXAMINATION

The EMG evaluation typically has four components:

1. Insertional activity
2. Activity at rest
3. MU analysis
4. Recruitment

Insertional Activity

Healthy muscle is electrically silent at rest. Insertional activity (1,5) refers to the brief electrical activity associated with the needle entering the sarcolemma, which causes muscle fiber injury. The associated sound should be crisp. Insertional activity is classified in three ways:

1. *Normal insertional activity* only lasts a few hundred milliseconds and is due to muscle depolarization.
2. *Increased insertional activity* occurs due to denervation or cell membrane irritability and lasts >300 ms. There may be evidence of initially positive deflection waveforms that do not persist. If these positive waveforms are sustained and fire regularly, they are considered abnormal spontaneous potentials (see the following text).
3. *Decreased insertional activity* occurs when the needle is placed into atrophied muscle, fat, or edema and lasts <300 m/s.

Activity at Rest

Normal Spontaneous Activity

A needle should be inserted into a muscle at three to four different depths and in three to four different directions (examining three or four electrically discrete areas of muscle) for insertional activity and activity at rest. The needle can be withdrawn almost to the skin and then redirected in a different direction, again stopping at three or four different depths in the muscle. This can be repeated so that the needle examines about 12 to 16 discrete areas of the muscle (depending on the patient's tolerance).

- After insertion of the needle into normal muscle at rest, there should be electrical silence (Figure 13.2A).
- Normal muscle may also display end plate activity. This occurs if a needle is placed in the region of the NMJ or end plate. The needle should be moved out of the end plate, as the clinician cannot get reliable information about the muscle. Either of two waveforms may occur: miniature end plate potentials (MEPPs) or end plate potentials (EPPs). The patient may complain of increased pain. It is important to recognize these potentials so that they are not misinterpreted as abnormal spontaneous potentials.

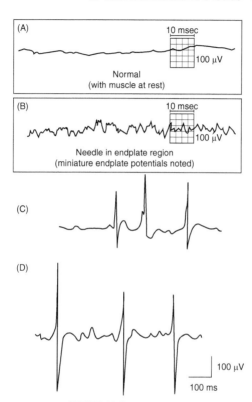

FIGURE 13.2 End plate activity.

Source: Parts A and B, adapted from Ref. (1) with permission from Elsevier.

- MEPPs - Represent spontaneous release of single quantum of acetylcholine (ACh) at the presynaptic terminal that manifests as end plate noise (Figure 13.2B).
- EPPs or "end plate spikes" - Represent single muscle fiber depolarizations at the presynaptic terminal with resultant release of large amounts of ACh (Figure13.2C).
- MEPPs and EPPs may or may not be present together (Figure13.2D).

Abnormal Spontaneous Activity

- Usually represents pathology (injury or denervation) that stems from a muscle or nerve. These spontaneous depolarizations have an abnormal morphology and firing pattern.

- Examples of *muscle fiber*–generated spontaneous potentials: Fibs—triphasic with initial positive (downward) deflection, PSWs—biphasic with positive deflection, myotonic discharges, and complex repetitive discharges (CRDs).
- Examples of *neural*-generated spontaneous potentials: Myokymic discharges, cramps, neuromyotonic discharges, tremors, fasciculations, and multiple MU potentials.
- Fibs and PSWs usually appear 1 to 3 weeks or more after injury.
- Abnormal spontaneous potentials are usually of small amplitude. Therefore, the gain on the EMG machine should be set to 50 to 100 μV for the best visualization (Figure 13.3).

Grading of fibs and PSWs is from 0 to 4+, with a sweep of 10 ms/division

> **(0)** No fibs or PSWs present
> **(1+)** One fib/PSW per screen persistent within two areas
> **(2+)** Fibs/PSWs in *greater than two areas*, about two per screen
> **(3+)** Fibs/PSWs in most muscle regions, greater than half of the screen
> **(4+)** Fibs/PSWs in all areas of the muscle and fill the entire screen

Fasciculation potentials originate from a single MU and may have an intermittent or a normal firing pattern. When associated with PSWs or fibs, they suggest pathology. In the absence of fibs or PSWs, they may be due to stress, fatigue, or caffeine (Figure 13.4).

CRDs frequently result from denervation and reinnervation through collateral sprouting. Their presence suggests a chronic process such as chronic radiculopathy, peripheral neuropathy, anterior horn disease, polymyositis, or myxedema (Figure 13.5).

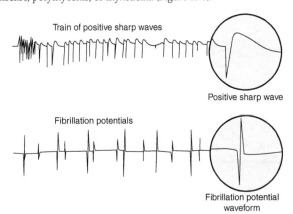

Train of positive sharp waves

Positive sharp wave

Fibrillation potentials

Fibrillation potential waveform

FIGURE 13.3 Fibs and PSWs.
Source: Adapted from Ref. (1) with permission from Elsevier.

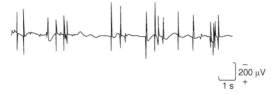

FIGURE 13.4 Fasciculation potentials.

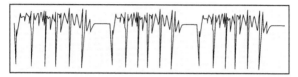

FIGURE 13.5 Complex repetitive discharges.
Source: Adapted from Ref. (1) with permission from Elsevier.

Myotonic discharges (Figure 13.6) originate in the muscle due to membrane instability. They have a typical waxing and waning character and have been compared with a dive-bomber sound. They are commonly seen in myotonic dystrophy, myotonia congenita, polymyositis, chronic radiculopathy, peripheral neuropathy, maltase deficiency, and hyperkalemic periodic paralysis (Table 13.2).

Other potentials that are nerve generated include cramp potentials, myokymia, and neuromyotonia. These are beyond the scope of our discussion here.

MU Analysis

After analysis of insertional activity and spontaneous activity, the next step is to analyze the motor unit action potentials (MUAPs). First assess the morphology (duration, amplitude, phases, and rise time). This should be done during a minimal contraction (sometimes positioning changes can bring this on). A trigger and delay line can be helpful in assessing MU stability.

MUAP morphology varies depending on the age of the patient and the muscle being tested.

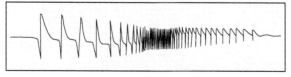

FIGURE 13.6 Myotonic discharges.
Source: Adapted from Ref. (1) with permission from Elsevier.

TABLE 13.2 Abnormal Spontaneous Potentials

	MMEPs	EPPs	Fib potentials	Positive sharp waves	Fasciculation potentials	Complex repetitive discharges	Myotonic discharges
Sound	Sea shells	Sputtering fat in a hot pan	Drops of rain on a tin roof	Dull thud	Varies	Misfired motorboat	Dive-bomber
Firing pattern	Irregular	Irregular	Regular	Regular	Irregular	Regular/starts and stops abruptly	Waxes and wanes
Duration (ms)	1–2	3–5	1–5	10–30	5–15	Variable	>5–20
Amplitude (pV)	10–20	100–200	20–1,000	20–1,000	>300 m	50–500	20–300
Rate (Hz)	150	50–100	0.5–15	0.5–15	0.1–10	10–100	20–100
Waveform/ deflection	Monophasic negative (upward)	Biphasic negative (upward)	Triphasic with initial positive (downward) deflection	Biphasic with initial positive (downward) deflection	Similar to motor unit action potential (MUAP)	Similar to MUAP, fibs, and PSWs	Similar to EPP, fibs, and PSWs

(continued)

TABLE 13.2 Abnormal Spontaneous Potentials (*continued*)

	MMEPPs	EPPs	Fib potentials	Positive sharp waves	Fasciculation potentials	Complex repetitive discharges	Myotonic discharges
Cause	MEPPs	Irregularly firing muscle fiber APs	Spontaneous depolarization of a muscle fiber	Spontaneous depolarization of a muscle fiber	Spontaneous involuntary discharge of single MU	Depolarization of single muscle fiber with ephaptic spread to adjacent denervated fibers	Spontaneous discharge of a muscle fiber
Seen in	Needle in the end plate	Needle in the end plate	Denervation (may be due to neurogenic muscle disorder or disorders of the NMJ)	Denervation (may be due to neurogenic muscle disorder or disorders of the NMJ)	Processes that affect the lower motor neuron (LMN). Also seen in benign fasciculations	Chronic neuropathic and myopathic disorders	Myotonic dystrophy, myotonia congenita and paramyotonia, some myopathies, hyperkalemic periodic paralysis, and rarely in denervation

AP, action potential; EPP, end plate potential; fib, fibrillation; MEPP, miniature end plate potential; MU, motor unit; NMJ, neuromuscular junction; PSW, positive sharp wave.
Source: Adapted from Ref. (4) with permission from Elsevier.

Duration is measured from the initial deflection from the baseline to the return to baseline (typically 5 to 15 ms) and reflects the synchrony of muscle fibers firing. The duration is increased with asynchronous firing of the fibers of an MU (as in reinnervation or other neuropathic processes) and is decreased in myopathic processes (fewer fibers contribute to the MU). *When listening to the MUs, duration correlates with pitch; thus, long duration is dull and thudding and short duration is crisp and static-like.*

Amplitude is measured from the most positive to the most negative peak of the MU and reflects fiber density. The criteria for normal amplitude depend on the type of needle used (several hundred μV to a few mV for concentric needles, 1 to 7 μV for a monopolar needle). Amplitude increases (a) as the needle approximates the MU, (b) as the number of muscle fibers of the MU is increased, (c) with increasing diameter of the muscle fibers (muscle fiber hypertrophy), and (d) with more synchronous firing of the muscle fibers. Also, amplitude may be increased after reinnervation (neuropathic injuries) and may be decreased in myopathies. *When listening to the MUs, amplitude correlates with volume (not pitch).*

Phases are determined by counting the number of baseline crossings and adding one. Polyphasia implies asynchronous firing of muscle fibers within an MU. Polyphasia is nonspecific and can be seen in both neuropathic and myopathic lesions. The MUAP is generally two to four phases. All muscles will normally exhibit about 10% polyphasia except the deltoid (up to 25% is normal). *When listening to the MUs, polyphasia results in a clicking sound.*

Serrations (or turns) are defined as changes in the direction of a potential that do not cross baseline. Serrations also imply asynchronous firing of muscle fibers within an MU. Often serrations will become phases with a slight movement of the needle.

Satellite potentials are seen only after denervation has occurred. Satellite potentials appear after collateral sprouting from adjacent intact MUs. The new sprouts are unmyelinated and conduct slower than the original MU. As the reinnervation matures and myelinates, the satellite potential moves toward the MUAP until it eventually becomes an additional phase of the MUAP (these may require a trigger and delay line to be appreciated).

Rise time is measured from the initial positive deflection to the first negative peak. It correlates with the proximity of the recording electrode to the MUAP being measured; thus, *as the discharging MU is approached, the sound will become sharper.* The electromyographer's qualitative analysis will be more accurate the closer he or she is to the MU. An acceptable rise time is 0.5 ms or less.

Stability – The morphology of an MU is stable in normal MUAPs. Unstable MUAP morphology (changes in amplitude or number of phases) occurs in primary NMJ disorders and disorders associated with new or immature NMJs (reinnervation). A trigger and delay function on the EMG machine may be helpful here.

Recruitment

MUAPs normally fire in a semirhythmic pattern with a slight variation in the time between MUAPs. There are two ways to increase force during a muscle contraction: *Increase the MU firing rate* or *recruit more MUs*. Normally, one MU fires semirhythmically around 5 Hz. If more force is needed, that unit increases its firing rate (activation) and a second unit is recruited. Most MUs will fire at about 10 Hz before recruiting a second MU. *Decreased recruitment* usually occurs in neuropathic disorders where the nerve is damaged. There are therefore fewer MUs available to fire. In order to increase the strength of a contraction, these MUs fire at a higher frequency. This is also described more accurately as an increase in MU firing frequency. *Early or increased recruitment* usually occurs in myopathic processes with a loss of muscle fibers. In order to increase the strength of a contraction, the remaining muscle fibers are quickly recruited. Many MUAPs are activated with minimal contraction. It is important not to confuse decreased recruitment (increased firing frequency of the MUs as seen in a neuropathic process) with early recruitment (recruitment of many MUAPs with slight contraction as seen in a myopathic process).

As a rule of thumb, myopathic MUAPs have early recruitment of short duration with low amplitude and an increased firing rate. Neuropathic MUAPs have late recruitment of increased duration and increased amplitude. MUAPs of central nervous system (CNS) disorders have normal morphology, but may have a decreased activation (1,4).

SPECIFIC DISORDERS

Median Neuropathy at the Wrist (Carpal Tunnel Syndrome)

Median neuropathy at the wrist presents with a combination of signs/symptoms known as carpal tunnel syndrome (CTS)—the most common entrapment neuropathy. Etiologies are multifactorial with varying contributions of local and systemic factors. The initial presentation is usually due to a demyelinating lesion of the median nerve sensory fibers. Demyelination may also affect the motor fibers early on. This may progress to axonal loss of both sensory and motor fibers.

Patient presentation is the most important aspect of the clinical diagnosis of CTS. The symptoms include numbness, tingling, and pain along the median nerve distribution (palmar surface of the first 3½ digits). Symptoms may be worst or most prevalent at night and may wake the patient from sleep. Weakness of grip strength (inability to open jars or dropping objects) may occur as symptoms progress and median motor fibers become involved. CTS can be bilateral, but the dominant hand is usually affected first. Physical examination involves sensory test (pinprick, 2-point discrimination, and/or *Semmes-Weinstein* pressure monofilaments) and motor test/inspection for abductor pollicis brevis (APB) atrophy and weakness. The special/provocative tests

TABLE 13.3 Provocative Tests and Their Descriptions

Provocative tests	Description
Carpal compression test	Direct application of pressure (150 mmHg) on the patient's wrist for 30 sec. Positive if pain, numbness, or paresthesia develops in a median distribution
Flick test	The patient shakes down hands (like a thermometer) to relieve the pain
Phalen's test	Reproduction of symptoms in a median distribution with prolonged (30 sec to 1 min) wrist flexion
Tinel's test	Pain, numbness, or paresthesia in a median nerve distribution elicited by mild taps along the course of median nerve at the wrist
Reverse Phalen's test	Reproduction of symptoms in a median distribution with prolonged (30 sec to 1 min) wrist extension

may assist in diagnosis (Table 13.3). The affected side should always be compared with the unaffected side.

Electrodiagnostic studies are helpful in confirming the diagnosis of CTS (85%–90% sensitivity) and determining the type of lesion (demyelinating, axonal, or both). However, one must keep in mind that all those with abnormal studies do not necessarily have CTS and all those with CTS do not necessarily have abnormal studies. Classic evaluation of CTS includes motor and sensory NCS of median nerve and its comparison with the ulnar nerve (ipsilaterally) and median nerve (contralaterally). A needle study may be helpful to assess for axonal damage or reinnervation and to rule out radiculopathy or other nerve lesions. Antidromic SNAPs are recorded with the active electrode over the proximal interphalangeal (PIP) joint of the second or third digit and stimulating the mid-palm (7 cm from electrode) and across the carpal tunnel (14 cm from electrode). *Note:* Larger/smaller distances can be used depending on the size of the patient's hand—it is important to change the distance in your recordings, as this will affect the velocity.

The electrodiagnostic analysis of CTS depends upon evidence of median nerve slowing, conduction block, or axon loss in the carpal tunnel. Commonly used criteria include prolonged absolute motor or sensory latency, sensory slowing across the carpal tunnel (or relatively prolonged or slowed in comparison with other nerves or the contralateral median nerve) as well as amplitude changes that would indicate axonal loss or a conduction block.

Sensory changes that may indicate CTS (note that all findings must be taken in the context of the global findings in all nerves):

- CV <44 m/s (median nerve across the carpal tunnel)
- Latency of >0.5 ms compared with the ipsilateral ulnar nerve

- Amplitude of the median response across the carpal tunnel <50% of the distal amplitude or the contralateral amplitude

  Motor changes that may indicate CTS (sensory fibers are usually affected first):

- Latency of >4.2 ms at a distance of 8 cm from the active electrode
- Latency of >1 ms greater than the ipsilateral ulnar motor nerve latency

The EMG test should include the APB muscle. If the APB is abnormal (PSW/fibs), more proximal median as well as nonmedian innervated muscles should be tested to rule out a more proximal median neuropathy, peripheral neuropathy, plexopathy, radiculopathy, or a lesion of the anterior horn cell.

A possible source of confusion in median nerve electrodiagnostic studies is a *Martin-Gruber anastomosis*. This relatively common anastomosis (found in 15% to 20% of population) occurs when ulnar fibers (destined for ulnar innervated muscles) travel with the median nerve. In the forearm, the nerve fibers travel with the anterior interosseous nerve and cross over to join the ulnar nerve (median to ulnar anastomoses). There are three classic electrodiagnostic findings:

1. The median CMAP has a positive (downward) initial deflection after median nerve stimulation at the elbow that is not seen with wrist stimulation. This deflection occurs because ulnar fibers (traveling at the elbow with median nerve fibers, before joining the ulnar nerve in the forearm) arrive at the thenar eminence first and stimulate the adductor muscle of the thumb causing downward deflection to be recorded over the APB.

2. The CMAP amplitude of median nerve stimulation at the elbow will be larger compared with the wrist stimulation. This can occur without median nerve entrapment. The amplitude is increased because at the elbow the ulnar nerve fibers traveling with the median nerve are stimulated and added to the median CMAP, whereas at the wrist, only median nerve fibers are stimulated and recorded.

3. There may be a false increase in median NCV in the forearm based on proximal (at the elbow) stimulation calculations. This is more prevalent in patients with CTS. Ulnar fibers stimulated with the median nerve at the elbow do not have to traverse the carpal tunnel and will therefore result in a faster proximal latency than normal.

Ulnar Neuropathy at the Elbow

Ulnar neuropathy at the elbow *(cubital tunnel syndrome)* is the second most common mononeuropathy of the upper extremity (second only to CTS). Patients usually complain of sensory changes in the fourth and fifth digits and/or weakness of the hand. Physical examination must include inspection for deformity and signs of muscle atrophy (first dorsal interosseous and abductor digiti minimi [ADM]), individual muscle strength testing, thorough sensory examination (including the dorsal ulnar cutaneous nerve), and special tests. Tinel's sign occurs when mild taps at the ulnar groove or cubital tunnel cause numbness or paresthesia in the hand along the ulnar nerve distribution. Froment's sign occurs when the patient is asked to hold a piece of paper between thumb and index finger and there is flexion of the thumb at the interphalangeal (IP) joint. The patient will substitute the flexor pollicis longus muscle (innervated by the median nerve) for the adductor pollicis muscle (innervated by the ulnar nerve).

Electrodiagnostic studies may help pinpoint the site of compression of the ulnar nerve, prognosticate, and distinguish ulnar neuropathy at the elbow from other pathologies. Depending on the severity, SNAPs may be affected, resulting in decreased amplitude. A side-to-side difference of more than 50% is considered significant. The dorsal ulnar cutaneous nerve should be tested in suspected ulnar neuropathy at the elbow. This cutaneous nerve branches off just before the ulnar nerve enters Guyon's canal and can help distinguish between ulnar neuropathy at Guyon's canal (the dorsal ulnar cutaneous response will be normal) and more proximal entrapment (the dorsal ulnar cutaneous nerve will be affected). If CMAPs are decreased and the SNAPs are normal, consider cervical radiculopathy.

Slowing of the ulnar motor response across the elbow may be noted. Slowing of more than 10 m/s (compared with distal CV) is considered significant. If the elbow is not flexed (90°–135°), the CV may be falsely decreased. The length of the segment should be measured by following the path of the nerve with the elbow bent. An amplitude drop of more than 20% to 30% compared with the distal segment may indicate conduction block. The "inching technique" (stimulating at 1-cm intervals and assessing for a drop in amplitude or excessive latency) can further help localize the site of entrapment.

Needle EMG testing can be difficult to interpret. Because the innervation of the flexor carpi ulnaris (FCU) sometimes occurs proximal and sometimes distal to the elbow, it is frequently spared in ulnar neuropathy at the elbow. NCS (including evaluation of the dorsal ulnar cutaneous nerve) must be taken into consideration when making a diagnosis.

Peroneal Neuropathy

The common peroneal nerve (also known as the fibular nerve) innervates the short head of biceps femoris that then proceeds to wind around the fibular head/neck where it becomes very superficial. This is the main site of entrapment of the common peroneal nerve, which then courses into the fibular tunnel and divides into superficial and deep peroneal nerves. The etiology of compression is usually trauma, habituation, iatrogenic, or work related. The pathophysiology can present as myelin, axon, or mixed damage, based on severity and etiology of compression. The clinical presentation is usually foot drop (steppage gait with inability to dorsiflex) and paresthesia/numbness on the dorsum of the foot and lateral leg.

The electrodiagnostic study remains the best test to assess the degree of nerve damage and pinpoint the location of entrapment. The classic NCS includes a sensory study of bilateral superficial peroneal nerves and a motor study of the peroneal nerves with recording electrode at extensor digitorum brevis (EDB; tibialis anterior muscle can be used as the recording electrode if the EDB is atrophied). The motor studies are performed with stimulation at the ankle, below the fibular head, and in the lateral popliteal fossa. These findings should be compared with the contralateral side. In general, a lower extremity motor CV of <40 m/s is considered abnormal. The proximal segment velocity should be greater than distal velocity due to greater axonal diameter in the proximal segment of the nerve. An accessory peroneal nerve should be suspected if the peroneal CMAP is larger on proximal (fibular head) stimulation than on distal (ankle) stimulation. This anomalous innervation can be found by stimulating posterior to the lateral malleolus. The amplitude of the CMAP stimulating at the ankle plus the amplitude of the CMAP stimulating posterior to the lateral malleolus will approximate the CMAP amplitude stimulating over the fibular head. Needle EMG helps confirm axonal loss, assess the degree of involvement of the muscles innervated by the peroneal nerve, localize the lesion, and rule out L5 radiculopathy/plexopathy. The examination of the short head of the biceps femoris muscle is very important, as this is the only peroneal nerve-innervated muscle above the knee. If this muscle demonstrates abnormality, the lesion is proximal to the fibular head.

PERIPHERAL NEUROPATHY

Peripheral neuropathy is a generalized dysfunction of the peripheral nerves. The distal segments of the nerves are usually more affected than the proximal segments (the longer the nerve, the more it is usually affected). Peripheral neuropathies typically occur in a "stocking and glove" distribution, affecting the feet and hands with numbness, pain, or paresthesias. Electrodiagnostic studies (NCS/EMG) are used to determine the presence of peripheral neuropathy and can help to identify its characteristics and severity. Peripheral neuropathy is classified based on the types of fibers involved (sensory or motor), the primary pathology affecting the component of the nerve (axonal or demyelinating), and its extent (segmental or uniform). When performing electrodiagnostic testing, both sensory and motor nerves must be tested in at least three extremities to differentiate between single entrapment neuropathy and a generalized process. Relevant findings must be found in at least three extremities to be diagnosed as a peripheral neuropathy. Early in the progression of peripheral neuropathy, changes may not be seen in the upper extremity.

Nerve Conduction Studies

1. *Sensory NCS:* SNAPs may be reduced
   a. If *axonal,* amplitude of SNAP will be reduced or unobtainable.
   b. If *demyelinating,* SNAP can have an increased latency and/or decreased CV; demyelination may result in loss of SNAP through conduction block (neurapraxia).

2. Motor NCS:
   a. If *axonal,* amplitude of CMAP may be affected or unobtainable.
   b. If *demyelinating,* CMAP may have increased distal latency or slowing of CV. (CV less than 80% of the lower limit of normal suggests a demyelinating neuropathy.) Conduction block may also cause decreased CMAP.

3. *Uniform versus segmental*: Assessed by location of slowing CV. If segmental, some fibers will travel slower than others and the CMAP will be dispersed, with a longer duration and lower amplitude (temporal dispersion). If uniform, all fibers are slowed, which will result in a uniform slowing of CV, prolonged latencies, and normal duration and amplitude NCS.

Note that late responses (F waves and H-reflexes) assess both the proximal and distal segments of a peripheral nerve and therefore may also be affected. However, findings are nonspecific.

EMG – Test proximal and distal muscles to assess for axonal neuropathy and rule out additional or concomitant pathology. Findings are usually negative in peripheral neuropathy except in a few cases:

1. *Axonal motor neuropathy:* Affected muscles (usually distal) may demonstrate spontaneous activity (fibs and PSW). If an axonal lesion is present, the duration of the disease can be assessed by evaluating chronic changes in MUAPs (increased duration, polyphasicity, or large amplitude reveals reinnervation and reorganization).

2. *Chronic neurogenic disorders:* May see CRDs.

There are many causes for peripheral neuropathy, including genetic and acquired disorders. These disorders are further typified based on separate classifications of peripheral neuropathy that can be derived using electrodiagnostic studies (Table 13.4; 1,3).

Plexopathy

The functional anatomy of the brachial plexus can be divided into supraclavicular (roots and trunks) and infraclavicular (cords and peripheral nerves or branches; Figure 13.7). The pattern of findings will help to localize the lesion. In general, infraclavicular lesions will cause weakness in a muscle group without affecting the antagonist muscles of that group, whereas supraclavicular lesions will affect both. Electrodiagnostic testing is a physiological examination, which can

TABLE 13.4 Common Disorders of Polyneuropathy

EMG Finding	Uniform demyelinating mixed sensorimotor	Segmental demyelinating	Axonal loss: motor > sensory	Axonal loss: sensory only	Axonal loss: mixed sensorimotor	Mixed axonal/ demyelinating sensorimotor
Common diseases	1. HMSN I, III, and IV 2. Metachromatic leukodystrophy 3. Krabbe's leukodystrophy 4. Adrenomyeloneuropathy 5. Congenital hypomyelinating neuropathy 6. Tangier disease 7. Cockayne syndrome 8. Cerebrotendinous xanthomatosis	1. AIDP: Guillain-Barre syndrome 2. CIDP 3. Leprosy (Hansen's disease) 4. Diphtheria 5. Lyme disease 6. Monoclonal gammopathy 7. Osteosclerotic myeloma 8. Carcinoma 9. AIDS 10. Acute arsenic polyneuropathy	1. Acute intermittent porphyria 2. Axonal Guillain-Barré syndrome 3. HMSN II and V 4. Paraneoplastic motor neuronopathy 5. Hypoglycemia 6. Lead neuropathy 7. Dapsone neuropathy	1. Sjogren's syndrome 2. Fisher variant Guillain-Barré syndrome 3. HMSN 1–IV 4. HSAN 5. Friedreich's ataxia 6. Chronic idiopathic ataxic neuropathy 7. Amyloidosis 8. Paraneoplastic sensory neuronopathy 9. Lymphomatous sensory neuronopathy 10. Spinocerebellar degeneration	1. Alcoholic polyneuropathy 2. Vitamin deficiency (B and folate) 3. Sarcoidosis 4. Multiple myeloma 5. Paraneoplastic syndrome 6. Gouty neuropathy 7. Connective tissue disorders (RA, SLE, and amyloidosis) 8. Myotonic dystrophy 9. Post gastrectomy and gastric bypass 10. Chronic liver disease 11. Hypothyroidism 12. Lyme disease	1. Diabetic polyneuropathy 2. Uremia

(continued)

TABLE 13.4 Common Disorders of Polyneuropathy *(continued)*

EMG Finding	Uniform demyelinating mixed sensorimotor	Segmental demyelinating	Axonal loss: motor > sensory	Axonal loss: sensory only	Axonal loss: mixed sensorimotor	Mixed axonal/ demyelinating sensorimotor
		11. Pharmaceuticals (amiodarone, perhexiline, and high-dose Ara-C)	8. Vincristine neuropathy	11. Abetalipoproteinemia (Bassen-Kornzweig disease) 12. Paraproteinemias 13. Primary biliary cirrhosis 14. Crohn's disease 15. Acute sensory neuronopathy (cis-platinum toxicity) 16. Pyridoxine toxicity	13. HIV 14. Critical illness neuropathy 15. Metal neuropathy (mercury, thallium, gold, etc.) 16. Vincristine neuropathy 17. Toxic neuropathy (acrylamide, carbon disulfide, and carbon monoxide)	

AIDP, acute inflammatory demyelinating polyneuropathy; CIDP, chronic inflammatory demyelinating polyneuropathy; HMSN, hereditary motor sensory neuropathy; HSAN, hereditary sensory and autonomic neuropathy; RA, rheumatoid arthritis; SLE, systemic lupus erythematosus.

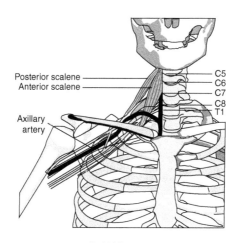

Posterior scalene
Anterior scalene

C5
C6
C7
C8
T1

Axillary
artery

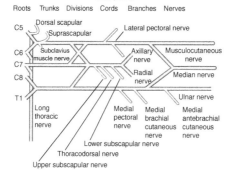

Brachial plexus

Roots   Trunks   Divisions   Cords   Branches   Nerves

C5 — Dorsal scapular
— Suprascapular
Lateral pectoral nerve

C6 — Subclavius
muscle nerve
Axillary
nerve
Musculocutaneous
nerve

C7

C8 — Radial
nerve
Median nerve

T1 — Ulnar nerve

Long
thoracic
nerve

Medial
pectoral
nerve

Medial
brachial
cutaneous
nerve

Medial
antebrachial
cutaneous
nerve

Lower subscapular nerve

Thoracodorsal nerve

Upper subscapular nerve

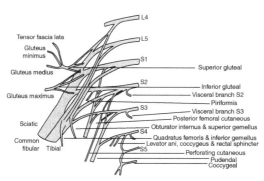

L4
L5
S1
S2
S3
S4
S5

Tensor fascia lata
Gluteus
minimus
Gluteus medius
Gluteus maximus
Sciatic
Common
fibular   Tibial

Superior gluteal
Inferior gluteal
Visceral branch S2
Piriformis
Visceral branch S3
Posterior femoral cutaneous
Obturator internus & superior gemellus
Quadratus femoris & inferior gemellus
Levator ani, coccygeus & rectal sphincter
Perforating cutaneous
Pudendal
Coccygeal

FIGURE 13.7 Brachial and lumbosacral plexus anatomy.
Source: Adapted from Ref. (1) with permission from Elsevier.

help to localize the site of a plexus lesion and provide an evaluation of the prognosis. The unaffected limb should be used as a control to compare nerve responses from the two sides tested.

Sensory Studies – Sensory NCSs are usually a more sensitive indicator of injury to the plexus than the motor nerve response. The distal latency and CV are usually normal. SNAP amplitude reflects the number of functioning axons in continuity with the sensory root cell body. Lesions proximal to the DRG, such as radiculopathy and nerve root avulsions, have normal SNAPs even though sensation may be affected clinically. Lesions distal to the DRG disconnect the sensory nerve cell body from its axons, resulting in decrement or absence of the SNAP. Therefore, differentiation between pre- and postganglionic lesions is extremely important.

Motor Studies – CMAPs are usually not affected unless the injury is severe. Motor latencies and conduction velocities are usually unaffected. Stimulation at Erb's point may reveal slowing if there is a demyelinating lesion in the brachial plexus. CMAP amplitudes may be decreased if there is severe axonal damage. In plexopathies, side-to-side amplitude differences can give an approximation of the degree of axonal injury during the first few months. A 70% decrement in CMAP amplitude correlates to 70% axon loss. Amplitude differences of less than 50% may not be significant.

Late Response – Most lesions are incomplete and the effect is diluted along the neural path of transmission of the F wave. In addition, the fastest fibers may not be affected. Therefore, F-wave prolongation is a nonspecific finding and F wave and H-reflexes are usually not helpful in the diagnosis of plexopathies.

EMG – Acute plexopathies usually show fibs and PSWs in the distribution of the nerve segment involved (see Tables 13.5 and 13.6). In chronic lesions where reinnervation has occurred, long-duration, increased-amplitude, or polyphasic MUAPs may be noted. It may take up to 3 weeks for electrodiagnostic abnormalities to develop. The paraspinal muscles, as well as muscles not in the distribution of the nerve segment involved, are expected to be normal.

Radiculopathy

Radiculopathy is a lesion of a specific nerve root that is generally caused by compression of that root. Electrodiagnostic studies aid in the diagnosis of radiculopathy, but they must be done in conjunction with a thorough history and physical examination. Imaging studies may be complementary, but they do not give information about nerve function. Physical examination findings suggestive of radiculopathy can include decreased reflexes, weakness in myotomal distribution, and/or decreased sensation in a dermatomal distribution. Despite the fact that sensory complaints are common in patients with suspected/

TABLE 13.5 Localization of Lesions in the Brachial Plexus

Area of injury	Affected sensory NCS	Affected motor NCS	Positive finding EMG
Root (radiculopathy)	Normal	CMAPs decreased	Cervical paraspinals and myotome pattern
Upper trunk	Lateral antebrachial cutaneous nerve Median nerve first digit Radial	Musculocutaneous nerve to biceps, suprascapular nerve to supraspinatus, and axillary nerve to deltoid	Supraspinatus, biceps, pronator teres, deltoid, brachioradialis, and extensor carpi radialis
Middle trunk	Median nerve to third and fourth digits	Radial nerve to extensor digitorum communis	Latissimus dorsi; teres major, extensor digitorum communis, pronator teres, and flexor carpi radialis
Lower trunk	Ulnar nerve to fifth digit Medial antebrachial cutaneous nerve	Ulnar nerve to ADM and median nerve to APB	APB, flexor digitorum superficialis, ADM, FCU, and flexor digitorum profundus
Lateral cord	Lateral antebrachial cutaneous nerve and median nerve to first digit	Musculocutaneous nerve to biceps	Biceps, pronator teres, and flexor carpi radialis
Posterior cord	Radial	Axillary nerve to deltoid and radial nerve to extensor carpi ulnaris	Latissimus dorsi, teres major, deltoid, and radial muscles
Medial cord	Ulnar nerve to fifth digit and medial antebrachial cutaneous nerve	Ulnar nerve to ADM and median nerve to APB	Ulnar muscles, flexor digitorum superficialis, flexor pollicis longus, and APB

ADM, abductor digiti minimi; APB, abductor pollicis brevis; CMAP, compound motor action potential; FCU, flexor carpi ulnaris.

TABLE 13.6 Localization of Lesions in the Lumbosacral Plexus

Nerve	Division	Roots	Affected sensory NCS	Affected motor NCS	Positive finding EMG
Iliohypogastric	Posterior	L1,2	None	None	Transversus abdominis and external and internal oblique
Lateral femoral cutaneous	Posterior	L2,3	Lateral femoral cutaneous nerve	None	None
Femoral	Posterior	L2,3,4	Saphenous nerve	Femoral nerve	Iliopsoas, pectineus, sartorius, and quadriceps
Obturator	Anterior	L2,3,4	None	Obturator nerve	Adductor longus, brevis, and magnus; gracilis; and obturator internus
Superior gluteal	Posterior	L4,5,S1	None	Superior gluteal nerve	Gluteus minimus and medius, TFL
Inferior gluteal	Posterior	L5,S1,2	None	Inferior gluteal nerve	Gluteus maximus
Sciatic (peroneal division)	Posterior	L4,5,S1,2	Superficial peroneal (and sural nerve)	Peroneal nerve	Short head of biceps femoris, tibialis anterior, EDB, peroneus tertius, and peroneus brevis and longus (brevis and longus are from the superficial branch)

(continued)

TABLE 13.6 Localization of Lesions in the Lumbosacral Plexus (continued)

Nerve	Division	Roots	Affected sensory NCS	Affected motor NCS	Positive finding EMG
Sciatic (tibial division)	Anterior	L4,5,S1,2,3	Sural nerve	Tibial nerve	Long head of biceps femoris, semimembranosus, semitendinosus, adductor magnus, plantaris, popliteus, gastrocnemius, tibialis posterior, soleus, flexor digitorum longus, and flexor hallucis longus
Sural (contains branches from the tibial and peroneal nerves)	Anterior and posterior	Mostly S1	Sural nerve	None	None

EDB, extensor digitorum brevis; NCS, nerve conduction study; TFL, tensor fasciae latae.

diagnosed radiculopathy, the SNAPs will be normal in amplitude and latency as the lesion is proximal to the DRGs. If there are abnormal SNAP findings, a different (or coexisting) lesion distal to the DRG should be considered.

CMAPs reflect the number of motor fibers activated upon stimulation. In most cases, the CMAP will also be normal in a radiculopathy. In a severe, multilevel radiculopathy, the CMAP amplitude may be reduced as a result of Wallerian degeneration distal to the lesion.

The H-reflex can be used to assess the afferent and efferent SI fibers and can be helpful in distinguishing an SI from an L5 radiculopathy. It is important to remember that H-reflexes are sensitive but not specific. Gastrocnemius-soleus H-reflex side-to-side latency differences of greater than 1.5 m/s are suggestive of SI radiculopathy (as is unilateral absence of an H-reflex). F-wave latencies and amplitudes are so variable that their use in evaluating a patient for radiculopathy is not recommended.

Needle EMG is the most useful study in the electrodiagnostic evaluation to both localize a radiculopathy and predict its prognosis. The presence of spontaneous activity on needle EMG is the most objective evidence of acute denervation. Fibs and PSWs can be seen in the paraspinal muscles within 5 to 7 days of initial injury. This is followed by findings in the peripheral muscles within 3 to 6 weeks. In order to diagnose radiculopathy, the corresponding paraspinal muscle and two peripheral muscles innervated by different peripheral nerves, but the same nerve root, should have positive findings (see Tables 13.7 and 13.8). With axon loss, MUs will fire with increasing frequency (>20 Hz); this is also known as "decreased recruitment." With reinnervation, the abnormal spontaneous activity may disappear (in the paraspinals at

TABLE 13.7 Clinical Presentation Associated With Levels of Radiculopathy

Root level	Muscle group	Clinical signs
C5	Rhomboid (dorsal–scapular n.) Supraspinatus/infraspinatus (suprascapular n.) Deltoid/teres minor (axillary n.) Biceps/brachialis (musculocutaneous n.)	1. Positive neck distraction/compression test 2. Decreased/absent biceps tendon reflex 3. Decreased/absent sensation to lateral arm (axillary n.) 4. Weakness of shoulder abduction
C6	Extensor carpi radialis longus/brevis (radial n.) Pronator teres/flexor carpi radialis (median n.) Deltoid/teres minor (axillary n.)	1. Decreased/absent brachioradialis reflex 2. Decreased/absent sensation to lateral forearm 3. Weakness of wrist extension

(continued)

TABLE 13.7 Clinical Presentation Associated With Levels of Radiculopathy (*continued*)

Root level	Muscle group	Clinical signs
C7	Triceps/extensor digitorum communis/extensor indicis/ extensor digiti minimi (radial n.) Flexor carpi radialis (median n.) FCU (ulnar n.)	1. Decreased/absent triceps reflex 2. Decreased/absent sensation to middle finger 3. Weakness of wrist flexion
C8	FCU (ulnar n.) Flexor pollicis longus/flexor digitorum superficialis (median n.) Flexor digitorum profundus (median/ulnar n.) Extensor indicis/extensor pollicis brevis (radial n.) First dorsal interosseous (ulnar n.)	1. Decreased/absent sensation to ring/little finger and to distal half of the forearm's ulnar side 2. Weakness of finger flexion 3. Intrinsic weakness/atrophy
T1	APB (median n.) ADM/first dorsal interosseous (ulnar n.)	1. Decreased/absent sensation to medial side of the upper half of the forearm and arm (medial brachial cutaneous n.) 2. Weakness of finger abduction/adduction

ADM, abductor digiti minimi; APB, abductor pollicis brevis; FCU, flexor carpi ulnaris; n., nerve.

TABLE 13.8 Clinical Presentation Associated With Levels of Radiculopathy

Root level	Muscle group	Clinical signs
L2, L3, L4	Iliacus/vastus medialis (femoral n.) L2, L3 and adductor longus/ gracilis (obturator n.) L2, L3, L4	1. Pain in the thigh 2. Weakness in hip flexion/ adduction
L4	Vastus lateralis and rectus femoris Tibialis anterior (deep peroneal n.) Vastus medialis/lateralis (L2–L4)	1. Decreased/absent patellar reflex 2. Knee extension weakness 3. Pain in the medial side of leg
L5	Gluteus medius/TFL (superior gluteal n., L4–S2) Flexor hallucis longus/flexor digitorum longus/lateral gastrocnemius/tibialis posterior (tibial n., L5–S2) Extensor hallucis longus/ extensor digitorum longus (deep peroneal n., L5)	1. Pain and paresthesias in lateral aspect of the leg and dorsum of the foot 2. Ankle dorsiflexor weakness

(continued)

TABLE 13.8 Clinical Presentation Associated With Levels of Radiculopathy (*continued*)

Root level	Muscle group	Clinical signs
S1*	Medial gastrocnemius/soleus/ flexor hallucis brevis (tibial n., L5–S2) Peroneus longus/brevis (superficial peroneal n., L5–S1), TFL/gluteus maximus (sup/inf gluteal n., L4–S1, L5–S2) Extensor hallucis longus and extensor digitorum longus (deep peroneal n., L4, L5, SI)	1. Decreased/absent ankle reflex 2. Pain and paresthesias at the lateral border of the foot 3. Weakness of foot plantar flexion and toe extension

*H-reflex may help to confirm the diagnosis and distinguish SI from L5 radiculopathy.
TFL, tensor fasciae latae.

6–9 weeks followed by proximal muscles at 2–5 months and distal muscles at 3–7 months). MUAPs will become polyphasic with a long duration (>15 ms). After 6 months to 1 year, large-amplitude (>7 mV using a monopolar needle) MUAPs may be noted.

MOTOR NEURON DISEASES

Motor neuron diseases may affect both the upper motor neurons (UMNs) and lower motor neurons (LMNs). These disorders specifically affect the motor cortex, corticospinal tracts, and/or anterior horn cells. Clinical signs of LMN lesions include atrophy, flaccidity, hyporeflexia, and fasciculations. UMN signs include weakness, spasticity, hyperreflexia, and upgoing plantar reflex (positive Babinski sign). There are usually no sensory changes. With EMG testing, only the LMN aspect of the disorder can be assessed.

Electrodiagnostic Findings – SNAP has *normal* amplitude and conduction velocities. CMAP conduction velocities are *normal or mildly decreased*. The amplitude of the CMAP may be *decreased* due to axonal loss if significant atrophy is present. EMG findings (in at least three limbs or two limbs and bulbar muscles) include abnormal spontaneous potentials (fibs and PSW), fasciculations, and CRDs. Decreased recruitment with increased firing frequency may be noted. Large-amplitude, long-duration polyphasic potentials may be noted if reinnervation has occurred.

  LMN: Poliomyelitis/post-polio syndrome (PPS) and spinal muscular atrophy (SMA)
  UMN and LMN: Amyotrophic lateral sclerosis (ALS)
  UMN: Primary lateral sclerosis (PLS)

ALS – Characterized by degeneration of anterior horn cell. UMN and LMN signs are usually present. Clinical presentation includes asymmetric atrophy, weakness and fasciculations, dysphagia, and dysarthria. Pseudobulbar signs may be noted. Bowel and bladder are typically spared. EMG findings include abnormal spontaneous potentials (fibs and PSWs). MUAPs demonstrate decreased recruitment with increased MUAP duration and amplitude.

PPS – Loss of anterior horn cell decades (typically 30 years) after polio. This disorder is hypothesized to be due to burnout of MUs from increased metabolic demand or normal axon loss with aging. *Halstead-Ross criteria* include the onset of two or more of the following: fatigue, arthralgia, myalgia, and cold intolerance with history of previous stable polio diagnosis. Electrodiagnostically, this may resemble poliomyelitis, so clinical findings must be considered. NCSs show normal SNAPs and abnormal CMAP. EMG shows increased amplitude and duration of MUAPs with decreased recruitment.

EMG FINDINGS IN MYOPATHIES

Electrodiagnostic testing is an important tool in the diagnosis of myopathies. EMG testing helps to make a diagnosis, determine the extent of a disease, prognosticate, and guide further studies, such as muscle biopsies. Generally, only one side of the body is tested on EMG, leaving the muscles on the other side preserved for muscle biopsy. It is important to rule out other diseases by performing at least one sensory and one motor nerve study in addition to the EMG study.

Typical Findings

NCS – Usually normal since myopathies typically affect proximal muscles initially (and in nerve studies, the active electrode is usually placed over a distal muscle). As the disease progresses, distal muscles may become involved and the motor NCS may be abnormal.

    SNAP: Normal (sensory fibers are not affected).

    CMAP: Amplitudes may be reduced due to muscle fiber atrophy; distal latency and CV are normal as the myelin is not affected.

EMG – MUs will usually show early recruitment, polyphasia (due to the variability in muscle fiber diameter), and small-amplitude (due to muscle fiber dropout) and short-duration potentials (see Figure 13.8).

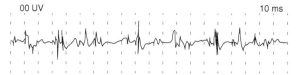

FIGURE 13.8 In this EMG of a patient with inclusion body myositis, many MUs are activated simultaneously at a low level of muscle contraction (early recruitment). Note the low amplitude and short duration of individual units.

Fib potentials and PSWs as well as myotonic discharges can be seen. In long-standing myopathies, there may be little activity at rest due to loss of muscle fiber. Increased insertional activity is also common in many myopathies.

Typically in myopathies, the proximal lower extremity muscles will show more positive EMG findings. It is important to sample a sufficient number of muscles to differentiate between a myopathy and a focal injury. Muscles should be sampled based on weakness as seen in the clinical examination. However, muscles that are extremely weak (<2/5 in manual testing) can be too deteriorated to provide a good signal.

In steroid myopathy, EMG testing would be normal, as it predominantly affects the type II muscle fibers (EMG tests primarily the type I fibers; 6–8).

NMJ DISORDERS

The NMJ is divided into the presynaptic terminal, the synaptic cleft, and a postsynaptic muscle end plate. Neuromuscular transmission involves (a) presynaptic terminal depolarization and ACh release, (b) ACh binding and ion channel opening, and (c) postsynaptic membrane depolarization and muscle AP generation. Disorders of the NMJ hinder the production, release, or uptake of ACh at the NMJ. The most well-known postsynaptic disorder is *myasthenia gravis (MG)*. Presynaptic abnormalities include *Lambert-Eaton myasthenic syndrome (LEMS)* and botulism. A *repetitive nerve stimulation (RNS)* study and *SFEMG* are useful electrodiagnostic tests when trying to evaluate for NMJ disorders.

Routine sensory and motor conduction studies will usually be normal. Only in profound weakness, as in myasthenic crisis, borderline or slightly decreased CMAP amplitudes will be observed. Routine EMG examination may demonstrate unstable MUAPs, where moment-to-moment variations in amplitude and configuration may be seen.

RNS after routine NCS is performed by delivering trains of supramaximal stimuli to a peripheral nerve while recording CMAPs. This depletes stores of releasable ACh from diseased NMJs, producing a progressive amplitude decrement from the first to the fifth waveform in patients with disorders of the NMJ. When RNS is performed at low rates (2–5 Hz), a decrement of >10% is considered abnormal. Although the proximal muscles are usually more affected than the distal muscles, the proximal muscles are more difficult to test (the limb must be restrained as the entire limb is often stimulated with proximal stimulation; Figure 13.9).

Postactivation facilitation occurs when there is recovery of the CMAP amplitudes on repeat slow RNS following a 10-second isometric contraction or rapid RNS (20–50 Hz) studies. This is due to calcium

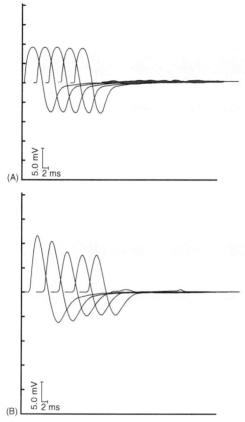

FIGURE 13.9 CMAPs recorded from the ADM of human subjects during repetitive stimulation of the ulnar nerve at three stimuli per second. (A) A recording from a normal individual shows no change in the amplitude of the muscle electrical response during the stimulation interval. (B) In a patient with MG, the same stimuli produce a 40% decrement in response amplitude over the first five stimuli, with a slow partial recovery during subsequent stimulations.

ADM, abductor digiti minimi; CMAP, compound motor action potential; MG, myasthenia gravis.
Source: Adapted from Ref. (1) with permission from Elsevier.

facilitation. Although present to a lesser degree in MG and botulism, it is a hallmark finding in LEMS where increments as high as 500% may be observed.

If initial studies are unrevealing and suspicion for an NMJ disorder is high, consider testing more proximal muscles (e.g., spinal accessory and facial nerves) and/or proceeding to SFEMG of at least one symptomatic muscle. SFEMG is the most sensitive test for NMJ disorders. Findings consistent with, but not specific for, NMJ disorders include increased *jitter*. Jitter refers to time variations between interpotential discharges of two different muscle fibers of the same MU. The most extreme abnormality of jitter is failed transmission, or *blocking*. In MG, jitter and blocking increase with increased firing rate. In LEMS and botulism, jitter and blocking decrease with increased firing rate (Figure 13.10).

Prerequisites for performing a reliable RNS study include immobilization of the limb and recording electrode, supramaximal stimulation, optimization of limb temperature (warming the limb), and withholding of acetylcholinesterase inhibitors 12 to 24 hours prior to testing (if not medically contraindicated). Distal nerves that can be easily tested for RNS are the median and ulnar nerves, with recording electrodes at APB and ADM, respectively. If proximal studies are indicated, spinal accessory nerve with the recording electrode on the upper trapezius muscle is commonly utilized. In patients suspected of having ocular MG, facial RNS recording at orbicularis oris can be performed (Tables 13.9–13.15).

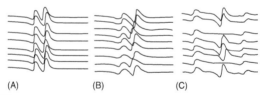

(A) (B) (C)

FIGURE 13.10 SFEMG recordings. Rastered view. (A) Normal. (B) Increased jitter. (C) Increased jitter with blocking.

TABLE 13.9 Upper Extremity–Motor

Nerve	Recording Electrode	Stimulation Site	Distance (cm) From Active to First Stimulation Site	Onset Latency (ms)	Amplitude (mV)*	Segment Name	Velocity (m/s)
Median	Abductor pollicis brevis	Wrist	8	<4.2	>4.0	Elbow–wrist	>50
		Elbow	TBD†		>4.0		
Ulnar	Abductor digiti minimi	Wrist	8	<3.4	>4.0		
		Below elbow (BE)	TBD†		>4.0	BE–wrist	>50
		Above elbow (AE)	TBD†		>4.0	AE–BE	>50
Radial	Extensor indicis proprius (EIP)	Forearm	4	<2.9	>3.0	AE–EIP	>50
		Erb's point	TBD†			Erb's point–AE	>55

Skin temperature should be maintained at 32°C. Distances may need to be modified based on size.
*Side-to-side amplitude difference of >50% is significant, or >20% amplitude drop distal to proximal is significant.
†TBD = distance to be determined by the surface measurement.

TABLE 13.10 Upper Extremity—Sensory

Nerve	Recording Electrode	Stimulation Site	Distance (cm)	Onset Latency (ms)	Amplitude µV	Segment Name	Velocity (m/s)
Median	Second digit	Mid palm	7	<1.9	>20	Mid palm–second digit	>45
		Wrist	14 (7 from palm)	<3.5	>20	Wrist-mid palm	>45
Ulnar	Fifth digit	Wrist	14	<3.1	>18	Wrist-fifth digit	>44
Radial	First digit	Wrist	10		>10		

Skin temperature should be maintained at 32°C.

TABLE 13.11 Lower Extremity—Motor

Nerve	Recording Electrode	Stimulation Site	Distance (cm)	Onset Latency (ms)	Amplitude (mV)	Segment Name	Velocity (m/s)
Fibular	Extensor digitorum brevis	Ankle fibular head	8	<5.5	>2.5	Fibular head–ankle	>40
		Popliteal				Popliteal–fibular head	>40
Tibial							
Medial plantar	Abductor hallucis	Ankle knee	10	<6.0	>3.0	Knee–ankle	>40
Lateral plantar	Abductor digiti minimi	Ankle	10	<6.0	>3.0		

Skin temperature should be maintained at 30°C. As in the hand, distances may need to be modified based on size.

TABLE 13.12 Lower Extremity—Sensory

Nerve	Recording Electrode	Stimulation Site	Distance (cm)	Onset Latency (ms)	Amplitude (μV)	Segment Name	Velocity (m/s)
Sural	Lateral malleolus	Calf	14	<3.8	>10.0	Calf–lateral malleolus	>36
Lateral femoral cutaneous	1 cm medial to the anterior superior iliac spine (ASIS)	Anterior thigh	12–16	2.6 ± 0.2	10–25	ASIS–anterior thigh	>44
Superficial fibular	Anterior to lateral malleolus	Anterolateral calf	14	3.4 ± 0.4	18.3 ± 8.0	Lateral malleolus to calf	51.2 ± 5.7

Skin temperature should be maintain at 30°C.

TABLE 13.13 H-Reflex

Site	Recording Electrode	Latency (msec)	Stimulation Site
Medial gastrocnemius soleus muscle	Halfway from mid popliteal crease to proximal flare medial malleolus	28.0–35.0	Popliteal (cathode proximal); use submaximal stimulation

Skin temperature should be maintained at 30°C.

TABLE 13.14 F-Waves and F-Ratio—Upper Extremities

Motor Nerve	Recording Electrode	F-Latency (msec)	F-Ratio*
Median	Abductor pollicis brevis	Wrist 29.1 ± 2.3	0.7 < F < 1.3
		Elbow 24.8 ± 2.0	
		Axilla 21.7 ± 2.8	
Ulnar	Abductor digiti minimi	Wrist 30.5 ± 3.0	0.7 < F < 1.3
		BE 26.0 ± 2.0	
		AE 23.5 ± 2.0	
		Axilla 11.2 ± 1.0	
Fibular	Extensor digitorum brevis	Ankle 51.3 ± 4 .7	0.7 < F < 1.3
		Knee 42.7 ± 4.0	
Tibial	Abductor hallucus	Ankle 52.3 ± 4.3	0.7 < F < 1.3
		Knee 43.5 ± 3.4	

*F-ratio = F-M-1/2M (as measured with elbow or knee stimulation), where F = F-wave latency and M = wave latency.

TABLE 13.15 Significant Differences (Side to Side or Nerve to Nerve)

Median-to-ulnar distal motor latency	>1 msec	Consider carpal tunnel syndrome.
Median-to-ulnar distal sensory latency	>0.5 msec	Consider carpal tunnel syndrome.
Combined sensory index (CSI)*	>0.9 msec	Consider carpal tunnel syndrome.
H-reflex side-to-side difference	>1.5 msec	Consider S1 radiculopathy.
Proximal-to-distal drop in motor amplitude	>20%	Consider conduction block or anomalous innervation.
CMAP or SNAP amplitude side-to-side difference	>50%	Consider axonal injury.

*Summation of the median and ulnar sensory antidromic conduction onset difference to the ring finger at 14 cm (ringdiff) + the median and radial sensory antidromic conduction difference to the thumb at 10 cm (thumbdiff) + the median and ulnar orthodromic conduction difference across the wrist with palmar stimulation at 8 cm (palmdiff).

REFERENCES

1. Weiss J, Weiss L, Silver J. *Easy EMG, 2nd ed.* London, UK: Elsevier; 2016.

2. Gooch CL, Weimer LH. The electrodiagnosis of neuropathy: basic principles and common pitfalls. *Neurol Clin.* 2007;25:1–28.

3. Canale ST, Beaty J. Peripheral nerve injuries. In: *Campbell's Operative Orthopaedics.* 11th ed. St. Louis, MO: Mosby.

4. Preston DC, ShapiroeBE, eds. *Electromyography and Neuromuscular Disorders: Clinical- Electrophysiologic Correlations,* 3rd ed. Elsevier, 2013.

5. Dumitru D, ed. *Electrodiagnostic Medicine.* 2nd ed. Philadelphia, PA: Hanley & Belfus; 2002.

6. Cifu DX. *Braddom's Physical Medicine and Rehabilitation.* 5th ed. Philadelphia, PA: Elsevier; 2016.

7. Cuccurullo SJ. *Physical Medicine and Rehabilitation Board Review.* 3rd ed. New York, NY: Demos Medical Publishing; 2015.

8. EMedicine - Medical Reference. Motor unit recruitment in EMG: EMedicine neurology. http://emedicine.medscape.c0m/article/1141359-overview

9. Stalberg E. Clinical electromyography in myasthenia gravis. *J Neurol Neurosurg Psychiatry.* 1980;43:622–633.

SUGGESTED READING

Ball RD. Electrodiagnostic evaluation of the peripheral nervous system (plexopathy). In: Delisa JA, Gans BM, eds. *Rehabilitation Medicine Principles and Practice.* Philadelphia, PA: Lippincott-Raven; 1998:358–359.

DeLisa JA. Physical Medicine & Rehabilitation Principles and Practice. *4th ed. Philadelphia, PA: Lippincott; 2005.*

Gaudino W. Brachial plexopathies. In: Weiss L, Silver JK, Weiss J, eds. *Easy EMG.* Philadelphia, PA; Butterworth-Heinemann; 2004:171–180.

Gaudino W. Lumbosacral plexopathies. In: Weiss L, Silver JK, Weiss J, eds. *Easy EMG.* Philadelphia, PA: Butterworth-Heinemann; 2004:181–187.

Katirji B. Electromyography in Clinical Practice: A Case Study Approach. *2nd ed. Philadelphia, PA: Mosby; 2007.*

Preston DC, Shapiro BE. Lumbosacral plexopathy. In: *Electromyography and Neuromuscular Disorder.* 2nd ed. Philadelphia, PA: Elsevier; 2005:471–489.

Weiss J, Weiss L, Silver J. *Easy EMG 2nd edition.* London: Elsevier; 2016.

Weiss LD, Weiss J, Pobre T. *Oxford American Handbook of Physical Medicine and Rehabilitation.* New York, NY: Oxford University Press; 2010:187.

CHAPTER 14

CARDIAC REHABILITATION

INTRODUCTION AND BENEFITS

Under the broadened scope of the Agency for Healthcare Research and Quality (AHRQ) guidelines, cardiac rehabilitation (CR) may include exercise programs, education, and risk factor modification for secondary prevention and psychosocial counseling (1). CR is indicated after acute myocardial infarction (MI), coronary revascularization, and cardiac transplantation or in patients with congestive heart failure (CHF) or chronic stable angina. CR improves max oxygen consumption (VO$_2$ max), peripheral O$_2$ extraction, ST depression, exercise tolerance, subjective sense of well-being, and return-to-work rates. It lowers BP, resting heart rate (HR), and myocardial O$_2$ demand. In addition, CR has been shown to improve glycemic control and cause favorable lipoprotein changes (e.g., reducing triglyceride [TG] and elevating high-density lipoprotein [HDL] levels). Long-term CR has been demonstrated to increase the quantity of mitochondrial enzymes in "slow twitch" muscle fibers and development of new capillaries in muscle. Angiographic studies have shown reduced atherosclerotic lesions in stable angina patients undergoing intensive physical exercise and consuming a low-fat diet over 1 year without lipid-lowering agents (2). It should be noted that, at least traditionally, it has been stated that CR does not improve anginal threshold, whereas angioplasty and coronary artery bypass graft (CABG) can (Figure 14.1).

Individual trials of CR after MI have not shown a statistically significant lower mortality rate in the CR groups, but a meta-analysis of 22 randomized trials (n = 4,554) has shown a benefit in overall mortality in the CR group (0.80 odds ratio vs. no CR) during a 3-year average post-MI period (4).

EPIDEMIOLOGY

As of 2015, roughly 935,000 Americans have a coronary event each year, with more than 30% having a second or potentially fatal event (5). Mortality reduction with CR participation is over 50% versus nonparticipation. CR can also reduce the likelihood of hospital readmissions for all causes by 25% (6,7). Fewer than 20% of all eligible patients, however, participate in a CR program (8,9). The utilization rate for eligible Medicare beneficiaries is only 12% (10). Women, the very elderly, minorities, and patients with multiple comorbidities are even less likely to receive CR (8,11,12). Low participation may be due to geographic factors and a failure of physicians to refer appropriate candidates.

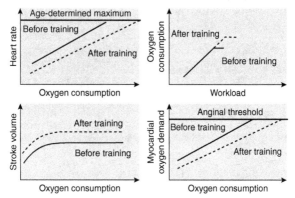

FIGURE 14.1 Benefits of cardiac rehabilitation. Compare before training *(solid lines)* with after training *(dashed lines)*.

Source: Adapted from Ref. (3).

PHASES OF CR

Phase I – The inpatient training phase can begin from days 2 to 4 of hospitalization and typically lasts ≈1 to 2 weeks. Disciplines involved typically include physical therapy, occupational therapy, social work, nutrition, and psychology. CR is generally performed with telemetry during this phase. Goals include prevention of the sequelae of immobilization, education regarding risk factor modification, independent self-care activities, and household distance ambulation on level surfaces. Protocol-limited submaximal stress testing is often done in uncomplicated patients prior to discharge as a guideline for outpatient ADLs and simple household activities.

Phase II – The outpatient training phase starts 2 to 4 weeks after discharge and typically lasts 8 to 12 weeks. Goals include increasing cardiac volume and gradually returning to normal activity levels. A functional exercise tolerance (stress) test is typically done 6 to 8 weeks following the cardiac event to allow for formation of a stable scar over the area of infarct. The stress test guides the exercise prescription and helps guide return to work and sexual activity. This phase of CR is supervised by trained therapists and typically does not require telemetry monitoring.

Phase III – The maintenance phase is ideally a lifelong program of home- or gym-based exercise, aimed at maintaining or adding onto benefits obtained during phases I and II, generally under minimal or no clinical supervision.

Absolute contraindications for functional stress testing include recent change in resting EKG or serious cardiac arrhythmias, unstable angina, acute or worsening left ventricular (LV) dysfunction, uncontrolled hypertension, systemic illness, severe aortic stenosis, or severe physical disability precluding treadmill or arm ergometry use. Relative contraindications include hypertrophic cardiomyopathy, electrolyte abnormalities, moderate valvular disease, or significant arterial or pulmonary hypertension. Note: The contraindications for exercise stress testing are similar to the contraindications for CR in general.

The 2006 Centers for Medicare & Medicaid Services expanded coverage for outpatient CR indications to include the following: acute MI within the preceding 12 months, CABG surgery, stable angina pectoris, heart valve repair/replacement, percutaneous coronary intervention (PCI) with or without stenting, and heart or lung transplant. Of note, heart failure as an indication for CR is often not covered by health insurance, although it is a recommended treatment in the American College of Cardiology (ACC)/American Heart Association (AHA) Heart Failure Guidelines.

EXERCISE PRESCRIPTION

The exercise prescription should address the type, intensity, content, duration, and frequency of exercise. Isotonic, aerobic, and rhythmic exercises involving large muscle groups should be emphasized. Isometrics and resistive exercise are relatively safe in patients with good LV function, but are contraindicated in patients with CHF, severe valvular disease, uncontrolled arrhythmias, or peak exercise capacity <5 METs. A MET (metabolic equivalent of task = 3.5 mL O_2 uptake/kg/min, or about 1 kcal/kg/hr) is a ratio of the energy expenditure of an activity relative to the resting metabolic rate (e.g., sitting quietly). Thus, a 5-MET activity uses 5 times the energy expended at rest. METs for common activities include sleeping 0.9, sedentary desk work ~1.5, slow walking on level ground ~2.3, fast walking ~3.6, sexual activity ~5.8, and jogging 7. Maximum MET capacity is usually achieved between the ages of 15 and 30 years and progressively decreases with age. It can, however, increase with exercise and conditioning. A maximum capacity of 10 METs is typical of healthy but nonathletic middle-aged men. Twelve METs is typical of maximal exercise in young men. Distance runners can average 18 to 24 METs.

The exercise content should include three phases. The first phase should involve a 5-to-10-minute warm-up. The warm-up should consist of flexible movements and stretching that gradually increase HR to target range. The subtle increase in O_2 demand reduces the risk of exercise-related cardiovascular complications. The second phase is the conditioning or training phase and should minimally last 20 minutes, up to the recommended 30 to 45 minutes of aerobic activity. The third phase is a low-intensity cooldown and should last 5 to 10 minutes. Omitting the third phase can cause complications such as hypotension, angina, and ventricular arrhythmias due to decreased coronary blood flow secondary to reduced venous return, during a state when myocardial oxygen consumption remains elevated.

Exercise intensity can be determined by a variety of methods, usually by calculating a "target" HR. The AHA method uses 70% to 85% of the maximum attained by stress testing. For young, healthy adults not undergoing formal exercise stress testing, 70% to 85% of (220 – age) can also be used for general exercise prescriptions, which is based on the assumption that 220 is the appropriate maximum for a newborn and that the maximum decreases ≈1 bpm/year. This latter formula, however, does not apply after MI. The standard deviation for this equation is 10 to 15 beats per minute. Since this formula was derived from studies of men, it may overestimate the HR in women. Therefore, it may be more appropriate to measure the peak exercise capacity or the maximum ability of the cardiovascular system to deliver O_2 to exercising skeletal muscle and its ability to extract O_2 from the blood. Peak exercise capacity can be measured clinically by O_2 uptake (Vo_2), CO_2 production (Vco_2), and minute ventilation via gas analyzers during exercise. Maximal O_2 uptake eventually plateaus despite increasing the workload. Anaerobic threshold (AT) is another index used to estimate exercise capacity. AT is defined as the point at which minute ventilation increases disproportionately relative to Vo_2 (often seen at 60% to 70% of Vo_2 max). AT is an indicator of increase in lactic acid produced by working muscles and can be used to distinguish cardiac and noncardiac (e.g., pulmonary or musculoskeletal) causes of exercise limitation.

The *Karvonen formula* (Target heart rate = ((HR_{max} – HR_{rest}) × % desired intensity) + HR_{rest}) is beneficial for calculating a target HR zone to achieve during therapy. HR_{max} can be estimated by subtracting patient age from 220. Usually, desired intensity for CR is between 40% and 85%. For more deconditioned patients, the exercise program should begin at the lower end of the spectrum (i.e., 40%–60%) and increase as fitness improves.

Borg's Rating of Perceived Exertion (RPE) Scale is particularly useful for cardiac transplant patients since denervation of the orthotopic heart makes HR parameters unreliable. The traditional Borg RPE scale is scored from 6 to 20, where 13 is rated as "somewhat hard" and corresponds with exercise intensity sufficient to provide training benefits but still allows conversation during exercise. A score of 12 to 13 corresponds to about 60% of max HR, while a score of 15 corresponds to 85% of max HR. The Borg scale is probably more psychological than physiological, but encourages independence in exercise (i.e., phase III CR) as external monitoring devices are weaned off.

For patients on beta-blockers, training at 85% of symptom-limited HR or 70% to 90% of the maximum workload determined by exercise testing is recommended (13). Pacemakers do not necessarily preclude exercise training in a CR program.

Usual exercise duration/frequency is 20 to 30 minutes three times a week × 12 weeks or more when training at 70% of the maximum HR.

Shorter durations of training on a daily basis for more severely decon-ditioned individuals may also be helpful.

The following risk stratification was developed by the AHA and is useful in determining the extent of medical supervision necessary for exercise training: Class A individuals are apparently healthy and have no evidence of cardiovascular risk with exercise. Class B individuals have established coronary heart disease that is clinically stable. They have low risk of cardiovascular complications with vigorous exer-cise. Class C individuals are at moderate risk of complications during exercise due to history of multiple MIs or arrest, the New York Heart Association (NYHA) class III or IV CHF, <6 METs exercise capacity, or significant ischemia on exercise test. Class D individuals have unstable cardiac disease and require restriction of activity; exercise is contrain-dicated. Patients referred to CR are typically in classes B or C.

POSTCARDIAC EVENT SEXUAL COUNSELING

Typical criteria for safe resumption of sexual activity after a cardiac event (e.g., MI or CABG) include a stable, asymptomatic patient and tolerance of exercise at 5 to 7 METs without abnormal EKG, BP, or HR changes. The time required is variable but is usually about 6 weeks after event, for sex with established partners in familiar positions. A useful clinical test is a two-flight stair climbing test: walking for 10 minutes at 3 mi/hr (~3.3 METs), then climbing two flights of stairs without stop-ping. Sexual activities associated with sudden death in a cardiac patient include illicit affairs and sex after heavy meals and alcohol intake.

MISCELLANEOUS

Sternal Precautions – Following sternotomy, typical instructions include no pushing, pulling, or lifting objects heavier than 5 to 10 lb. for 6 to 8 weeks. A "side-rolling" maneuver for getting out of bed is typi-cally taught, and manual wheelchair propulsion is usually prohibited during this time as well.

Cardiac Precautions for Persons With Coronary Artery Disease (CAD) in Nonacute Inpatient Settings – Activity should be terminated if any of the following develops: new-onset cardiopulmonary symptoms; HR decreases >20% of baseline; HR increases >50% of baseline; SBP increases to 240 mmHg; SBP decreases ≥30 mmHg from baseline or to <90 mmHg; or diastolic blood pressure (DBP) increases to 120 mmHg (14). These guidelines were developed by studying 64 physically dis-abled male patients with CAD using arm ergometers (14). Individ-ualized parameters for maximum or minimum HR and BP are also frequently used.

Considerations for CR/Exercise in the Elderly – There is a greater emphasis on warm-up activities including flexibility and ROM exercises, which help prepare the musculoskeletal and cardiovascular systems for exercise. Cooldown activities are of heightened importance to gradually decrease the peripheral vasodilation that can lead to hypotension, especially due to the delayed baroreceptor responsiveness associated with aging. The elderly also require a longer rest period in between exercises because of the slower return of exercise HR to resting HR. Aging is associated with decrease in skin blood perfusion, lowering the efficiency to sweat and regulate heat dissipation during exercise. Thus, a lower intensity exercise should be considered for the elderly in hot/humid environments.

NYHA Classification (for CHF and Angina) – I. >7 METs tolerated asymptomatically, without functional limitation. II. <6 METs tolerated, but higher levels of activities cause symptoms. III. Asymptomatic at rest and with most ADLs; >4 METs not tolerated. IV. Symptomatic at rest and with minimal physical activities.

REFERENCES

1. Wenger NK. Clinical Guideline No. 17, AHCPR Publication No. 96-0672, 1995 (reviewed by the AHRQ, 2000).

2. Schuler G. Regular physical exercise and low-fat diet: effects on progression of CAD. *Circulation*. 1992;86:1–11.

3. Braddom RL, ed. *Braddom's Physical Medicine and Rehabilitation*. Philadelphia, PA: WB Saunders; 1996.

4. O'Connor GT. An overview of randomized trials of rehabilitation with exercise after MI. *Circulation*. 1989;80:234–244.

5. Mozaffarian D, Benjamin EJ, Go AS, et al. Heart disease and stroke statistics-2015 update: a report from the American Heart Association. *Circulation*. 2015;131(4):e29–e322.

6. Dunlay SM, Pack QR, Thomas RJ, et al. Participation in cardiac rehabilitation, readmissions, and death after acute myocardial infarction. *Am J Med*. 2014;127(6):538–546.

7. Plüss CE, Billing E, Held C, et al. Long-term effects of an expanded cardiac rehabilitation programme after myocardial infarction or coronary artery bypass surgery: a five-year follow-up of a randomized controlled study. *Clin Rehabil*. 2011;25(1):79–87.

8. Suaya JA, Shepard DS, Normand SL, et al. Use of cardiac rehabilitation by Medicare beneficiaries after myocardial infarction or coronary bypass surgery. *Circulation*. 2007;116(15):1653–1662.

9. Hammill BG. Relationship between cardiac rehabilitation and long-term risks of death and myocardial infarction among elderly Medicare beneficiaries. *Circulation*. 2009;121(1):63–70.

10. Suaya JA, Stason WB, Ades PA, et al. Cardiac rehabilitation and survival in older coronary patients. *J Am Coll Cardiol*. 2009;54(1):25–33.

11. Colella JF, Gravely S, Marzolini S, et al. Sex bias in referral of women to outpatient cardiac rehabilitation? A metaanalysis. *Eur J Prev Cardiol*. 2015;22(4):423–441.

12. Menezes AR, Lavie CJ, DeSchutter A, Milani RV. Gender, race and cardiac rehabilitation in the United States: Is there a difference in care? *Am J Med Sci*. 2014;348(2):146–152.

13. Flores AM, Zohman LR. Rehab of the cardiac patient. In: DeLisa J, ed. *Rehabilitation Medicine: Principles and Practice*. 3rd ed. Philadelphia, PA: Lippincott-Raven; 1998:1347–1349.

14. Fletcher BJ. Cardiac precautions for non-acute inpatient settings. *Am J Phys Med Rehabil*. 1993;72:140–143.

SUGGESTED READING

Ades PA. Cardiac rehabilitation and secondary prevention of coronary heart disease. *N Engl J Med*. 2001;345:892–902.

CHAPTER 15

PULMONARY REHABILITATION

Pulmonary rehabilitation (PR) is a multidisciplinary program that aims to alleviate symptoms, optimize function, and promote adaptation to chronic lung disease. In chronic obstructive pulmonary disease (COPD), PR has been shown to improve dyspnea, exercise capacity, and health-related quality of life, while reducing health care utilization (1). When considering PR, the respiratory disorders can be generally characterized as ventilatory restrictive disorders (CO_2 retention) or obstructive disorders (oxygen impairment). Forced expiratory volume in one second/forced vital capacity (FEV_1/FVC) in particular helps distinguish between ventilatory and obstructive disorders (Figure 15.1).

VENTILATORY DISORDERS (RESTRICTIVE OR MECHANICAL DISORDERS)

Ventilatory disorders are generally caused by neuromuscular or skeletal disorders (e.g., myopathy, motor neuron disease, myelopathy, multiple sclerosis [MS], and chest wall deformity), and are characterized by a decrease in vital capacity (VC), residual volume (RV), functional residual capacity (FRC), and total lung capacity (TLC). Key clinical monitoring tools include spirometry (for VC and max insufflation capacity), cough flow meters, and noninvasive CO_2 monitoring. Insufflation is the forced inhalation of volumes greater than that which can be inhaled naturally using the muscles of respiration. Glossopharyngeal breathing is a technique that can be used to maximize

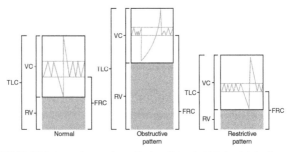

FIGURE 15.1 Lung volumes and capacities in ventilatory (restrictive) and obstructive disorders.

FRC, functional residual capacity; FVC, forced vital capacity; RV, residual volume; TLC, total lung capacity; VC, vital capacity.

TABLE 15.1 Characteristic Physiologic Changes Associated With Pulmonary Disorders

Measure	Obstructive Disorders	Restrictive Disorders	Mixed Disorders
FEV_1/FVC	Decreased	Normal or increased	Decreased
FEV_1	Decreased	Decreased, normal, or increased	Decreased
FVC	Decreased or normal	Decreased	Decreased or normal
TLC	Normal or increased	Decreased	Decreased, normal, or increased
RV	Normal or increased	Decreased	Decreased, normal, or increased

FEV_1/FVC, Forced expiratory volume in one second/forced vital capacity;
RV, residual volume; TLC, total lung capacity.
Source: Adapted from Ref. (2).

insufflation and should be taught as a life-saving backup measure in the event of mechanical ventilation failure. Respiratory muscles can be aided by devices such as mouthpiece or nasal intermittent positive pressure ventilation (IPPV) and intermittent abdominal pressure ventilation (IAPV). The latter can augment tidal volume (TV) by 250 to 1,200 mL (Table 15.1).

Peak cough flow (PCF) <160 L/min (~2.7 L/s) has been associated with failure to close a tracheostomy, and PCF <270 (4.5 L/s) indicates a high risk of ineffective cough in acute respiratory disease. These values have been shown to be clinically useful in patients who are healthy or have neuromuscular disease (3). In a clinically stable state, when VC is <1,000 to 1,500 mL or when PCF <4.5 L/s, interventions to assist cough are warranted (3). Manually assisted cough (MAC), for example, "quad cough," can be provided by a caregiver via an abdominal thrust, with or without patient assist, and with or without insufflation prior to the MAC. Commercial insufflator–exsufflator devices (e.g., CoughAssist, Respironics) may also be beneficial. Invasive suctioning is a less ideal alternative and must be used with caution (4). With paralyzed abdominal muscles due to an upper motor neuron (UMN) lesion, cough can also be produced by functional electrical stimulation (FES; 4). Additional methods to mobilize secretions include positive expiratory pressure mask therapy and autogenic drainage (a technique involving specific breathing maneuvers aimed at expelling secretions independently; 4).

In general, intubation, tracheostomy, and supplemental oxygen therapy are probably overutilized in patients with ventilatory disorders, whereas noninvasive assisted ventilation and assisted cough are probably underutilized.

OBSTRUCTIVE DISORDERS (INTRINSIC DISORDERS)

These include COPD, asthmatic bronchitis, and cystic fibrosis (CF), and are characterized by a decrease in VC and forced expiratory volume (FEV), and an increase in RV, FRC, and TLC. A PR program for intrinsic disorders should be comprehensive to include nutritional management, pharmacologic management, appropriate supplemental O_2 use, breathing method education (e.g., pursed lip breathing to help manage dyspnea), airway secretion management techniques, and an exercise program. Lower limb strengthening exercises and ambulation/endurance programs can improve exercise tolerance and activities of daily living outcomes and are strongly recommended for patients with COPD. Psychological interventions such as relaxation therapy may be helpful with adjustment and coping.

Supplemental home O_2 may be indicated when PO_2 is consistently <55 to 60 mmHg. Medicare guidelines for coverage of home O_2 generally require documentation of resting, sleep, or exercise PO_2 ≤ 55 mmHg or SaO_2 <88% (on room air; 5). Patients with PO_2 of 56% to 59% or SaO_2 of 89% may be eligible with concomitant congestive heart failure (CHF), pulmonary HTN, or other criteria. Long-term O_2 therapy has been shown to improve survival and quality of life in COPD.

Surgical options include lung volume reduction surgery and organ transplant. Candidates for volume reduction surgery have advanced emphysema and have had inadequate clinical improvement following a trial of PR. Typically, 20% to 30% of one or both lungs is removed. Lung volume reduction surgery has been shown to reduce hyperinflation and improve FEV_1, forced vital capacity (FVC), and quality of life. Lung transplant is an option in the setting of conditions such as CF, pulmonary HTN, COPD, and pulmonary fibrosis. Ongoing tobacco/substance abuse, active HIV infection, and current/recent malignancy (other than nonmelanoma skin cancer) are absolute contraindications. History of older malignancy, psychiatric diagnoses, obesity, and correctable coronary artery disease are relative contraindications. The self-paced 6-minute walk test (6MWT) is frequently employed to assess candidates for lung transplant, both as a measure of urgency and predicting survival. Because of the high risk of mortality of lung transplant surgery, a minimum 6MWT score of 600 feet is commonly used by programs to screen out candidates who are not expected to survive surgery and tolerate postoperative rehabilitation.

REFERENCES

1. Ries AL. Pulmonary rehabilitation: Joint American College of Chest Physicians/American Association of Cardiovascular and Pulmonary Rehabilitation evidence- based guidelines. *Chest.* 2007;131:4S–42S.
2. The Merck Manuals Online Medical Library. The Merck Manual for Healthcare. Professionals. Retrieved from http://www.merckmanuals.com

3. Servera E, et al. Cough and neuromuscular diseases. Noninvasive airway secretion management. *Arch Bronconeumol*. 2003;39(9):418–427.
4. Alba A, et al. Pulmonary rehabilitation. In: Braddom R, ed. *Physical Medicine and Rehabilitation*. 3rd ed. Philadelphia, PA: Saunders Elsevier; 2007;739–753.
5. Medicare Carriers Manual. *Claim Processing, Part 3*. HCFA Publication. 1994; 14–3: PB 94–954799.

CHAPTER 16

BURN REHABILITATION

Burn injuries are due to external agents. Heat is the most common agent. Cold, chemicals, electricity, and radiation are others. In the United States, the majority of patients admitted to acute burn centers are males. Burns are among the leading causes of accidental death in younger children. Severe burn injuries can lead to a hypermetabolic state, increased hormone production, and muscle wasting. Predictors of mortality are older age (where 60–70 years old appears to be a threshold), higher total body surface area (TSBA) affected, and presence of inhalation injury.

DEGREE/SEVERITY

First-degree burns (e.g., sunburns) affect the epidermis only and are characterized by red, painful areas without blisters or open areas. There is, at most, some exudate. Treatment options include soaking in cool water (effective only when performed within the first 2 minutes of injury) and over-the-counter analgesics. Ice application is contraindicated because it may compound the thermal injury. Healing occurs spontaneously over ~3 to 7 days.

Partial-thickness (second-degree) burns are divided into superficial and deep burns. Superficial partial-thickness burns affect the epidermis and upper third of dermis and are characterized by serous fluid-filled blisters and mild-to-moderate exudate. The basal layer remains intact and there is no neurovascular damage. Healing occurs within ~7 to 14 days. The risk of scarring is low, but some pigmentation changes may be seen. Deep partial-thickness burns affect the epidermis and most of the dermis, with neurovascular damage present. There is moderate-to-severe exudate, but fewer blisters than superficial partial-thickness burns. Deep partial-thickness burns may heal in ~14 to 21 days. There is an increased risk of scarring. Surgical intervention (e.g., early burn wound excision, tissue coverage/skin grafting) frequently plays a role in management.

Full-thickness (third-degree) burns involve the epidermis and full dermal layer, with possible fat, muscle, or bone involvement as well. Eschar eventually covers the burned area if skin grafting is not performed. Eschar requires debridement, followed by skin grafting (Figure 16.1).

Burn severity is classified by the American Burn Association as minor (<10% TBSA for adult; <5% TBSA for young/old; or <2% full-thickness burn), moderate (10%–20% TBSA for adult; 5%–10% TBSA for young/old; or 2%–5% full-thickness burn), or major (>20% TBSA for adult; >10% TBSA for young/old; or >5% full-thickness burn). Any burn involving the eye, face, ear, or perineum, or any

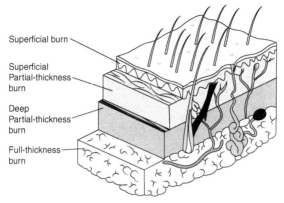

FIGURE 16.1 Burn severity.

electrical or inhalation injury is classified as a major burn. Affected TBSA may be estimated using the "Rule of 9s." (also see Figure 16.2).

RULE of 9s

	Adult TBSA (%)	Infant TBSA (%)
Head	9	18
Each upper extremity	9	9
Each lower extremity	18	14
Anterior trunk	18	18
Posterior trunk	18	18
Perineum	1	—

REHABILITATION GOALS

The goals of rehabilitation include preventing/minimizing contractures with positioning/splinting, scar management, pain control, psychosocial well-being, and functional restoration (e.g., activities of daily living, social reintegration, and return to work).

Patients who sustain burn injuries naturally tend to seek and maintain positions of greatest comfort, often with joints in a flexed position, which can result in contractures in this position. Burns on the flexor surfaces of a joint/limb are at greatest risk for developing contractures. Positioning joints in extension and abduction, as well as early mobilization, helps limit contracture development. The classic positioning for a patient with burn injuries is diagrammed in Figure 16.3. Dependent edema should be avoided by ensuring that all of the extremities spend

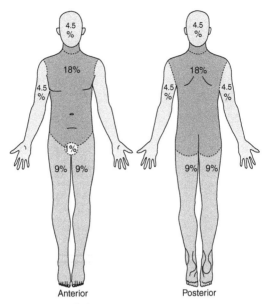

FIGURE 16.2 Diagram of the rule of 9s.

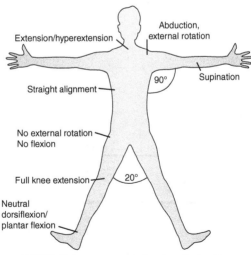

FIGURE 16.3 Proper positioning for patient with a burn injury.
Source: Adapted from Ref. (1).

sufficient time in elevated positions. In selected cases, elevating the head and chest may be important to decrease swelling of the upper airway and optimize respiration. Specialty hospital beds may facilitate positioning.

The ideal material for a *splint* is a low-temperature thermoplastic due to its light weight and moldability/remoldability. These splints can be softened in hot water and placed directly on the skin, to conform to the contour of the extremity in the desired position. A splinting program must be applied in conjunction with mobilization.

Hypertrophic scarring is a scar that is present at ≥3 months after burn injury with at least 2-mm thickness. Hypertrophic scars are more likely to occur if wounds take >2 to 3 weeks to heal. Maturation is usually seen at ~1½ years. These scars increase the risk of contracture development. *Compression garments* may be worn to prevent or treat hypertrophic scarring. The mechanism of action is not fully elucidated, but it is believed that these garments reduce scar formation by reducing the blood flow into the capillaries responsible for the scar formation. It has also been proposed that the silicone material of the garments influences collagen remodeling in the wound, softening and flattening the wound. Compression garments for burn injury are best worn 23 out of 24 hours per day. Local steroid injections may also help reduce scarring.

Nutritional management in the patient with significant burn injury is critical. Patients with >30% TBSA burns are at high risk for loss of lean body mass and bone mineral density. The daily caloric goal is 25 kcal/kg of body weight, plus 40 kcal for each 1% TBSA affected. Supplements commonly added to the diet include vitamin C, vitamin A, zinc, copper, and manganese. Optimizing nutrition has been shown to accelerate wound healing, decrease infection rates, and decrease length of hospital stay.

PHARMACOTHERAPY

Burn injuries can alter drug pharmacokinetics, for example, by increasing the effective distribution volume. Dose adjustments are frequently required for efficacy or to avoid toxicity.

Opioids remain the mainstay of treatment for pain relief for burn injury. Opioid tolerance and altered pharmacokinetics, however, may significantly increase the dosage of opioids required to effectively manage pain.

Patients with high TBSA burns may have increased insulin resistance. Close monitoring of blood sugars should be considered, particularly for patients with large burns and patients older than 60 years old. Insulin administration may decrease healing time by decreasing protein catabolism and increasing muscle protein synthesis. Administration of the synthetic testosterone oxandrolone has been shown to increase lean body mass and to improve overall outcomes, including wound healing. Beta-blockers may help by reducing the catecholamine and stress responses to burn injury, which mitigates protein and lean body mass loss. Beta-blockers may also play a role in reducing the risk for post-traumatic stress disorder.

Venous thromboembolism (VTE) risks are recognized to be elevated following burn injury, particularly with high TBSA injuries. Although there is no strong consensus regarding VTE prophylaxis, the data would generally suggest that burn patients with higher levels of VTE risk (e.g., >40% TBSA burns and need for intensive care unit [ICU] level care) would benefit from early and aggressive chemoprophylaxis (2).

COMPLICATIONS

Besides contractures, other significant complications following burn injury include infections, peripheral neuropathy, multiple mononeuropathies, bony osteophyte formation, heterotopic ossification (the posterior elbow is the most common site), spinal deformity (e.g., scoliosis and kyphosis), joint subluxation/dislocation, and pressure ulcers (particularly in the heel and sacral regions).

REFERENCES

1. Cuccurullo SJ, ed. Associated topics in physical medicine and rehabilitation. In: *Physical Medicine and Rehabilitation Board Review*. 3rd ed. New York, NY: Demos Medical Publishing; 2015:925.
2. Pannucci CJ, Osborne NH, Wahl WL, et al. Venous thromboembolism in thermally injured patients: Analysis of the National Burn Repository. *J Burn Care Res*. 2011;32(1):6–12.

SUGGESTED READING

Esselman PC, Moore ML. Issues in burn rehabilitation. In: Braddom, RL, ed. *Physical Medicine and Rehabilitation*. 3rd ed. New York, NY: W.B. Saunders; 2006: 1399–1413.

Esselman PC, Thombs BD, Magyar-Russell G, Fauerbach JA. Burn rehabilitation: state of the science. *Am J Phys Med Rehabil*. 2006;85:383–413.

Evidence-based Guidelines Group, American Burn Association. Practice guidelines for burn care. *J Burn Care Rehabil*. 2001.

Gabriel V, et al. Burns. In Cifu DX, ed. *Braddom's Physical Medicine and Rehabilitation*. 5th ed. Philadelphia, PA. Elsevier; 2016:557–569.

Procter F. Rehabilitation of the burn patient. *Indian J Plast Surg*. 2010;43(Suppl): S101–S113.

Rowan MP, Cancio LC, Elster EA, et al. Burn wound healing and treatment: review and advancements. *Critical Care*. 2015;19:243.

CHAPTER 17

CANCER REHABILITATION

Cancer rehabilitation is a subspecialty of Physical Medicine and Rehabilitation that aims to improve function and quality of life throughout the continuum of cancer care, including treatment and survivorship.

FUNCTIONAL ASSESSMENT TOOLS

In the oncology setting, the Karnofsky Performance Scale (KPS) is the most widely used tool for assessing and describing physical function (Table 17.1). It is a clinician-rated, 11-point ordinal scale and can be used to help assess the need for treatment, for example, chemotherapy dose adjustments, the need and intensity of rehabilitation services, the need for supportive care, or the need for palliative care (1). The Eastern Cooperative Oncology Group (ECOG) Scale of Performance is another commonly used tool, which is a 6-point ordinal scale that is simpler to administer but less descriptive than the KPS.

CNS AND SPINE TUMORS

Brain Tumors

The most commonly diagnosed brain tumor is metastatic, and it usually arises from tumors of the breast and lung and from melanoma (2). Primary brain tumors are classified based on their cellular origin and histologic grade. The most common primary brain tumors are malignant gliomas (derived from astrocytes, oligodendrocytes, and ependymal cells). Glioblastoma multiforme (GBM) is the most common type of glioma and carries the worst prognosis. Meningiomas, which arise from the meninges covering the brain and spinal cord, are the most common benign brain tumor (20% of primary brain tumors; 3).

Clinical presentation of brain tumors includes headache, nausea, vomiting, cognitive dysfunction, and seizures. Treatment of brain tumors can involve surgery, chemotherapy, and radiation. In comparison to patients with a stroke or traumatic brain injury (TBI), challenges in the oncology setting include progressive disease course and complications during cancer treatment, for example, side effects of radiation therapy (XRT), chemotherapy, steroids, and antiseizure medications. Patients may have residual deficits from their disease and treatment, including gait abnormality, hemiparesis, cognitive/speech deficits, and dysphagia. Cognitive dysfunction can result from the tumor, surgery, chemotherapy, XRT, and medications such as seizure prophylaxis and is considered a negative prognostic indicator (4).

TABLE 17.1 Karnofsky Performance Scale

General category	Specific criteria	Index
Able to carry out normal activity, no special care needed	Normal, no complaints, no evidence of disease	100
	Able to care on normal activity, minor signs or symptoms of disease	90
	Normal activity with effort, some signs or symptoms of disease	80
Unable to work, able to live at home and care for most personal needs, variable amount of assistance needed	Cares for self, but unable to carry on normal activities or work	70
	Requires occasional assistance from others, but able to care for most self needs	60
	Requires considerable assistance from others and frequent medical care	50
Unable to care for self, requiring hospital care, disease may be rapidly progressing	Disabled, requires special care and assistance	40
	Severely disabled, hospitalization indicated, death not imminent	30
	Very sick, hospitalization required, requiring active supportive treatment	20
	Terminal, death imminent	10
	Death	0

Source: Adapted from Ref. (1).

Spinal Cord and Spine Tumors

Tumors of the spinal cord can be primary or metastatic. Primary tumors account for 2% to 4% of all central nervous system (CNS) tumors (5). Tumors are classified by location (intramedullary, intradural, extramedullary, and extradural). Ependymomas and astrocytomas are the most common intramedullary tumors. Schwannomas, meningiomas, and gliomas are the most common intradural extramedullary tumors. Leptomeningeal metastases are diffuse metastases that surround the spinal cord and brain and present with polyradicular involvement with pain, weakness, paresthesias, and areflexia (6). Extradural tumors are usually in the vertebral body and are typically metastatic. While any tumor can metastasize to the spine, the most common are breast, lung, prostate, colon, thyroid, and kidney tumors. Primary malignant tumors of the spine are very rare (7).

Cancer-related spinal cord compression occurs in up to 5% of cancer patients. Back pain is the most common presenting symptom, and neurologic deficits such as weakness, sensory loss, and sphincter dysfunction warrant urgent evaluation and treatment (8). Pain from spinal metastases and pathological fractures due to metastases is most common in the thoracic spine and is worse at night and when lying down (7). The finding of a spine or spinal cord lesion warrants further evaluation, that is, of the whole spine and brain, as lesions can be non-congruous. Treatment for spinal cord compression usually begins with high-dose corticosteroids, which are started for patients with neurologic deficits (9). Radiation, decompressive surgery, or both are used to treat cord compression from metastatic disease.

PARANEOPLASTIC SYNDROMES

Paraneoplastic syndromes occur when the immune system produces antibodies against tumor cells and proteins and cross-reacts with healthy tissue. Paraneoplastic syndromes are most commonly associated with lung, breast, hematologic, and gynecologic cancers (10). Suspicion of a paraneoplastic syndrome should trigger a workup for a primary malignancy if none has already been identified.

Paraneoplastic syndromes often affect the central and/or peripheral neurological systems and are often characterized by a rapid neurologic deterioration (e.g., over days to weeks) that is faster than typical noncancer-related pathologies. Examples of neurological paraneoplastic syndromes include limbic encephalitis (CNS), cranial nerve pathologies, Lambert-Eaton syndrome (neuromuscular junction [NMJ]), and myasthenia gravis (NMJ). Workup includes serology for onconeural antibodies, imaging, nerve conduction study/electrodiagnostic study (NCS/EMG), and cerebrospinal fluid (CSF) studies. Treatment options include IV Ig, steroids, and immunosuppressants (10).

CHEMOTHERAPY-INDUCED PERIPHERAL NEUROPATHY

Chemotherapy-induced peripheral neuropathy (CIPN) is a common and often debilitating side effect of cancer treatment. Risk increases with dose, duration, and intensity of chemotherapy. Clinical presentation can vary depending on the agent. The dorsal root ganglion, nerve terminals of primary sensory neurons, and motor and/or autonomic systems can be affected. Nerve conduction studies most often show decreased or absent sensory nerve action potentials (11). Duloxetine, nortriptyline, gabapentin, and pregabalin can be used for symptoms of paresthesias. Physical and occupational therapy is recommended when there are functional deficits. If the manifestations of CIPN become severe, alteration of the chemotherapy itself (dose, duration, or agent) may need to be considered (Table 17.2; Figure 17.1).

TABLE 17.2 Manifestations of Chemotherapy-Induced Peripheral Neuropathy by Drug Class

Drug class	Sensory	Motor	Reflexes	Autonomic
Taxanes (paclitaxel, docetaxel)	Stocking glove distribution, feet greater than hands	Occasional weakness in feet	Reduced ankle plantar flexion	Rare
Platinum compounds (cisplatin)	Stocking glove distribution	No motor deficits	Normal	Rare
Vinca alkaloids (vincristine)	Distal sensory loss in lower extremities. Rare upper extremity involvement	Occasional symmetric weakness in lower extremities	Reduced/absent	Constipation, orthostatic hypotension
Proteasome inhibitors (bortezomib)	Stocking glove distribution	Occasional weakness in lower extremities	Reduced/absent	Constipation, diarrhea, orthostatic hypotension
Immunomodulating agents (thalidomide, lenalidomide, pomalidomide)	Stocking glove distribution	Mild weakness in affected extremities	Reduced/absent	Constipation

Source: Adapted from Refs. (12,13).

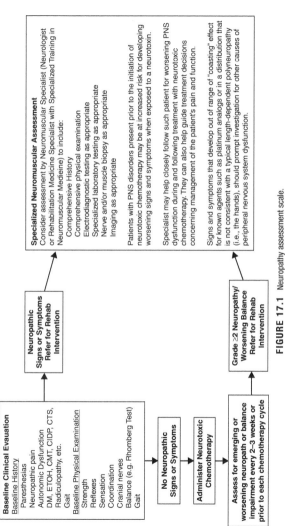

Baseline Clinical Evaluation

Baseline History
Paresthesias
Neuropathic pain
Autonomic Dysfunction
DM, ETOH, CMT, CIDP, CTS,
Radiculopathy, etc.
Gait
Baseline Physical Examination
Strength
Reflexes
Sensation
Coordination
Cranial nerves
Balance (e.g. Rhomberg Test)
Gait

No Neuropathic Signs or Symptoms

Administer Neurotoxic Chemotherapy

Assess for emerging or worsening neuropath or balance impairment every 2–3 weeks or prior to each chemotherapy cycle

Neuropathic Signs or Symptoms Refer for Rehab Intervention

Grade ≥2 Neuropathy/ Worsening Balance Refer for Rehab Intervention

Specialized Neuromuscular Assessment

Consider assessment by Neuromuscular Specialist (Neurologist or Rehabilitation Medicine Specialist with Specialized Training in Neuromuscular Medicine) to include:

Comprehensive History
Comprehensive physical examination
Electrodiagnostic testing as appropriate
Specialized laboratory testing as appropriate
Nerve and/or muscle biopsy as appropriate
Imaging as appropriate

Patients with PNS disorders present prior to the initiation of neurotoxic chemotherapy may be at increased risk for developing worsening signs and symptoms when exposed to a neurotoxin.

Specialist may help closely follow such patient for worsening PNS dysfunction during and following treatment with neurotoxic chemotherapy. They can also help guide treatment decisions concerning management of the patient's pain and function.

Signs and symptoms that develop out of range of "coasting" effect for known agents such as platinum analogs or in a distribution that is not consistent with a typical length-dependent polyneuropathy (i.e., the hands), should prompt investigation for other causes of peripheral nervous system dysfunction.

FIGURE 17.1 Neuropathy assessment scale.
Source: Adapted from Ref. (41).

PLEXOPATHY

XRT for malignancies occurring in proximity to the brachial plexus, for example, breast cancer and chest wall melanoma, can result in brachial plexopathy. Most cases occur within 3 years of XRT (14). The typical presentation is upper limb weakness, usually painless, in the distribution of the upper trunk of the brachial plexus (affecting the shoulder). The weakness can progress to affect the whole upper limb. There may be concurrent lymphedema. Treatment is largely supportive (15).

Neoplastic brachial plexopathy typically affects the lower trunk and presents with acute pain and sensory loss. MRI and NCS/EMG can help differentiate between neoplastic and XRT-induced plexopathy. Myokymic discharges on EMG are consistent with XRT plexopathy. Neoplastic brachial plexopathy is best managed by treating the underlying malignancy with XRT and chemotherapy (16).

BONY METASTASES

Bony metastases are typically a complication of advanced cancer. Cancers of the breast, prostate, lung, kidney, and thyroid account for 80% of metastases (17). Bony metastases are seen most commonly in the axial skeleton, followed by the femur, humerus, skull, ribs, and pelvis. For patients with a known history of cancer presenting with bone pain, metastatic disease must be ruled out (18). Evaluation of suspicious bony metastases on x-rays should be confirmed by bone scan. Spinal metastases are best evaluated by MRI (19). The more common complications of bony metastases include pain, hypercalcemia, spinal cord compression, and pathologic fractures.

Medical therapy for bony metastatic disease includes chemotherapy, hormone therapy, bisphosphonates (e.g., zoledronic acid), and RANK ligand inhibitors (e.g., denosumab). They significantly reduce complications such as fractures, need for XRT or surgery, hypercalcemia, and spinal cord compression (20). Complications of bisphosphonate use include nephrotoxicity, hypocalcemia, osteonecrosis of the jaw, and atypical fractures. During rehabilitation, patients with bony metastatic lesions should only perform active range of motion exercises with the involved limb and avoid resistive exercises (18). Radiation and surgical stabilization are highly effective in treating pain as well as neurological deficits (21).

RADIATION FIBROSIS SYNDROME

Radiation activates the body's coagulation and inflammatory pathways, leading to increased vascular permeability and an abnormal accumulation of thrombin and fibrin leading to progressive tissue fibrosis. Risk and severity of radiation fibrosis syndrome (RFS) is related to the total dose of XRT, fraction size, and duration of treatment.

RFS is most frequently seen in patients who have had treatment for head and neck cancer and those who have received mantle XRT for Hodgkin's lymphoma. Onset of RFS is classified into three phases: acutely after treatment, early–delayed (3 months after completion), or delayed (more than 3 months after completion of XRT). Pathology can occur anywhere in the neuromuscular axis and can present as pain, weakness, and/or spasticity. Pain is caused by ectopic activity in the sensory nerves within the radiation field, while weakness is secondary to fibrosis of the nerves and muscles. Painful spasms of the sternocleidomastoid and trapezius muscles can cause cervical dystonia. Spasms of the muscles of mastication can cause trismus, which may lead to decreased PO intake, poor nutritional status, impaired oral hygiene, and impaired verbal expression, negatively impacting quality of life (22).

Treatment of RFS depends on the tissues affected. Jaw-opening splints (e.g., TheraBite and Dynasplint) may help improve jaw range of motion (23). Orthoses may address cervical spine extensor weakness or foot drop (24). Neuropathic pain may be managed with agents such as gabapentin, pregabalin, or duloxetine. Baclofen or tizanidine can help address painful spasms, while botulinum toxin injection may be an option for cervical dystonia or trismus (25).

LYMPHEDEMA

The body's lymphatic system absorbs, filters, and transports lymphatic fluid, which can be disrupted after trauma, surgery, or radiation. While most commonly associated with breast cancer and melanoma, lymphedema may occur with any type of cancer following lymphadenectomy. Risk factors include the location of tumor, type of surgery, the number of lymph nodes removed, number of nodes returned positive for disease, treatment with XRT, and increased body mass index (BMI; 26). Lymphedema is staged using the International Society of Lymphology's descriptive system (27).

Stage 0 – Subclinical or latent condition; swelling is not evident, despite impaired lymphatic transport. Most patients are asymptomatic, but some report a feeling of heaviness in the limb.

Stage 1 – Spontaneously reversible that is soft, pitting, and resolves after elevation.

Stage 2 – Affected limb is firmer due to fibrotic tissue and scarring. Prolonged elevation temporarily reduces swelling.

Stage 3 – Affected limb is grossly enlarged, with hardening and thickening; no reduction of lymphedema with prolonged elevation.

Presentation includes swelling, feeling of heaviness, and functional impairment of the affected area. A difference in circumference of 2 cm or greater between involved and uninvolved limbs is considered diagnostic for mild lymphedema (28). Primary treatment includes complete decongestive therapy (CDT) performed by a lymphedema therapist and consists of two phases. Phase I (reductive CDT) focuses on manual lymphatic drainage (MLD), compression bandaging, therapeutic exercises, and education on skin care. When maximum volume reduction is achieved, the patient transitions to Phase II (maintenance CDT), which includes the use of compression garments, self-massage, and exercises. Research has shown CDT to be a safe and well-tolerated treatment for lymphedema. Compression bandaging combined with MLD has the potential to reduce lymphedema by 30% to 40% from baseline (29).

UPPER BODY PAIN DISORDERS

Cervical Radiculopathy
The primary cause of radiculopathy in individuals with cancer is degenerative joint disease; however, impingement due to the cancer itself should be included in the differential. MRI is recommended for any patient with known malignancy and worsening neck pain. Patients with head and neck cancer may have damage to nerve roots from XRT.

Shoulder Joint Pain
Cancer patients who have undergone a mastectomy or thoracotomy are at an increased risk for developing rotator cuff dysfunction (30). Patients with premorbid C5/C6 radiculopathy or XRT-induced plexopathy are also at higher risk for rotator cuff pathology. Pain secondary to rotator cuff dysfunction often presents as an ache extending over the anterior shoulder and deltoid muscle. Overhead activities and movements requiring internal rotation may exacerbate pain. On physical exam, range of motion will be limited, motor strength will be reduced secondary to pain, and impingement tests will be positive. Treatment options include analgesics, modalities, range of motion/strengthening exercise, and intra-articular injections. Axillary web syndrome, also known as axillary cording, may limit forward flexion of the shoulder secondary to pain and may respond to myofascial release.

Post-Mastectomy Pain Syndrome
Post-mastectomy pain syndrome (PMPS) is a chronic neuropathic pain condition that can occur after any surgical procedure of the breast, including mastectomy, lumpectomy, axillary lymph node dissection (ALND), and reconstruction (31). PMPS refers to persistent pain lasting greater than 3 months postoperatively when all other causes, such as infection or tumor recurrence, have been ruled out. Pathophysiology includes damage to the intercostobrachial nerve, axillary nerve, or

chest wall during surgery (32). Risk factors include extensive ALND, severe pain in the acute postoperative period, treatment with adjuvant XRT, younger age at diagnosis, lower socioeconomic status, and anxiety (33).

PMPS typically presents as electric, burning, or stabbing pain in the axilla at the operative site or within the ipsilateral arm (34). Physical exam includes examination of the breasts and surgical incision for signs of infection, adhesions, or neuromas. The axilla should be palpated for axillary cording and masses. The shoulder should be examined for asymmetry, passive and active range of motion, and provocative testing of the rotator cuff (35). Neurologic exam should focus on motor testing of the muscles of the shoulder joint innervated by the thoracodorsal, long thoracic, and medial and lateral pectoral nerves. Treatment includes aggressive perioperative and postoperative pain management. Neuropathic pain medications and compounded creams may be helpful. Physical therapy prescription should focus on improving ROM of the shoulder muscles, including the pectoralis minor and major, and latissimus dorsi as well as myofascial release of axillary cording (16).

Post-Thoracotomy Pain Syndrome

Patients with lung cancer requiring thoracotomy are at risk for developing post-thoracotomy pain syndrome (PTPS). PTPS is defined as pain that persists along the thoracotomy scar for greater than 2 months after surgery. The pain is thought to be due to intraoperative damage to the intercostal nerves. Due to a lack of formalized diagnostic criteria, the reported incidence of PTPS ranges from 30% to 50% (36).

Risk factors include poorly controlled preoperative and acute postoperative pain, and the use of video-assisted thoracoscopic surgery (VATS) procedure (37). Studies have shown that thoracic epidural anesthesia administered prior to surgery may help reduce PTPS. Pharmaceutical agents commonly used in treating neuropathic pain, such as gabapentin, pregabalin, tricyclic antidepressants, serotonin–norepinephrine reuptake inhibitors (SNRIs), lidocaine patches, and analgesic creams may help. Intercostal nerve blocks may help with refractory pain (38).

CHEMOTHERAPY- AND RADIATION THERAPY–INDUCED CYTOPENIAS

XRT and chemotherapy can cause neutropenia and thrombocytopenia, which can increase the risks of infection or bleeding. When platelet counts fall below 25,000/µL, holding therapies should be considered (39). Chemotherapy-induced neutropenia typically occurs 3 to 7 days following the administration of chemotherapy. Survivors with leucopenia and compromised immune function should avoid public gyms and other public places until their white blood cell (WBC) counts return to safe levels. Anemia, unless it is very severe, is generally less of a concern than thrombocytopenia due to the latter's associated risk of complications such as intracranial hemorrhage and uncontrolled bleeding (40).

REFERENCES

1. Mor V, Laliberte L, Morris JN, Wiemann M. The Karnofsky performance status scale: an examination of its reliability and validity in a research setting. *Cancer*. 1984;53(9):2002–2007.

2. Johnson JD, Young B. Demographics of brain metastasis. *Neurosurg Clin N Am*. 1996;7(3):337–344.

3. Strong MJ, Garces J, Vera JC, et al. Brain tumors: epidemiology and current trends in treatment. *Brain Tumors Neurooncol*. 2015;1:102. doi:10.4172/jbtn.1000102

4. Taphoorn MJ, Klein M. Cognitive deficits in adult patients with brain tumours. *Lancet Neurol*. 2004;3(3):159–168.

5. Duong LM, McCarthy BJ, McLendon RE, et al. Descriptive epidemiology of malignant and nonmalignant primary spinal cord, spinal meninges, and cauda equina tumors, United States, 2004–2007. *Cancer*. 2012;118:4220.

6. Custodio CM. Electrodiagnosis in cancer treatment and rehabilitation. *Am J Phys Med Rehabil*. 2011;90(5 Suppl 1):S38–S49.

7. Graber JJ, Nolan CP. Myelopathies in patients with cancer. *Arch Neurol*. 2010;67(3):298–304.

8. Helweg-Larsen S, Sørensen PS. Symptoms and signs in metastatic spinal cord compression: a study of progression from first symptom until diagnosis in 153 patients. *Eur J Cancer*. 1994;30A(3):396–398.

9. George R, Jeba J, Ramkumar G, et al. Interventions for the treatment of metastatic extradural spinal cord compression in adults. *Cochrane Database Syst Rev*. 2008;(4):CD006716.

10. Pelosof LC, Gerber DE. Paraneoplastic syndromes: an approach to diagnosis and treatment. *Mayo Clin Proc*. 2010;85(9):838–854.

11. Hershman DL, Lacchetti C, Dworkin RH, et al. Prevention and management of Chemotherapy-induced peripheral neuropathy in survivors of adult cancer: American Society of Clinical Oncology clinical practice guidelines. *J Clin Oncol*. 2014;32(18):1941.

12. Argyriou AA, Kyritsis AP, Makatsoris T, Kalofonos HP. Chemotherapy-induced peripheral neuropathy in adults: a comprehensive update of the literature. *Cancer Manag Res*. 2014;6:135–147.

13. Cheville AL. Cancer rehabilitation. In: Cifu DX, ed. *Braddom's Physical Medicine & Rehabilitation*. 5th ed. Philadelphia, PA: Elsevier; 2016:627–652.

14. Fathers E, Thrush D, Huson SM, Norman A. Radiation-induced brachial plexopathy in women treated for carcinoma of the breast. *Clin Rehabil*. 2002;16(2):160–165.

15. Kori SH, Foley KM, Posner JB. Brachial plexus lesions in patients with cancer: 100 cases. *Neurol*. 1981;31(1):45–50.

16. Stubblefield M, O'Dell M, eds. Upper extremity disorders in cancer. In: *Cancer Rehabilitation: Principle and Practice*. New York, NY: Demos Publishing; 2009:693–710.

17. Buckwalter JA, Brandser EA. Metastatic disease of the skeleton. *Amer Fam Phys*. 1997;55(5):1761–1768.

18. Stubblefield M, O'Dell M, eds. Bone metastases. In: *Cancer Rehabilitation: Principle and Practice*. New York, NY: Demos Publishing; 2009:773–785.

19. Rosenthal DI. Radiologic diagnosis of bone metastases. *Cancer*. 1997;80(8 Suppl):1595–1607.

20. Saad F, Gleason D, Murray R, et al. Long-term efficacy of zoledronic acid for the prevention of skeletal complications in patients with metastatic hormone-refractory prostate cancer. *J Natl Cancer Inst*. 2004;96(11):879–882.

21. Ziellinski S. Shorter course of radiotherapy effective for palliation of painful bone metastases. *J Natl Cancer Inst*. 2005;97(11):785.

22. Sciubba JJ, Goldberg, D. Oral complications of radiotherapy. *Lancet Oncol*. 2006;7(2):175.

23. Stubblefield MD, Manfield L, Riedel ER. A preliminary report on the efficacy of dynamic jaw opening device (Dynasplint Trismus System) as part of multimodal treatment of trismus in patients with head and neck cancer. *Arch Phys Med Rehabil*. 2010;91(8):1278–1282.

24. Hojan K, Milecki P. Opportunities for rehabilitation of patients with radiation fibrosis syndrome. *Rep Pract Oncol Radiother*. 2014;19(1):1–6.

25. Stubblefield MD. Radiation fibrosis syndrome. In: Cooper G, ed. *Therapeutic Uses of Botulinum Toxin*. Totowa, NJ: Humana Press; 2007:19–38.

26. Andrews KL, Wolf LL. Vascular diseases. In: Cifu DX, ed. *Braddom's Physical Medicine & Rehabilitation*. 5th ed. Philadelphia, PA: Elsevier; 2016:553–555.

27. The Diagnosis and Treatment of Peripheral Lymphedema. The International Society of Lymphology 2013. http://www.u.arizona.edu/~witte/ISL.htm

28. Warren AG, Brorson H, Borud LJ, Slavin SA. Lymphedema: a comprehensive review. *Ann Plast Surg*. 2007;59(4):464–472.

29. Ezzo J, Manheimer E, McNeely ML, et al. Manual lymphatic drainage for lymphedema following breast cancer treatment. *Cochrane Database of Syst Rev*. 2015;(5):CD003475. doi:10.1002/14651858.CD003475.pub2

30. Yang EJ, Park WB, Seo KS, et al. Longitudinal change of treatment-related upper limb dysfunction and its impact on the late dysfunction in breast cancer survivors: a prospective cohort study. *J Surg Oncol*. 2010;101(1):84–91.

31. Macdonald L, Bruce J, Scott NW, et al. Long-term follow-up of breast cancer survivors with post-mastectomy pain syndrome. *Br J Cancer*. 2005;92(2):225–230.

32. Vilholm OJ, Cold S, Rasmussen L, Sindrup SH. The Postmastectomy pain syndrome: an epidemiological study on the prevalence of chronic pain after surgery for breast cancer. *Br J Cancer*. 2008;99:604–610.

33. Gärtner R, Jensen MB, Nielsen J, et al. Prevalence of and factors associated with persistent pain following breast cancer surgery. *JAMA*. 2009;302(18):1985–1992

34. Miguel R, Kuhn AM, Shons AR, et al. The effect of sentinel node selective axillary lymphadenectomy on the incidence of postmastectomy pain syndrome. *Cancer Control*. 2001;8(5):427–430.

35. Lauridsen MC, Overgaard M, Overgaard J. Shoulder disability and late symptoms following surgery for early breast cancer. *Acta Oncologica*. 2007;47(4):569–575.

36. Khelemsky Y, Noto C. Preventing post-thoracotomy pain syndrome. *Mt Sinai J Med*. 2012;79:133–139.

37. Wildgaard K, Ravn J, Kehlet H. Chronic post- thoracotomy pain: a critical review of pathogenic mechanisms and strategies for prevention. *Eur J Cardiothorac Surg*. 2009;36:170–180.

38. Senturk M, Ozcan PE, Talu GK, et al. The effects of three different analgesia techniques on longterm postthoracotomy pain. *Anesthesia Analg.* 2002;94:11–15.

39. Cifu DX. *Braddom's Physical Medicine and Rehabilitation.* 5th ed. Chapter 29: Cancer Rehabilitation. Philadelphia, PA: Elsevier; 2016:627–652.

40. Rock CL, Doyle C, Demark-Wahnefried W, et al. Nutrition and physical activity guidelines for cancer survivors. *CA Cancer J Clin.* 2012;62(4):243–274.

41. Stubblefield MD, McNeely ML, Alfano CM, Mayer DK. A prospective surveillance model for physical rehabilitation of women with breast cancer: chemotherapy-induced peripheral neuropathy. *Cancer.* 2012;118(8 Suppl):2250–2260.

CHAPTER 18

SPINAL CORD INJURY

EPIDEMIOLOGY OF TRAUMATIC SCI

There are nearly 17,000 new spinal cord injury (SCI) cases in the United States each year (1). Since 2015, the mean age at time of injury is 42 years. The male-to-female ratio remains roughly 4:1. Incomplete tetraplegia is the most common category (45.0%), followed by incomplete paraplegia (21.3%), complete paraplegia (20%), and complete tetraplegia (13.3%).

Since 2010, the most common etiologies are vehicular crashes (38%), followed by falls (30.5%), acts of violence (13.5%), sports/recreation (9.0%), medical/surgical causes (5%), and other causes (4%). The proportion of injuries from falls has increased and that from sports has decreased, with falls being the fastest rising category (2, 3).

SELECTED TRACTS

The majority of descending *motor fibers* from the brain cross at the medulla to become the lateral corticospinal tract (CST). A small number of CST fibers do not decussate at the medulla and descend via the anterior CST before crossing at the level of the anterior white commissure. Although often depicted in many representations of the spinal cord (see Figure 18.1), the existence of a somatotopic organization of the lateral CST has been challenged (4).

The ascending *dorsal white columns, made up of the fasciculus gracilis and fasciculus cuneatus,* cross in the medulla, via the medial lemniscus, then ascend to the thalamus. These fibers carry joint position, vibration, and light touch (LT) sensation. The *spinothalamic tracts,* which carry pain, temperature, and nondiscriminative tactile sensations, cross to the contralateral side shortly after entry to the cord in the ventral white commissure of the spinal cord.

CLASSIFICATION OF SCI

As per the International Standards for Neurological Classification of SCI (ISNCSCI), examine the patient in the supine position in the following order:

1. Perform a sensory examination of the 28 dermatomes at key sensory points on each side for pinprick (PP; poke once, not repeatedly) and LT (use a cotton-tipped applicator, stroke ≤1 cm). Sensory levels are scored as 0 (absent), 1 (impaired, including hyperesthesia), 2 (normal), or not testable (NT). When scoring PP, the inability to discriminate PP from LT is scored 0.

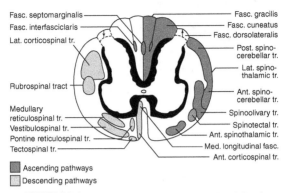

FIGURE 18.1 Ascending and descending pathways of the spinal cord.
Source: Adapted from Ref. (5).

The sensory examination also includes evaluation of deep anal pressure, as determined by a reliable ability to feel the examiner's finger applying gentle pressure to the anorectal wall (graded as present or absent). The sensory level is the most caudal level with intact sensation for both PP and LT on each side, where all rostral sensory levels are also intact.

Selected American Spinal Injury Association (ASIA) Key Sensory Points

C2	At least 1 cm lateral to occipital protuberance	T1	Medial epicondyle elbow	L3	Medial femoral condyle above knee
C3	Supraclavicular fossa at midclavicular line	T2	Apex of the axilla	L4	Medial malleolus
C4	Over the acromioclavicular joint	T4	Medial to nipple at midclavicular line	L5	Dorsum of foot at 3rd metatarsophalangeal joint
C5	Lateral antecubital fossa	T10	Lateral to umbilicus at midclavicular line	S1	Lateral heel (calcaneus)
C6	Dorsal thumb (proximal phalanx)	T12	Midpoint of the inguinal ligament	S2	Midpoint of popliteal fossa
C7	Dorsal middle finger (proximal phalanx)	L1	Halfway between T12 and L2	S3	Ischial tuberosity or infragluteal fold
C8	Dorsal little finger (proximal phalanx)	L2	Midpoint between T12 and L3 (anteromedial thigh)	S4-5	Perineal area <1 cm from anal mucocutaneous junction

2. Perform a motor examination of the 10 key muscle groups on each side, as well as voluntary anal contraction (instruct the patient to squeeze the examiner's finger as if holding back a bowel movement). Muscles are graded from 0 (total paralysis) to 5 (full active ROM against full resistance), or not testable (NT). A palpable or visible contraction is graded 1. Muscles limited only by pain or deconditioning are graded 5* instead of 4. Plus and minus designations are not used in ISNCSCI. If contracture limits more than 50% of the expected ROM, the muscle is NT. The motor level for each side is the most caudal myotome with grade 3 or more, where all muscles rostral to it are grade 5. Voluntary anal contraction is graded as present or absent and must be distinguished from reflex contraction (e.g., due to Valsalva maneuver).

American Spinal Injury Association (ASIA) Key Muscles

C5	Elbow flexors	T1	Little finger abductors	L5	Extensor hallucis longus
C6	Wrist extensors	L2	Hip flexors	S1	Ankle plantar flexors
C7	Elbow extensors	L3	Knee extensors		
C8	Flexor digitorum profundus of third digit	L4	Ankle dorsiflexors		

3. Determine the single neurologic level of injury (NLI), which is the most caudal level with normal sensory and at least antigravity (3/5) motor function bilaterally, provided there is normal sensory and motor function rostrally.

4. Classify injury as complete or incomplete. Complete injuries have no motor or sensory function, including deep anal sensation, preserved in segments S4–5. Somatosensory evoked potentials (SSEPs) may be useful in differentiating complete versus incomplete SCI in patients who are uncooperative or unconscious.

5. Categorize the injury using the American Spinal Injury Association (ASIA) Impairment Scale (AIS) A to E: (6).

    A. **Complete**—No sensory or motor function is preserved in segments S4–S5.

    B. **Sensory Incomplete**—Sensory function is preserved below the single NLI and *must* include segments S4–S5. No motor function is preserved on either side of the body more than three levels below the motor level.

    C. **Motor Incomplete**—Motor function is preserved below the single NLI*, and more than half of the key muscles below the NLI have a muscle grade less than 3/5.

D. **Motor Incomplete**—Motor function is preserved below the single NLI*, and at least half the key muscles below the NLI have a muscle grade greater than 3/5.

E. **Normal**—Sensory and motor function of the key dermatomes and myotomes per ISNCSCI is normal in all segments.

Note. To receive a grade of AIS C or D, there must be voluntary anal contraction OR sensory sparing at the S4–S5 level with sparing of motor function more than three levels below the motor level. According to ISNCSCI, preservation of motor control of non-key muscles below the motor level may be used to determine sensory versus motor incomplete status (i.e., AIS B vs. C).

6. The zone of partial preservation (ZPP) is used only for AIS A and is defined as the most caudal partially innervated sensory and motor segments (requires volitional contraction of a key muscle) below the sensory and motor levels, respectively (documented as four distinct levels: R-sensory, L-sensory, R-motor, and L-motor).

SCI CLINICAL SYNDROMES

Central Cord – Incomplete SCI syndrome is typically seen in persons with preexisting cervical spondylosis who experience neck hyperextension injuries, typically due to falls. There is inward bulging of the ligamentum flavum into a stenotic canal, resulting in cord compression. Clinically, there is greater upper limb weakness than lower limb, variable sensory loss, and variable effects on the bowel, bladder, and sexual function. Penrod retrospectively studied 51 patients with central cord syndrome and noted better overall recovery of ambulation, self-care, and bowel/bladder function in patients aged less than 50 years compared to their older counterparts at time of discharge from rehabilitation (7).

Brown-Séquard – This occurs when a hemisection of the spinal cord is damaged (classically due to knife trauma or tumor), resulting in ipsilateral hyperreflexic spastic paralysis and loss of tactile discrimination, vibration sense, and proprioceptive sense at and below the level of injury. Contralaterally, typically starting at two segments below the level of injury, there is loss of PP and temperature sense due to lateral spinothalamic tract damage. At the level of injury, PP and loss of temperature sense is ipsilateral because the tracts have already crossed. The prognosis for functional ambulation is best when compared to other incomplete SCI syndromes. Pure Brown-Sequard syndrome is rare. Brown-Sequard-Plus syndrome includes features of central cord syndrome and is more frequently seen clinically.

Anterior Cord – The etiology is typically a vascular lesion in the territory of the anterior spinal artery. Other causes include retropulsed disks/vertebral fragments and radiation myelopathy. Intraoperative SSEPs, which primarily monitor the posterior column pathways, may miss the development of an anterior cord syndrome. There is variable loss of motor function and PP sensation, with relative preservation of proprioception and LT. Bladder and bowel function are usually affected because the descending autonomic tracts to the sacral centers are typically involved. Prognosis for motor recovery is generally poor.

Cauda Equina – Cauda equina syndrome (CES) may be due to neural canal compression or fractures of the sacrum or spine at L2 or below. While the damage occurs within the spinal canal, CES can be described as "multiple lumbosacral radiculopathies," because the lesion is at the level of the nerve roots. Sequelae depend on the roots involved, but primarily manifest as lower motor neuron deficits. Bladder retention (followed by overflow incontinence), bowel dysfunction, sexual dysfunction, flaccid lower limb weakness, and saddle anesthesia are the characteristics. Radicular neuropathic pain is common and can be severe. CES is considered an emergency, thus urgent surgical consultation is indicated. Recovery is possible because the nerve roots can recover.

Conus Medullaris – A pure conus medullaris lesion (e.g., intramedullary tumor) results in saddle anesthesia and bowel, bladder, and sexual dysfunction due to cord injury at the S2–S4 segments. While this syndrome may appear similar to CES, anal cutaneous and bulbocavemosus reflexes (S2–S4), and ankle deep tendon reflexes (S1, S2) may be preserved if the lesion is "high" in the conus. Conus lesions due to trauma (e.g., L1 vertebral body fracture) are typically accompanied by injury to some of the lumbosacral nerve roots, resulting in a mixed upper and lower motor neuron lesion presentation. Prognosis for recovery is poorer than for CES.

ACUTE TREATMENT OF SCI

Currently, there is no proven cure for SCI. Mega-dose steroids were previously reported to be neuroprotective in acute SCI by inhibiting lipid peroxidation and scavenging free radicals. The use of IV methylprednisolone (MP) in acute nonpenetrating traumatic SCI was supported by the second *National Acute Spinal Cord Injury Study* (NASCIS), which demonstrated improved neurologic outcomes if steroids were administered within 8 hours of injury (8). This study, however, was found to have methodologic flaws and the results have been largely discredited (9, 10). Currently, high-dose MP is considered an optional treatment for acute SCI (11).

Other interventions, for example, IV GM-1 *ganglioside*, intralesional activated autologous macrophages, and intralesional stem cells, have been investigated as potentially neuroprotective or neuroregenerative agents, but none has been proven to date to be clinically effective for acute SCI. At present, the standard of care for acute SCI involves expert medical and surgical care, followed by multidisciplinary restorative rehabilitation. The optimal timing for surgery after SCI is unknown, although early surgery may be superior to delayed surgery because it allows for earlier mobilization and reduction of medical complications. Retrospective data suggest a role for urgent decompression in the setting of bilateral facet dislocation or incomplete SCI with evidence of progressive neurologic deterioration (12).

PROGNOSIS AND RECOVERY IN TRAUMATIC SCI

Complete SCI – Only 2% to 3% of patients who are AIS A at 1 week post-SCI make significant neurologic recoveries; that is, improve to AIS D by 1 year (13). In persons with complete tetraplegia, more than 95% of key muscles in the ZPP with grade 1 or 2 power at 1 month post-SCI will reach grade 3 at 1 year (16). About 25% of the most cephalad grade 0 muscles at 1 month will recover to at least grade 3 at 1 year (13), with those having PP sensation being the most likely to recover motor function. Most upper limb recovery occurs during the first 6 months, with the greatest rate of change during the first 3 months. Motor level is superior to the neurologic or sensory level in correlating with function. In patients who have complete paraplegia at 1 week post-SCI, NLI has been found to remain unchanged at 1 year in 73%, improve one level in 18%, and improve two or more levels in 9% (14). Waters reported that only 5% of persons with complete paraplegia eventually achieve community ambulation (15).

Incomplete SCI – Persons with incomplete tetraplegia often recover multiple levels below the initial level, with the majority of recovery occurring within the first 6 months. Waters reported that 46% of incomplete tetraplegics recover sufficient motor function to ambulate at 1 year (15). As much as 80% of persons with incomplete paraplegia regain hip flexors and knee extensors (grade ≥3) by 1 year, thus improving their likelihood of community-based ambulation (13).

In a review of 27 patients who were initially sensory incomplete, Crozier reported that partial (or greater) preservation of PP sensation below the zone of injury was predictive of eventual functional ambulation (16). Patients with AIS B injuries with PP sparing converted to AIS D status nearly as frequently as those with AIS C injuries, thus having a favorable prognosis for ambulation.

Miscellaneous – The 72-hour post-SCI neurologic examination may predict recovery more reliably than an examination performed on the day of injury. Absence of the bulbocavernosus reflex beyond the first few days can signify a lower motor neuron lesion and have implications on bowel, bladder, and sexual function. On MRI, presence of hemorrhage and length of edema are independent negative predictors of motor function at 1 year (13). Strength 3/5 or more in the bilateral hip flexors and the knee extensors on at least one side correlates with community ambulation (17).

EXPECTED FUNCTIONAL OUTCOMES

(I, independent; A, assist; D, dependent; predicted outcomes are based on patients of typical age for traumatic SCI with complete injuries–older patients have overall poorer expected outcome)

C1–3 – Dependent for secretion management. Independent with power WC mobility and pressure relief with enhanced equipment; otherwise dependent for all care but Independent for directing care.

C4 – May be able to breathe without a ventilator. May use a mobile arm support for limited ADLs if there is some elbow flexion and deltoid strength. May be able to use a sip-puff or head-control WC.

C5 – May require A to clear secretions. May be I for feeding after setup and with adaptive equipment, for example, a long opponens orthosis with utensil slots and mobile arm support. Requires A for most upper-body ADLs. Most patients will be *unable* to perform self-intermittent catheterization. I with power WC; some users may be I with manual WC with hand rim projections on noncarpeted, level, indoor surfaces. Some may drive specially adapted vans.

C6 – May use a tenodesis orthosis and short opponens orthosis with utensil slots. I with feeding except for cutting food. I for most upper-body ADLs after setup and with modifications (e.g., Velcro straps on clothing); A to D for most lower-body ADLs, including bowel care. Some males may be I with self-intermittent catheterization (IC) after setup; females are usually D. Some patients may be I for transfers using a sliding board and heel loops, but many will require A. May be I with manual WC, but power WCs are often used, especially for longer distances and outdoors. May drive an adapted van.

C7 – Essentially I for most ADLs, often using a short opponens splint and universal cuff. May require A for some lower-body ADLs. Women may have difficulty with IC. Bowel care may be I with adaptive equipment, but suppository insertion may still be difficult. I for mobility at a manual WC level, except for uneven transfers. Patients may be I with a nonvan automobile with hand controls if the patient can transfer and load/ unload the WC.

C8 – Completely I with ADLs including bowel and bladder care and mobility using manual WC and adapted car.

Paraplegia – Trunk stability improves with lower lesions. Those with upper and mid-thoracic injuries may stand and ambulate with b/l knee ankle foot orthosis (KAFOs) and Lofstrand crutches (i.e., using a swing-through or swing-to gait), but the intent is usually exercise, not functional mobility. Patients with lower thoracic or L1 SCI may be able to ambulate in the household using orthoses and gait-assistive devices, and rarely in the community. Patients with L2–S5 SCI may be community ambulators with or without orthoses (i.e., KAFOs or AFOs) and/or gait-assistive devices. (AFOs generally compensate for the ankle weakness, while canes, crutches, and walkers primarily compensate for hip abduction and extension weakness.)

SELECTED ISSUES IN SCI

Autonomic Dysreflexia (AD) – It can occur in 48% to 85% of patients with SCI at T6 or above (18). Since resting systolic blood pressures (SBPs) can be 90 to 110 mmHg in this population, SBPs of 20 to 40 mmHg more than the baseline may signify AD (18). A noxious stimulus below the level of injury causes reflex sympathetic vasoconstriction (BP ↑). Due to the SCI, higher CNS centers cannot directly modulate the sympathetic response. The body attempts to lower BP by carotid and aortic baroreceptor/vagal-mediated bradycardia, but this is usually ineffective (Figure 18.2).

The primary treatment of AD is removal of the noxious stimulus, which is most commonly related to bladder dysfunction. The second most common cause is bowel distention (e.g., high fecal impaction). Other causes can include abdominal emergencies, urinary tract infections (UTIs), testicular torsion, epididymitis, endometriosis, undiagnosed fractures, DVTs, pressure injury, gout, cellulitis, ingrown toenails, and tight clothing/stockings or splints, and body positioning.

Bone Metabolism – The risk of osteoporosis and fractures is increased below the level of injury following SCI, especially in long bones. The exact pathogenesis is unknown but is thought to be related to disuse and neural factors. Trabecular bone has been found to be involved more than cortical bone. A new steady state is achieved between bone resorption and formation about 2 years following SCI. Clinical management can include treatment with calcium phosphate, Vitamin D, calcitonin, and bisphosphonates, as well as functional stimulated exercises (20).

Heterotopic ossification (HO) is an acquired extraskeletal formation of bone, typically near large joints. HO is common after SCI, affecting up to half of patients, beginning at approximately 12 weeks following injury. Those with complete lesions, and those who experience other complications such as spasticity, UTIs, and pneumonia have a higher risk of developing HO (21). The hip is the most common site of HO in SCI. Symptoms occur in less than 20% of patients and can include pain, decreased ROM, and inflammation. A triple-phase bone scan is highly sensitive and may be positive well before plain radiographs. Initial treatment includes gentle passive ROM of the affected joint and NSAIDs. Some studies have shown bisphosphonates may also be useful. Surgical excision is an option (after HO maturation), but recurrence rates are high (22).

Cardiovascular Disease (CVD) – As long-term survival has improved, CVD is an increasingly common complication of SCI. Risk factors such

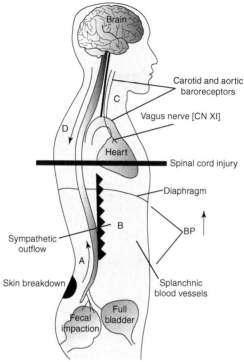

FIGURE 18.2 (A) A strong sensory input (not necessarily noxious) is carried into the spinal cord through intact peripheral nerves. The most common origins are bladder and bowel. (B) This strong sensory input travels up the spinal cord and evokes a massive reflex sympathetic surge from the thoracolumbar sympathetic nerves. This sympathetic surge causes widespread vasoconstriction, most significantly in the subdiaphragmatic (or splanchnic) vasculature. Thus, peripheral arterial hypertension occurs. (C) The brain detects this hypertensive crisis through intact baroreceptors in the neck delivered to the brain through cranial nerves IX and X (vagus). (D) The brain attempts two maneuvers to halt the progression of this hypertensive crisis. First, the brain attempts to shut down the sympathetic surge by sending descending inhibitory impulses. Unfortunately, these inhibitory impulses do not reach most sympathetic outflow levels because of the spinal cord injury at T6 or above. Therefore, inhibitory impulses are blocked in the injured spinal cord. The second maneuver orchestrated by the brain, in an attempt to bring down peripheral blood pressure, slows the heart rate through an intact vagus (parasympathetic) nerve. This may result in a compensatory bradycardia but is inadequate, and hypertension continues. In summary, the sympathetic nerves prevail below the level of neurologic injury, and the parasympathetic nerves prevail above the level of injury. Once the inciting stimulus is removed, the reflex hypertension resolves.

Source: Adapted from Ref. (19).

as obesity, abnormal lipid profiles, and impaired glucose metabolism are more prevalent in the chronic SCI versus general population. Morbidity and mortality from CVD exceed those caused by pulmonary or renal conditions in the chronic SCI population (23). Preventive measures and regular screening for CVD are warranted.

Long-Term Routine Urinary Tract Surveillance – Upper-tract follow-up can include renal scan with glomerular filtration rate (GFR) or renal scan with 24-hour Cr clearance yearly to follow renal function. Renal and bladder ultrasound can be done annually to detect hydronephrosis and stones. Lower-tract evaluation can include urodynamics once the bladder starts exhibiting uninhibited contractions (or at around 3 to 6 months post-injury) and then as determined by the clinician (often done annually). Routine cystoscopy to potentially diagnose neoplasm at an earlier rather than a later stage should be performed annually as patients approach 10 years of chronic indwelling (urethral or suprapubic) catheter use, or sooner (e.g., after 5 years) if there are additional risk factors (heavy smoker, age > 40 years, and history of many UTIs).

Posttraumatic Syringomyelia – It may be seen clinically in nearly 3% to 8% of posttraumatic SCI patients, or in up to 20% on autopsy. It can develop as early as 2 months post-SCI. Symptoms include pain (often worsened by coughing or straining, but not by lying supine) and worsening neurological function (e.g., ascending sensory loss, progressive weakness including bulbar muscles, increased sweating, orthostasis, and Horner's syndrome). Treatment is usually observational, with surgical interventions considered for large, progressive lesions.

Sexual Function and Fertility – *Females:* About 44% to 55% of women with SCI can achieve orgasm (24). Menses typically returns within 6 months post-SCI, and reproductive function is preserved. Pregnancy in women with SCI is usually classified as high risk due to high rates of complications, which include AD, infections, and spasticity. Incidence of prematurity and small-for-date infants is high, but there is no increase in spontaneous abortions. Spinal anesthesia is recommended during delivery for patients with SCI at T6 or above to prevent AD as 85% of patients with SCI at these levels have been observed to develop AD during labor (25).

Males: With complete upper motor neuron SCI, reflexogenic erections can usually be achieved, although ejaculation is rare. With incomplete SCI, reflexogenic erections are usually attainable; ejaculation is less rare than for those with complete SCI; and some patients can achieve psychogenic erections. Complete or incomplete injuries below T11 may result in erections of poor quality and duration. Treatment options for erectile dysfunction (ED) can include medications, assistive devices, and surgical prosthetic implants. Phosphodiesterase-5 (PDE-5) inhibitors (e.g., sildenafil, tadalafil, and vardenafil) have been shown to improve ED and patient satisfaction (26). While PDE-5 inhibitors are well tolerated in general, contraindications exist, including use of organic nitrates and some alpha blockers. Direct self-injection of alprostadil (prostaglandin E1) into the corpus cavernosum is highly effective for ED, but is invasive and carries risks of priapism and penile fibrosis. Infertility after SCI is common, due to factors such as retrograde ejaculation and poor sperm quantity and motility. Penile vibratory stimulation for ejaculation requires resolution of spinal shock and an intact ejaculatory reflex (sympathetic fibers from superior hypogastric plexus/T10-L2 for emission; and somatic fibers from the pudendal/S2–S4 for expulsion). Electroejaculation (seminal vesicle and prostatic stimulation through the rectum) is another option, which requires general anesthesia for those without a complete SCI. The ejaculate is collected and processed for intrauterine or in vitro fertilization.

Tendon Transfer Surgery in Tetraplegia – Triceps function can be restored in the patient with C5 or C6 SCI using a posterior deltoid-to-triceps or a biceps-to-triceps transfer. Lateral key grip can be restored in a patient with C6 SCI via the modified Moberg procedure, which involves attachment of the brachioradialis (C5, C6) to the flexor pollicis longus (C8, T1) and stabilization of the thumb carpometacarpal and IP joints.

REFERENCES

1. NSCISC National Spinal Cord Injury Statistical Center. The University of Alabama at Birmingham. https://www.nscisc.uab.edu

2. Devivo M. Epidemiology of traumatic SCI. In: Kirshblum S, ed. *Spinal Cord Medicine*. Philadelphia, PA: Lippincott Williams & Wilkins; 2002:69.

3. Spinal Cord Injury (SCI). Facts and Figures at a Glance. 2016 SCI Data Sheet. National Spinal Cord Injury Statistical Center, Birmingham, AL

4. Levi AD. Clinical syndromes associated with disproportionate weakness of the upper versus the lower extremities after cervical spinal cord injury. *Neurosurgery*. 1996;38:179–183.

5. Adams M, ed. Adams & Victor's Principles o f Neurology. 7th ed. McGraw-Hill, 2001

6. American Spinal Injury Association. *International Standards for Neurological Classification of SCI, Revised 2013*. Chicago, IL: ASIA; 2013.

7. Penrod LE. Age effect on prognosis for functional recovery in acute, traumatic central cord syndrome. *Arch Phys Med Rehabil*. 1990;71:963–968.

8. Bracken MB. NASCIS 2. *N Engl J Med*. 1990;322:1405–1411.

9. Nesathurai S. Steroids and SCI: revisiting NASCIS 2 and 3. *J Trauma*. 1998;45:1088–1093.

10. Hurlbert RJ. Methylprednisolone for acute SCI: an inappropriate standard of care. *J Neurosurg*. 2000;93(1 suppl):l–7.

11. Wing, P. et al. Early acute management in adults with spinal cord injury: a clinical practice guideline for health-care professionals. *J Spinal Cord Med*. 2008;31(4):403–479.

12. Fehlings MG. The role and timing of decompression in acute SCI. *Spine*. 2001;26(suppl):101–109.

13. Ditunno JF. Predicting outcome in traumatic SCI. In: Kirshblum S, ed. *Spinal Cord Medicine*. Philadelphia, PA: Lippincott Williams & Wilkins; 2002:87.

14. Waters RL. Donald Munro lecture: functional and neurologic recovery following acute SCI. *J Spinal Cord Med*. 1998;21:195–199.

15. Waters RL. Motor and sensory recovery following incomplete tetraplegia. *Arch Phys Med Rehabil*. 1994;75:306–311.

16. Crozier KS. SCI: prognosis for ambulation based on sensory examination in pts who are initially motor complete. *Arch Phys Med Rehabil*. 1991;72:119–121.

17. Hussey RW. SCI: requirements for ambulation. *Arch Phys Med Rehabil*. 1973;54:544–547.

18. Campagnolo D. Autonomic and CV complications of SCI. In: Kirshblum S, ed. *Spinal Cord Medicine*. Philadelphia, PA: Lippincott Williams & Wilkins; 2002:123–132.

19. American Spinal Injury Association. Standards for Neurological and Functional Classification of SCI. 3rd ed. Chicago, IL: ASIA; 1990

20. Jiang SD. Osteoporosis after spinal cord injury. *Osteoporos Int*. 2006;17(2):180.

21. Citak M. Risk factors for heterotopic ossification in patients with spinal cord injury: a case–control study of 264 patients. *Spine*. 2012;37(23):1953–1957.

22. Teasell RW. A systematic review of the therapeutic interventions for heterotopic ossification after spinal cord injury. *Spinal Cord*. 2010;48(7):512.

23. Myers J, Lee M, Kiratli J. Cardiovascular disease in spinal cord injury: an overview of prevalence, risk, evaluation, and management. *Am J Phys Med Rehabil*. 2007;86(2):142.

24. Sipski ML. Sexual arousal and orgasm in women: the effects of SCI. *Ann Neurol*. 2001;49:35–44.

25. Westgren, N. Pregnancy and delivery in women with a traumatic spinal cord injury in Sweden, 1980–1991. *Obstet Gynecol*. 1993;81(6):926.

26. Giuliano F. Vardenafil improves ejaculation success rates and self-confidence in men with erectile dysfunction due to spinal cord injury. *Spine*. 2008;33(7):709.

CHAPTER 19

TRAUMATIC BRAIN INJURY

INTRODUCTION AND EPIDEMIOLOGY

Traumatic brain injury (TBI) is a serious public health problem in the United States. In 2010, ~2.5 million people sustained a TBI, where 2% died, 11% were hospitalized, and 87% were treated and released from an emergency department (1). These figures do not include those who did not receive medical care, had outpatient or office-based visits, or received care at a federal facility. Per the most recent report to Congress in 2015 (1), the most common causes were falls (40.5%), unintentional blunt trauma (15.5%), motor vehicle accidents (MVAs) (14.3%), and assaults (10.7%). Adults aged ≥75 years had the highest rates of hospitalization and death. Alcohol use is one of the most preventable causes for TBI.

PATHOPHYSIOLOGY

The primary injury occurs on impact and within the first few hours of the injury. *Diffuse axonal injury* (DAI) is the shearing of axons secondary to acceleration-deceleration, rotational forces, and differences in tissue density between the white and gray matter on impact. It may cause petechial hemorrhages primarily in the white matters of the brain (corpus callosum, parasagittal white matter, midbrain, pons; 2). It is likely to cause loss of consciousness, arousal, and cognitive deficits. A *cerebral contusion* is the result of coup–contrecoup injury involving rapid acceleration/deceleration. It primarily affects the orbital/inferior frontal and anterior temporal lobes. *Subdural hemorrhages* (SDHs) are crescent shaped and are the most common bleed in TBI. SDHs may be due to shearing of bridging veins or arterial vessel damage. SDHs are more common in the elderly due to cerebral atrophy. An *epidural hemorrhage* is elliptical in shape and commonly due to injury of the middle meningeal artery and a related temporal fracture. There may be a lucid interval, which may be clinically misleading. This is a surgical emergency. A *subarachnoid hemorrhage* (SAH) occurs between the pia and the arachnoid space and can lead to hydrocephalus. *Penetrating injuries* may be due to localized injuries such as gunshots or shrapnel.

Secondary injury occurs in response to the primary injury, in hours to days after the TBI. There may be biochemical changes, inflammatory changes, ischemia, hypoxia, or anoxia related to hypoperfusion. Vasogenic (extracellular) and cytogenic (intracellular) edema may be a result of disruption of the blood–brain barrier, damaged blood vessels, and cytoskeletal membrane integrity. These secondary injury processes are interrelated, each exacerbating the other. Biomarkers are currently being developed to identify the presence or extent of brain injury.

CLASSIFICATION OF TBI SEVERITY

TBI severity can be classified using various scales; see Tables 19.1 and 19.2.

TABLE 19.1 Classification of TBI Severity

	Mild	Moderate	Severe
Structural Imaging	Normal	Normal or abnormal	Normal or abnormal
Loss of Consciousness	<30 minutes	30 minutes–24 hours	>24 hours
Alteration of Consciousness/Mental State	<24 hours	>24 hours	>24 hours
Glasgow Coma Scale (best in 24 hours)	13–15	8–12	3–8
Post-Traumatic Amnesia	0–1 day	1–7 days	>7 days

Source: Adapted from Ref. (3).

TABLE 19.2 Glasgow Coma Scale

	Response	Score
Eye opening	Spontaneously	4
	To speech	3
	To pain	2
	None	1
Verbal Response	Oriented	5
	Confused	4
	Inappropriate	3
	Incomprehensible	2
	None	1
Motor Response	Obeys commands	6
	Localizes to pain	5
	Withdraws from pain	4
	Flexion to pain (decorticate posturing)	3
	Extension to pain (decerebrate posturing)	2
	None	1

Source: Adapted from Ref. (4).

TABLE 19.3 Rancho Los Amigos Cognitive Functioning Scale

Rancho level	Clinical correlate
I	No response
II	Generalized response
III	Localized response
IV	Confused, agitated response
V	Confused, inappropriate response
VI	Confused, appropriate response
VII	Automatic, appropriate response
VIII	Purposeful, appropriate response

Source: Adapted from Ref. (5).

Post-traumatic amnesia (PTA) is the inability to retain memory after the TBI, such as day-to-day information or ongoing events. It is measured by using the Galveston Orientation Amnesia Test (GOAT) or the Orientation Log (O-Log). The GOAT is a series of questions related to orientation and recall of recent events. The O-Log was developed as an alternative to the GOAT and appears to be a better predictor of outcome. The end of PTA is marked by a score of ≥75 on the GOAT or ≥25 on the O-Log on two consecutive days.

The *Rancho Los Amigos Cognitive Functioning Scale* (Table 19.3) helps provide generalized descriptions of behaviors commonly seen in TBI patients as recovery progresses.

RECOVERY AND OUTCOMES

Neuroplasticity may influence recovery through processes such as the unmasking of existing connections, long-term potentiation, long-term depression, axonal and dendritic sprouting, and synaptogenesis (6). Maladaptive changes can result in negative consequences such as spasticity and seizures. Diaschisis is a decrease in function of an area of uninjured brain that is connected with an area of injured brain due to functional deafferentation. Gradual reduction in diaschisis occurs through natural neuroplasticity and improved cerebral blood flow. Compensation is the use of alternative strategies to restore lost function.

Outcomes following TBI are commonly measured using the Disability Rating Scale (DRS). The DRS is intended to measure general functional changes over the course of recovery. It is a 30-point scale that scores impairment, disability, and handicap.

Factors associated with worse outcomes include age ≤4 years and ≥65 years; presence of brain stem reflexes such as dilated pupils, impaired Doll's eye, no deviation with caloric testing, and decerebrate > decorticate posturing; lower Glasgow Coma Scale (GCS) score;

bilateral > unilateral findings on brain imaging (brain stem > cere-bral); longer duration in a poor arousal state; longer duration of PTA; flaccidity and spasticity; incontinence; lower Functional Independent Measure (FIM) Score; and absence of N20 response on somatosensory evoked potential (SEP). Severe disability is unlikely when PTA is <2 months and good recovery unlikely when >3 months.

DISORDERS OF CONSCIOUSNESS

Consciousness is a state of arousal where there is awareness of self and environment, as well as responses to the environment. Coma and vegetative state are clinical manifestations of damage to the arousal center, the reticular activating system (RAS), and its projections to the cortex. A longer duration of coma is associated with a worse outcome. Severe disability is unlikely when coma lasts less than 2 weeks. Good recovery is unlikely when coma lasts longer than 4 weeks.

Distinguishing between vegetative state and minimally conscious state (MCS; see Table 19.4) is particularly important because the prog-noses are sufficiently different to affect long-term management plans. The JFK Coma Recovery Scale-Revised (CRS-R) was designed to help differentiate between the vegetative state and MCS. It is a 23-item scale

TABLE 19.4 Coma, Vegetative State, Minimally Conscious State

	Consciousness	Sleep/wake cycle on EEG	Functional response
Coma	None, eyes closed	Absent	None, only reflexive responses
Vegetative State	None, eyes open	Present	Nonpurposeful movement No command following Inconsistent or reflexive responses
Minimally conscious state	Partially aware of self and environment, but limited in response Localizes pain	Present	Inconsistent command following Visual fixation/pursuit (tracks moving objects) Automatic movements/manipulation Communication is unreliable
Confused State	Aware of self and environment and able to respond consistently	Present	Consistently follows commands Functional object manipulation Purposeful movements Able to communicate reliably

that measures function across six subscales (auditory, visual, motor, oromotor/verbal, communication, and arousal responses), which are hierarchically arranged to correspond to brain stem, subcortical, and cortical functions.

ACUTE MANAGEMENT OF TBI

Intracranial pressure (ICP) monitoring may play a role in early TBI care, although there is a lack of high-quality data indicating that routine ICP monitoring in TBI improves clinical outcomes. The rationale of ICP monitoring is that increased ICPs cause decrease in cerebral perfusion pressure (CPP = mean arterial pressure − ICP). ICP may be increased by temperature, stress, stimuli, elevated BP, lying supine, suctioning, or aggressive physical therapy (PT). An external ventricular drain is placed in the setting of severe brain injury (e.g., GCS ≤8) when accompanied by edema, compressed basilar cisterns, or clinical decline. Increased ICPs (>20 mmHg; normal is 2–5 mmHg) can be managed by elevating the head, using diuretics (mannitol) or hypertonic saline, barbiturates/sedatives, neurosurgical decompression with a craniectomy/craniotomy (morbidity can be higher in the elderly), or hyperventilation (used cautiously). Hypothermia is inconsistently beneficial in reducing ICP.

Steroids are not recommended as routine treatment for acute TBI given the data from the large (n = 10,008), randomized, multicenter Corticosteroid Randomisation After Significant Head Injury (CRASH) trial, the results of which were published in 2004 and 2005 (7). CRASH showed significantly increased mortality in the group receiving steroids versus the no-steroids group.

TREATMENT OF COMA AND VEGETATIVE STATE

Treatment generally focuses on sensory stimulation (auditory, sensory, vibratory, etc.) and the use of stimulants (methylphenidate, amantadine, dopamine agonists, selective serotonin reuptake inhibitors [SSRIs], etc.). There is a dearth of high-grade evidence demonstrating improved clinical outcomes with these treatments, but they are often performed anyway given the lack of viable alternatives. Secondary complications (skin breakdown, contractures, etc.) should be prevented.

TREATMENT OF MEDICAL COMPLICATIONS OF TBI

Sleep disturbance is one of the most common symptoms after a TBI. Proper sleep hygiene is first-line management. Regular sleep–wake cycles should be reestablished by maintaining a schedule, avoiding caffeine and exercise late in the day, and promoting a quiet, restful environment. Medication side effects, pain, and other factors inhibiting sleep should be addressed. Second-line management is medication, starting with melatonin (3–9 mg), which is over-the-counter

(OTC). Ramelteon, a melatonin receptor agonist, is more expensive and requires a prescription, but is not necessarily more effective. Trazodone is another common alternative (25–150 mg). Zolpidem and other "Z-drugs" have benzodiazepine-like sedative/hypnotic effects and should not be used. Antihistamines (e.g., diphenhydramine) should also be avoided, as they can interfere with memory and new learning.

Poor arousal is also very common and requires that sleep is managed appropriately. Stimulants such as amantadine (100–200 mg) and methylphenidate (5–20 mg), given at breakfast and lunch, are commonly used. Methylphenidate does not lower the seizure threshold and is safe for patients at risk for seizure. Bromocriptine (typically 2.5–7.5 mg bid), modafinil, carbidopa, and donepezil can also improve alertness and memory.

Agitation is a subtype of delirium present during PTA, manifested by behavioral excesses such as aggression, akathisia, disinhibition, emotional lability, destructiveness, or combativeness (8). Such behaviors are expected in frontotemporal lobe injuries. Agitation can be measured and tracked using the Agitated Behavior Scale (which rates 14 behaviors such as restlessness, impulsivity, uncooperative, mood, etc., each on a scale of 1 to 4; a higher score indicates more agitation). Management focuses on optimizing the environment and ruling out underlying causes of agitation (i.e. medications, hunger, pain, fatigue, seizure, and infection). Visitors should be limited and treating staff should be consistent. The patient should be redirected and reoriented frequently. A 1:1 observer may help guide behaviors. Pharmacotherapy is a second-line intervention when environmental management is insufficient. Mood stabilizers (valproic acid, lamotrigine, carbamazepine), atypical antipsychotics (risperidone, ziprasidone, olanzapine, quetiapine), antidepressants (SSRIs, buspirone), and lipophilic beta-blockers (propranolol, carvedilol, labetalol) can be used with careful consideration of their side effects and interactions. Medications should be started at low doses and increased slowly while monitoring for cognitive side effects. Benzodiazepines and haloperidol can cause significant side effects, but may be used in select cases, particularly those complicated by premorbid psychiatric disease. Neurostimulants such as amantadine and methylphenidate can improve agitation by improving the confusion related to poor attention and executive function. Physical restraints should be restricted to situations where there is risk of injury to self or others.

Neuroendocrine dysfunction is related to hypothalamic/pituitary injury and may present months after TBI. This may contribute to malaise, hypothermia, bradycardia, hypotension, or stagnation of rehabilitation progress. An estimated 30% to 50% of patients who survive TBI have endocrine abnormalities, which often goes unidentified. Screening is recommended at 3 to 6 months and 1 year (e.g., AM cortisol, follicle-stimulating hormone [FSH], luteinizing hormone [LH], testosterone, prolactin, insulin-like growth factor 1[IGF-1], estradiol, thyroid panel, prolactin). Treatment generally involves hormone replacement.

Sodium abnormalities may be secondary to the syndrome of inappropriate antidiuretic hormone (SIADH), cerebral salt wasting (CSW), or diabetes insipidus (DI). ADH binds to the renal collecting tubules to allow water reabsorption. Without ADH, the tubules are impermeable to water. ADH excess, therefore, causes water retention and Na+ excretion. SIADH results in hyponatremia, low serum osmolality, and high urine osmolality, with euvolemia to mild extracellular fluid (ECF) expansion. SIADH is treated with free water restriction (e.g., 1 L/day). In more severe cases, hypertonic saline infusion may be required (noting risk of pontine myelinolysis, if corrected too quickly). Chronic SIADH can be treated with demeclocycline, an ADH inhibitor. CSW is the renal loss of Na+ due to cerebral causes, resulting in hyponatremia, low serum osmolality, and high urine osmolality. The key distinguishing feature between SIADH and CSW is the dehydration/hypovolemia (ECF loss) seen in CSW. Treatment for CSW (a dehydrating and Na+ wasting condition) is hydration with isotonic saline. DI is caused by severe damage to the pituitary, with ADH deficiency resulting in reduced total body water (intracellular plus ECF) and hypernatremia, although ECF status is euvolemic. Dehydration with DI may be severe if fluid intake is not maintained. DI is treated with vasopressin.

A *post-traumatic seizure* may be classified as simple partial (localized with no LOC), complex partial (localized, with +LOC), or generalized/grand mal. The risk is higher with more severe TBIs, with penetrating injury, bleed, foreign bodies, dural tear, compressed skull fracture, or midline shift. Valproic acid or levetiracetam is recommended for prophylaxis for 1 week after moderate-to-severe TBI to prevent seizures. Prophylaxis beyond 1 week is not recommended and can negatively impact neurological function and recovery. Immediate seizures (occurring within 24 hours) are considered to be caused directly by the trauma and are not predictive of having future seizures. Management following TBI associated with an immediate seizure is also 1 week of prophylaxis. The optimal management of early post-traumatic seizures (occurring between post-TBI day 1 and 7) has yet to be established. Typically, patients are treated with anticonvulsants for a period of at least several months. About 25% of persons who have an early post-traumatic seizure will have a subsequent seizure. Late seizures (occurring after day 7 post-TBI) should be managed with long-term anticonvulsants. Carbamazepine is recommended for partial seizures and valproic acid for generalized seizures. These medications are preferred due to their favorable side effect profiles in the setting of TBI. Other commonly used medications include levetiracetam, gabapentin, phenytoin, and lamotrigine. Multiple concomitant antiseizure drugs must be used with caution because of interactions. Phenobarbital use should be avoided. Anticonvulsants are used as long as seizures persist. Tapering off of medication may be considered if seizure-free for at least 2 years. EEGs are often performed prior to cessation of anticonvulsants. Surgical options include vagal nerve stimulation and stereotactic resection of seizure locus.

Paroxysmal autonomic instability with dystonia (PAID) syndrome is a constellation of symptoms consisting of tachycardia, elevated BP, tachypnea, fever, diaphoresis, and dystonia. Treatment includes minimizing stressors (e.g., pain or noise), addressing underlying medical issues and complications (e.g., urinary tract infections [UTIs], wound infections, comorbid conditions), and using cooling blankets. Medications commonly used include NSAIDs, lipophilic beta-blockers, bromocriptine, and amantadine for their effect on the hypothalamus, lioresal for spasticity, and dantrolene for malignant hyperthermia.

Hemodynamic Disorders – Tachycardia and hypertension may be related to catecholamine release and/or deconditioning. Treatment with beta-blockers is an option.

Spasticity – Early and aggressive range of motion therapy is recommended to preserve joint mobility and prevent secondary complications. Use of typical oral antispasticity medications should be avoided due to their side effects. Botulinum toxin is an option for local antispasticity treatment.

Cranial Nerve Injuries – CN I (olfactory) is the most common and is the most commonly missed. All patients with a TBI should be tested for this injury because it can affect eating/nutrition. A third will regain full CN I function; a third will recover some function; while a third will not recover. CN VII (facial) and VIII (vestibulocochlear) are also commonly injured.

REFERENCES

1. Centers for Disease Control and Prevention. Report to Congress on Traumatic Brain Injury in the United States: Epidemiology and Rehabilitation. Atlanta, GA: National Center for Injury Prevention and Control; Division of Unintentional Injury Prevention; 2015.

2. Yokobori S, Bullock R. Pathobiology of primary traumatic brain injury. In: Zasler N, Katz D, Zafonte R, eds. *Brain Injury Medicine: Principles and Practice.* New York, NY: Demos Medical Publishing; 2013:137–147.

3. Brasure M, Lamberty GJ, Sayer NA, et al. *Multidisciplinary Postacute Rehabilitation for Moderate to Severe Traumatic Brain Injury in Adults.* Rockville, MD; 2012.

4. Teasdale G, Jennett B. Assessment of coma and impaired consciousness. A practical scale. *Lancet.* 1974;2(7872):81–84.

5. Hagen C, Malkmus D, Durham P. *Levels of Cognitive Functioning.* Downey, CA: Rancho Los Amigos Hospital; 1972.

6. Nudo R, Dancause N. Neuroscientific basis for occupational and physical therapy interventions. In: Zasler N, Katz D, Zafonte R, eds. *Brain Injury Medicine: Principles and Practice.* New York, NY: Demos Medical Publishing; 2013.

7. Edwards P, Arango M, Balica L, et al. Final results of MRC CRASH, a randomised placebo-controlled trial of intravenous corticosteroid in adults with head injury-outcomes at 6 months. *Lancet*. 2005;365:1957–1959.
8. Sandel ME, Mysiw WJ. The agitated brain injured patient. Part 1: Definitions, differential diagnosis, and assessment. *Arch Phys Med Rehabil*. 1996;77(6):617–623.

SUGGESTED READING

Centers for Disease Control and Prevention. Nonfatal traumatic brain injuries related to sports and recreation activities among persons aged </=19 years–United States, 2001–2009. *Morb Mortal Wkly Rep*. 2011;60(39):1337–1342.

Champion HR, Holcomb JB, Young LA. Injuries from explosions: physics, biophysics, pathology, and required research focus. *J Trauma*. 2009;66(5):1468–1477.

CHAPTER 20

STROKE

EPIDEMIOLOGY AND RISK FACTORS

Stroke is classically characterized as a neurological deficit attributed to an acute focal injury of the central nervous system (CNS) by a vascular cause, including cerebral infarction, intracerebral hemorrhage (ICH), and subarachnoid hemorrhage (SAH) (1). The two major types of stroke are ischemic (87%) and hemorrhagic (13%; 2). Thirty-two percent are embolic, 31% large vessel thrombotic, 20% small vessel thrombotic, 10% ICH, and 3% SAH (2).

Risk factors for stroke are classified as modifiable and non-modifiable. Non-modifiable factors include age, race (African Americans > Whites), and family history. Some modifiable risk factors include HTN, transient ischemic attack (TIA) or prior stroke, heart disease, atrial fibrillation, smoking, hyperlipidemia, carotid disease, DM, hypercoagulable states, substance abuse, and physical inactivity. The risk of stroke is higher for men compared to women in those younger than 75 years of age, but it becomes more common in women at age 75 years and greater. Stroke remains the leading cause of long-term disability in the United States.

SELECTED ISCHEMIC STROKE SYNDROMES

Middle Cerebral Artery

Deficits can include contralateral (c/1) hemiplegia/hypesthesia (face and arm worse than leg), c/1 homonymous hemianopia, and ipsilateral (i/1) gaze preference. With *dominant* hemisphere involvement, receptive aphasia (inferior division of middle cerebral artery [MCA] to Wernicke's area) and/or expressive aphasia (superior division of MCA to Broca's area) can occur. With *nondominant* hemisphere involvement, spatial neglect may be seen. Anosognosia, defined as lack of awareness or insight, is often present (likely to need supervision). *Gerstmann's syndrome* (parietal lobe) consists of dyscalculia, finger agnosia, dysgraphia, and inability to distinguish between right and left side of one's body.

Anterior Cerebral Artery

Deficits can include c/1 hemiplegia/hypesthesia (leg worse than arm; face and hand spared), alien arm/hand syndrome, urinary incontinence, gait apraxia, abulia (lack of will or initiative), perseveration, amnesia, paratonic rigidity *(Gegenhalten,* or variable resistance to passive ROM), and transcortical motor aphasia (with a dominant hemisphere anterior cerebral artery [ACA] lesion).

Posterior Cerebral Artery

Deficits can include c/1 homonymous hemianopia, c/1 hemianes-thesia, c/1 hemiplegia, c/1 hemiataxia, and vertical gaze palsy. *Dom-inant-sided* lesions can lead to amnesia, color anomia, dyslexia without agraphia, and simultagnosia. *Non-dominant-sided* lesions can lead to prosopagnosia (cannot recognize familiar faces). A bilateral (b/1) pos-terior cerebral artery (PCA) stroke can cause *Anton syndrome* (cortical blindness, with denial) or *Balint's syndrome*, which consists of optic ataxia, loss of voluntary but not reflex eye movements, and an inabil-ity to understand visual objects (asimultagnosia). The *central poststroke pain (Déjerine-Roussy or thalamic pain) syndrome* can occur with involve-ment of the thalamogeniculate branch. *Weber's syndrome* (penetrating branches to the midbrain) consists of i/1 cranial nerve III palsy and c/1 limb weakness.

Brainstem

The *lateral medullary (Wallenberg) syndrome* (posterior inferior cerebellar artery) consists of vertigo, nystagmus, dysphagia, dysarthria, dyspho-nia, i/1 Horner's syndrome, i/1 facial pain or numbness, i/1 limb ataxia, and c/1 pain and temporary sensory loss. The *"locked-in" syndrome* (basilar artery) is due to b/1 pontine infarcts affecting the corticospinal and bulbar tracts, but sparing the reticular activating system. Patients are awake and sensate, but paralyzed and unable to speak. Voluntary blinking and vertical gaze may be intact. The *Millard-Gubler syndrome* is a unilateral lesion of the ventrocaudal pons that may involve the basis pontis and the fascicles of cranial nerves VI and VII. Symptoms include c/1 hemiplegia, i/1 lateral rectus palsy, and i/1 peripheral facial paresis.

Lacunar

The more common syndromes include *pure motor hemiplegia* (poste-rior limb internal capsule [IC]), *pure sensory stroke* (thalamus or pari-etal white matter), the *dysarthria-clumsy hand syndrome* (basis pontis), and the *hemiparesis-hemiataxia syndrome* (pons, midbrain, IC, or pari-etal white matter). "Pseudobulbar palsy" is caused by anterior IC and corticobulbar pathway lacunes (loss of volitional bulbar motor control [e.g., dysarthria, dysphagia, dysphonia, and face weakness], but invol-untary motor control of the same muscles is intact, e.g., can yawn or cough). Emotional lability may be seen.

ISCHEMIC STROKE PHARMACOTHERAPY AND INTERVENTION

Guidelines for Acute Stroke Pharmacotherapy

IV *tissue plasminogen activator* (tPA) is indicated for acute ischemic stroke within 3 hours of symptom onset. In 2009 and 2013, the Amer-ican Heart Association (AHA)/American Stroke Association (ASA) guidelines for the administration of tPA following acute stroke were revised to expand the window of treatment from 3 hours to 4.5 hours to give more patients an opportunity to benefit from tPA, albeit with additional exclusion criteria. Intra-arterial fibrinolysis is also considered in a highly selective group of patients with major ischemic strokes of <6 hours duration caused by occlusion of the MCA.

Absolute contraindications for the use of tPA are head CT positive for blood; severe uncontrolled HTN, BP >185/110; head trauma or stroke in the previous 3 months; thrombocytopenia, platelet count <100k; coagulopathy, international normalized ratio (INR) >1.7, or protime (PT) >15 seconds; treatment with therapeutic dose of low-molecular-weight heparin (LMWH), direct thrombin inhibitors or Factor Xa inhibitors within the past 24 hours; and blood sugar <50 or >400. Relative contraindications are age >80 years; mild/improving stroke symptoms; severe stroke/coma; major surgery within the past 14 days; gastrointestinal (GI) or genitourinary (GU) bleed within the past 21 days; seizure at time of stroke onset; myocardial infarction (MI) within the past 3 months; and history of CNS structural lesion, for example, intracranial neoplasm, arteriovenous malformation (AVM), or aneurysm.

Aspirin is recommended within 24 to 48 hours for patients with acute ischemic strokes not receiving thrombolytics or anticoagulation (3). The administration of acetylsalicylic acid (ASA) or other antiplatelet agents as an adjunctive therapy within 24 hours of intravenous thrombolysis is not recommended. Aspirin can be safely used with low-dose SC heparin or LMWH for DVT prophylaxis. Anticoagulation is considered in the appropriate clinical settings. However, it is not recommended within 24 hours after administration of tPA (3).

Elevated BPs may have a protective role initially after a stroke by improving perfusion to the ischemic (but un-infarcted) penumbra. The goal of "permissive hypertension" is to optimize blood flow during this period (4). Per the AHA/ASA guidelines, antihypertensive therapy within the first 24 hours after symptom onset is not recommended unless SBP >220 and/or diastolic BP (DBP) >120 for this reason (3). After this 24-hour period, however, AHA/ASA guidelines recommend that antihypertensive therapy be resumed or started, but an ideal BP goal has not been established (3). The literature (e.g., the PROGRESS trial; 5) generally indicates that tighter BP control after the initial 24-hour period prevents recurrent stroke.

Recommendations for Secondary Prevention

Education on applicable lifestyle and risk factor modifications is critical. For non-cardioembolic cerebral ischemic events, antiplatelet agents including ASA, clopidogrel, or a combination of ASA and diprimadole (Aggrenox) are considered. For cardioembolic cerebral ischemic events, oral anticoagulation with a target INR of 2.5 (range 2.0–3.0) is recommended (3). Novel oral anticoagulants (NOACs) are now available for secondary stroke prophylaxis in appropriate clinical settings. Statins are considered as first-line treatment in secondary stroke prophylaxis, with high-dose statin therapy recommended for select populations based on overall risk profile, and not solely on serum lipid results (6).

The North American Symptomatic Carotid Endarterectomy Trial (NASCET; 7) demonstrated a 6 to 10 times reduction in the long-term risk of stroke following carotid endarterectomy (CEA) versus medical management alone for patients with recent stroke or TIA with extracranial internal carotid artery stenosis of 70% to 99%. The benefit, however, was largely dependent on the skill of the surgeon. CEA for stenosis <70% was not supported. Guidelines for incidentally discovered asymptomatic carotid stenosis are less clear.

Patent foramen ovale (PFO) is relatively common in the general population, but its prevalence is higher in patients with cryptogenic stroke (i.e., stroke with no identifiable cause). Importantly, paradoxical embolism through a PFO should be strongly considered in young patients with cryptogenic stroke. There is no consensus on the optimal management strategy, but treatment options include antiplatelet agents, warfarin, percutaneous device closure, and surgical closure.

POSTACUTE MEDICAL COMPLICATIONS

The major causes of death after stroke are the stroke itself (i.e., recurrent stroke, progressive cerebral edema, and herniation), pneumonia, cardiac disease, and pulmonary embolism (PE). Complications can arise due to the stroke itself or from the ensuing disability or immobility. Complications noted during the postacute stroke rehabilitation period include pneumonia and pulmonary aspiration, falls, urinary incontinence, DVT, musculoskeletal pain, and central poststroke pain. *Urinary incontinence* typically improves but may still be present in 15% to 20% after 6 months (8). Treatment can include timed voiding, fluid intake regulation, and treatment of urinary tract infections (UTIs). *Glenohumeral subluxation,* seen in 30% to 50% of patients, may play a role in poststroke shoulder pain. Arm trough or lapboard use while sitting, stretching of the shoulder depressors/internal rotators, and avoiding pulling on the affected arm during transfers can be key aspects of management during the early rehabilitation phase. Functional electrical stimulation is also frequently used as a treatment. If spasticity becomes severe, a subscapularis phenol/botulinum toxin injection can sometimes be helpful.

MOTOR RECOVERY FOLLOWING STROKE

Twitchell gave the first systematic clinical description of motor recovery following stroke (9). In particular, tone and "stereotypic" movements, characterized by a tight coupling of movement at adjacent joints (later termed "synergy" by Brunnstrom) were noted to develop before isolated voluntary motor control was reestablished. In addition, it was noted that motor control returned proximally before distally and lower limb function recovered earlier and more completely than upper limb function. Full recovery, when it occurred, was usually complete within 12 weeks (Figure 20.1).

THERAPY APPROACHES

Traditional physiotherapeutic approaches (e.g., neurodevelopmental treatment [NDT]/Bobath approach, proprioceptive neuromuscular facilitation [PNF], and the Brunnstrom approach) have been in use for decades and are still commonly used in practice today. Using "hands on" techniques, these approaches focus on stimulating movement when there is weakness/inactivity, inhibiting excessive tone/primitive patterns of movement, and facilitating functional movement patterns. Recent systematic reviews, however, have not shown superiority of these approaches over more "modern" stroke rehabilitation approaches (11). For gait training, these traditional approaches have shown non-superiority to inferiority to techniques such as electromyography (EMG) biofeedback, functional training, and body weight–supported treadmill training (11). The strongest therapy recommendations in the 2016 AHA/ASA Guidelines for Adult Stroke Rehabilitation and Recovery (which is endorsed by the American Academy of Physical Medicine and Rehabilitation [AAPM&R]) are for intensive, repetitive,

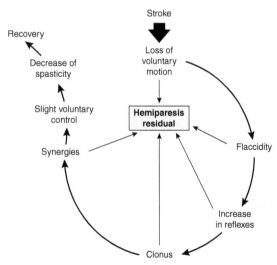

FIGURE 20.1 Stroke recovery pattern, per Cailliet.

Source: Adapted from Ref. (10).

task-specific training; activities of daily living (ADL) and instrumental
activities of daily living (IADL) training tailored to individual needs;
and the implementation of appropriate orthoses and other adaptive
equipment (11). Strengthening exercises complement task-specific
training. *Constraint-induced movement therapy* (CIMT), which forces a
patient to use the affected limb by restraining the unaffected one, and
neuromuscular electrical stimulation (NMES) training use elements of
task-specific training and are generally recommended.

FUNCTIONAL OUTCOMES FOLLOWING STROKE

The prognosis for a stroke survivor, overall, is generally good. Approximately 80% of stroke survivors walk within a year following stroke,
85% recover normal swallowing, 40% are able to return to work, and
90% are able to return home. The *Auckland Stroke Outcomes Study*
showed that of 418 five-year stroke survivors, two thirds had good
functional outcome (defined as a Modified Rankin Scale [MRS] score
<3) (12). The MRS is a commonly used outcomes measure for neu-
rological conditions. It is a 7-point (0–6) ordinal scale, where 0 is no
symptoms; 1 is some symptoms but no significant disability; 2 is a
"slight disability" but independent; 3 is a moderate disability requiring some help, but able to walk independently; 4 is a moderately severe
disability; 5 is a severe disability requiring constant nursing care; and
6 is dead. Nevertheless, in the Auckland Study, 22.5% had cognitive
impairment indicative of dementia, 20% had experienced a recurrent
stroke, almost 15% were institutionalized, and 29.6% had symptoms
suggesting depression (12). Stroke does remain the leading cause of
long-term disability among adults.

Initial stroke recovery is generally the most important factor in
both neurologic and functional recovery. Neurological recovery precedes functional recovery by 2 weeks on average (13). The best neurologic recovery is seen by 11 weeks for 95% of patients; most ADL
recovery (by Barthel Index) is by 12.5 weeks with therapy (13). The
greatest proportion of recovery in ischemic strokes occurs in 3 to 6
months, though a proportion of patients may experience improvement for up to 18 months (14). Prognosticating the recovery of specific neurologic deficits such as weakness, aphasia, dysphagia, sensory
loss, spatial neglect, and hemianopsia is challenging. The time course
and amount of improvement varies, but as a general rule, mild deficits
improve more rapidly and completely than severe deficits.

A number of factors affect outcome after stroke, including age,
stroke locus, stroke type/severity, comorbidities, complications, acute
interventions received (e.g., tPA), and whether an individual received
stroke unit care and rehabilitation. Paolucci et al. reported a better
functional prognosis in stroke survivors with hemorrhagic stroke versus ischemic stroke (15). *The Copenhagen Stroke Studies* have reported
that morbidity/mortality and rehabilitation outcomes are positively
affected by special stroke units (vs. general medical or neurologic

units; 13,16). *A Very Early Rehabilitation Trial (AVERT)*, a phase II randomized controlled trial (RCT), reported that earlier and more intensive mobilization after stroke is both feasible and improves walking and functional recovery (17). A follow-up RCT by the AVERT group, however, reported that a high-dose very early mobilization protocol was associated with reduced odds of a favorable outcome at 3 months (where favorable outcome was defined as MRS <3; 18).

REFERENCES

1. Sacco RL, Kasner SE, Broderick JP, et al. An updated definition of stroke for the 21st century. A statement for healthcare professionals from the American Heart Association/American Stroke Association. *Stroke*. 2013;44:2064–2089.

2. Cuccurullo. *Physical Medicine and Rehabilitation Board Review*. 3rd ed. New York, NY: Demos Medical Publishing; 2015:7.

3. Jauch EC, Saver JL, Adams HP Jr, et al. Guidelines for the early management of patients with acute ischemic stroke: A guideline for healthcare professionals from the American Heart Association/American Stroke Association. *Stroke*. 2013;44:870–947.

4. McManus M, Liebeskind DS. Blood pressure in acute ischemic stroke. *J Clin Neurol*. 2016;12(2):137–146.

5. Arima H, Chalmers J, Woodward M, et al. Lower target blood pressures are safe and effective for the prevention of recurrent stroke: the PROGRESS trial. *J Hypertens*. 2006;24(6):1201–1208.

6. AHA/ASA guidelines. Guidelines for prevention of stroke in patients with stroke or transient ischemic attack: A guideline for healthcare professionals from the American Heart Association/American Stroke Association. *Stroke*. 2014;45(7):2160–236.

7. North American Symptomatic Carotid Endarterectomy Trial Collaborators. Beneficial effect of carotid endarterectomy in symptomatic patients with high-grade carotid stenosis. *N Engl J Med*. 1991;325:445–453.

8. Stein J. *Stroke Recovery and Rehabilitation*. New York, NY: Demos Medical Publishing; 2009.

9. Twitchell TE. The restoration of motor function following hemiplegia in man. *Brain*. 1951;74:443–480.

10. Cailliet R. *The Shoulder in Hemiplegia*. Philadelphia, PA: FA Davis; 1980.

11. Winstein CJ, et al. Guidelines for adult stroke rehabilitation and recovery: A guideline for healthcare professionals from the American Heart Association/American Stroke Association. *Stroke*. 2016;47(6):e98–e169.

12. Feigin VL, Barker-Collo S, Parag V, et al. ASTRO study group. Auckland stroke outcomes study. Part 1: gender, stroke types, ethnicity, and functional outcomes 5 years poststroke. *Neurology*. 2010;75(18):1597–1607.

13. Jorgensen HS. The effect of a stroke unit: reductions in mortality, discharge rate to nursing homes, length of hospital stay, and cost. *Stroke*. 1995;26:1178–1182.

14. Hankey GJ, Spiesser J, Hakimi Z, et al. Rate, degree, and predictors of recovery from disability following ischemic stroke. *Neurology*. 2007;68(19):1583–1587.

15. Paolucci S, Antonucci G, Grasso MG. Functional outcome of ischemic and hemorrhagic stroke patients after inpatient rehabilitation: a matched comparison. *Stroke*. 2003;34:2861–2865.

16. Jorgensen HS. Outcome and time course of recovery in stroke. *Arch Phys Med Rehabil*. 1995;76:406–412.

17. Cumming TB, Thrift AG, Collier JM, et al. Very early mobilization after stroke fast-tracks return to walking: further results from the phase II AVERT randomized controlled trial. *Stroke*. 2011;42(1):153–158.

18. The AVERT Trial Collaboration group: Efficacy and Safety of very early mobilization within 24h of stroke onset (AVERT): Randomised Control Trial. *Lancet*. 2015;386:46–55.

CHAPTER 21

PHYSIOLOGICAL CHANGES WITH AGING

Frailty is an age- and disease-related loss of adaptation. Multiple-organ systems decline and lose functional reserve. Events that caused minor stress earlier in life can later have significant biomedical and social consequences as age-related changes accumulate.

Sarcopenia is an age-related decrease in skeletal muscle mass and function. It is also seen with non-age-related conditions such as disuse or cachexia. With aging, motor unit numbers decrease. Fast-twitch fibers are lost at a greater rate than slow-twitch fibers. There is a general association with increased fat mass and abdominal girth.

Bone is a dynamic tissue that undergoes continual remodeling, with osteoclasts resorbing old bone (that has become weaker/defective due to fatigue damage and microfractures) and osteoblasts forming new bone in its place. With aging, there is a reduction in bone turnover rate, evidenced by a reduction in bone turnover markers. The bone matrix half-life is increased, which increases its exposure to damage and reduces its structural integrity. There is also a disruption in the bone turnover balance with aging, with bone resorption favored over formation. This results in cortical and trabecular thinning, a decline in bone mass, and an increased risk of fractures.

Articular cartilage absorbs compressive loads at joints and withstands shear forces. Its function is derived from the extracellular matrix (ECM). The ECM contains large hydrophilic proteoglycans, which release water when compressed but quickly resorb the water back with pressure release, as well as a superficial lubricating layer of hyaluronic acid and lubricin, which allows for smooth and efficient joint motion. With aging, there is loss of ECM volume and changes in its composition, including the loss and degradation of proteoglycans, increases in collagen cross-links, changes in the superficial lubricating layer, and deposition of calcium crystals. The net biomechanical result is increased stiffness, susceptibility to mechanical failure, and the other clinical manifestations of osteoarthropathy/articular degenerative joint disease (DJD). DJD is a very common manifestation of aging because the ECM is maintained by chrondrocytes, cells that are known to have a low replication rate, which makes them highly susceptible to the accumulation of cellular damage and dysfunction over time.

The **neurologic system** experiences multiple changes with aging. Common age-related anatomical changes include reduced brain size and weight, primarily due to cortical volume loss. There is neuronal loss and loss of synaptic interconnectivity. There is reduced neurotransmitter production. Brain function generally remains stable for most of adulthood, but generally declines after a certain age, which is variable. Short-term memory and new learning are typically affected first. Other changes include slower reaction times, speed of learning, and decreased acuity of the special senses (i.e., vision, hearing, balance, smell, and taste). Age-related visual impairment may be due to decreased lens adaptability and/or an accumulation of age-related conditions such as macular degeneration, cataracts, and glaucoma. Presbycusis is a sensorineural hearing loss caused by aging characterized by a decreased ability to perceive and discriminate sounds, with higher pitched frequencies typically lost first. Some deterioration in central nervous system (CNS) function may be difficult to differentiate from conditions that are common in the elderly, including depression and hypothyroidism. Protective mechanisms against functional loss include redundancy of cells and synaptic connections, synaptogenesis, and neuronogenesis, particularly in the hippocampus and basal ganglia. Physical exercise can be protective against neuronal loss in areas of the brain involved in memory. Alcohol, smoking, and cerebrovascular disease are likely to cause faster/greater neuronal loss, which may have clinical implications, including the risk of early dementia. With aging, the peripheral nervous system may conduct impulses more slowly, causing decreased sensory function, slower reflexes, and clumsiness.

Gait decline is common in older adults. Changes in gait characteristics associated with aging include increased double limb support, slower speed, shorter stride length, flexed posture, and broader base of support. Other factors potentially contributing to gait decline, such as visual impairment, orthostatic hypotension, cardiovascular disease, peripheral arterial disease, Parkinson's disease, cerebellar degeneration, normal pressure hydrocephalus, vertebrobasilar insufficiency, vestibular disorders, myelopathy, peripheral neuropathy, arthropathy, fear of falling, and medication side effects, should be considered and addressed. The Timed Up and Go (TUG) test is a reliable and commonly used screen to assess gait and fall risk. Examinees are timed as they arise from a chair without using the upper limbs, walk 3 meters, turn around, return to the chair, and sit down. A time of 14 seconds or more is considered abnormal and is associated with an increased risk for falls. Examinees demonstrating difficulty performing the TUG should be followed up with a formal physical therapy evaluation. Environmental hazards in the home, such as poor lighting and slippery surfaces, should be addressed. Gait speed has been positively associated with survival in the elderly.

Cardiovascular changes associated with aging include decreased arterial compliance and increased systolic blood pressure. The left ventricle stiffens and hypertrophies. Myocyte numbers decrease. There is a decrease in the intrinsic heart rate. Sinoatrial node conduction time is increased. The tachycardic response to exercise is diminished. Maximal heart rate (HR) decreases by 6 to 10 beats per minute per decade. Maximal oxygen consumption decreases 5% to 15% per decade after the age of 25 years. Decreased baroreceptor sensitivity results in orthostatic hypotension.

Pulmonary changes associated with aging include decreased lung surface area, resulting in diminished gas exchange and ventilation/ perfusion mismatch. Lung compliance increases, thoracic wall mobility decreases, and respiratory muscle strength decreases, resulting in greater residual volume and functional residual capacity.

Gastrointestinal changes associated with aging include decreased basal pepsin and gastric hydrochloric acid production. The latter impairs absorption of vitamin B12, Ca, Fe, Zn, and folic acid. Food intake can decrease due to weakened taste and odor senses, early satiety, prolonged postprandial satiety, and reduced central feeding drive. Hepatic mass and blood flow progressively decrease, which affects drug clearance.

Renal and urological changes associated with aging include decreases in renal mass, nephron number, renal blood flow, glomerular filtration rate (GFR), and bladder distensibility. Despite the decrease in GFR, serum creatinine levels typically remain within normal limits because of the concurrent loss of muscle mass. These normal creatinine levels can be misleading, masking an underlying compromise of renal function. Reduced GFR affects the drug clearance of many agents such as water-soluble antibiotics, water-soluble beta-blockers, digoxin, diuretics, and NSAIDs. The ability to concentrate urine when water deprived is decreased. Urinary incontinence is common, although this is not part of the normal aging process.

Endocrine changes associated with aging include a significant decrease in the reproductive hormones, a mild decrease in many other hormones, and a reduced sensitivity of hormone receptors in the end organs to circulating hormones. Hormones that typically decrease with age include aldosterone, renin, growth hormone, insulin-like growth factor-1, calcitonin, melatonin, prolactin, estrogen, and testosterone. Decreased glucose tolerance is seen due to increased peripheral insulin resistance, as well as some decreased insulin secretion. Cortisol, epinephrine, T3, and T4 levels typically remain unchanged or decrease slightly. Hashimoto's thyroiditis is the most common cause of hypothyroidism in the elderly. Norepinephrine and parathyroid hormone levels may increase with age.

Skin becomes frailer with aging. There is a loss of moisture, blood supply, sensation, and elasticity in connective tissue, as well as thinning of the epidermis, decreased cell replacement, impaired immune response, and wound healing. As a result, the elderly are more prone to skin injury.

SUGGESTED READING

Jones CM, Boelaert K. The endocrinology of ageing: A mini-review. *Gerontology.* 2015;61(4):291–300.

Lotza M, Loeserb RF. Effects of aging on articular cartilage homeostasis. *Bone.* 2012;51(2):241–248.

Mangoni AA, Jackson SHD. Age-related changes in pharmacokinetics and pharmacodynamics: basic principles and practical applications. *Br J Clin Pharmacol.* 2004;57(1):6–14.

CHAPTER 22

RHEUMATOLOGY

OSTEOARTHRITIS

Osteoarthritis (OA), the most prevalent form of arthritis in the United States, is caused by a disruption of the normal process of degradation and synthesis of articular cartilage and subchondral bone (1). Biomechanical and biologic factors are implicated. Age, trauma, obesity, and female gender are among the risk factors; joint involvement is typically asymmetric. Weight-bearing joints are usually involved. In case of an underlying systemic disease or local injury, the cartilage destruction is considered as secondary OA. The pathogenesis of primary OA suggests an intrinsic disease of cartilage in which biochemical and metabolic alterations result in its breakdown. There are several genetic associations of primary OA, and in this type, the small distal joints of the hands may be affected. The pathogenesis primarily affects the cartilage but involves the entire joint, including subchondral bone, ligaments, capsule, synovial membrane, and periarticular muscles. The progression of OA is related to signaling molecules and pro-inflammatory cytokines that induce the production of matrix-degrading enzymes while suppressing matrix synthesis. The focus of research has been mainly on the mechanism of cartilage degradation and treatments to alter this process (2).

Characteristically, pain is worsened by joint use (end of day), and stiffness occurs with inactivity (gelling). Classification criteria exist for OA of the hand, hip, and knee and include various combinations of clinical and radiologic features (2). Generally, evidence of pain at the specified joint, with bony swelling and lack of inflammatory markers (erythrocyte sedimentation rate [ESR] <20, morning stiffness <30 minutes, non-erythematous, and cool to touch) in a patient >50 years, is a consistent feature of the disease. Radiologic confirmation on the basis of joint space narrowing and osteophyte formation can be made.

Nonpharmacologic Management

Strengthening and aerobic exercises (e.g., fitness walking) have been shown in numerous trials to reduce pain and disability while improving quality of life. The Fitness Arthritis and Seniors Trial (FAST) confirmed the beneficial effects of quadriceps strengthening and aerobic exercise in patients with knee OA (3). Felsen reported that a decrease of 2 body mass index (BMI) units (~11.2 lb.) over 10 years in a group of women above median BMI decreased the odds of developing OA by over 50% (4).

To promote self-efficacy, psychological well-being, and improved pain levels, patients should be encouraged to participate in programs such as the Arthritis Foundation Self-Help Course (5). For patients who are poorly tolerant of weight-bearing exercises due to their OA, aquatic exercises may be an alternative. (Swimming, however, may worsen lumbar facet arthritis symptoms.) Physical modalities and judicious rest between sessions may also improve tolerance and compliance with exercises.

A cane held in the hand contralateral to a painful hip can help unload the joint and make ambulation more bearable. For a painful knee, the cane can be held in either hand (6). Knee unloading braces and lateral heel wedges can reduce stress in the medial knee compartment and relieve pain. Environmental adaptations include raising toilet and chair heights.

The American College of Rheumatology (ACR) recommendations for nonpharmacologic management of knee and hip OA include participating in cardiovascular and/or resistance land-based exercise, participating in aquatic exercise, losing weight (if applicable), using walking aids (as needed), and using thermal agents (7).

Pharmacologic Management

In 2012, the ACR updated their pharamacologic recommendations for knee and hip OA (7). Initial options include acetaminophen, oral NSAIDs, tramadol and intra-articular (IA) corticosteroids. NSAIDs are to be avoided with stage IV or V chronic kidney disease; and used selectively with stage III chronic kidney disease, based on risks and benefits. Topical NSAIDs are recommended as an option for initial management of knee OA, particularly for persons aged ≥75 years. Glucosamine, chondroitin sulfate and topical capsaicin are conditionally not recommended. The ACR only recommends opioid analgesics (i.e., stronger than tramadol) for patients who have symptomatic knee or hip OA not adequately responding to both nonpharmacologic and pharmacologic therapies, and who are unable or unwilling to undergo joint replacement. Practitioners are advised to follow American Pain Society/American Academy of Pain Medicine guidelines for chronic nonmalignant pain management (8).

Older reviews generally concluded that IA hyaluronan viscosupplementation is a second line consideration for knee OA after IA corticosteroids (first line). More recent reviews have raised questions about IA hyaluronan's efficacy. In 2014, the OA Research Society International (OARSI) concluded that IA hyaluronan is a treatment of "uncertain" appropriateness (9). In a 2015 meta-analysis, Jevsevar et al. noted that when all trial data (including from improperly designed trials) were reviewed, a bias towards stronger treatment effects was observed. A review of only the high quality studies, however, showed no clinically important differences of hyaluronan treatment over placebo (10).

Alternative and Investigational Treatments

Complementary and alternative medicine treatments abound. Although preliminary studies of glucosamine/chondroitin appeared promising at providing modest short-term symptomatic improvement, a recent National Institutes of Health (NIH)-sponsored multicenter trial (GAIT) did not show benefit in pain, function, or radiologic progression in over 1,500 patients with knee OA (11). Research on the efficacy of acupuncture in OA is likewise promising but qualitatively suboptimal. Other complementary treatments currently under investigation include supplementation with vitamin D and the antioxidant vitamins A, C, E, and coenzyme Q10, and the curcumin–phosphatidylcholine complex.

A recent development in the surgical treatment of knee OA is the UniSpacer, which is FDA approved for isolated, moderate, medial compartment OA. The kidney bean–shaped lightweight metallic alloy device is a self-centering bearing that requires no shaving of bone or screw/cement fixation to the native anatomy. Long-term efficacy is under investigation, though early clinical studies are disappointing, with high revision rates and only modest relief of pain (12).

Greater understanding of chondrocyte biology and the inflammatory mediators of this disease has already led to novel investigational therapeutic targets, known as disease-modifying osteoarthritis drugs (DMOADs), for example, iNOS inhibition, pentosan, and IA administration of autologous conditioned serum. A recent meta-analysis of IA platelet-rich plasma (PRP) for knee OA concluded that IA-PRP is a viable treatment and could potentially lead to symptomatic relief for up to 12 months (13). IA-PRP was noted to offer better symptomatic relief to patients with early degenerative changes. An increased risk of local adverse reactions after multiple PRP injections was noted.

RHEUMATOID ARTHRITIS

Rheumatoid arthritis (RA) is a chronic systemic inflammatory disorder affecting women more than men, with ~1% prevalence in the United States. RA can cause an erosive, polyarticular, typically symmetric synovitis with or without extra-articular manifestations. Extra-articular manifestations are less common than articular manifestations (see Table 22.1; 1,14,15). Classic late physical examination findings include Boutonniere's, swan neck, or mallet finger deformities, joint deformities, Baker's cysts, metacarpophalangeal (MCP) subluxation with ulnar deviation of the fingers, and distal interphalangeal (DIP) joint sparing.

Modified ACR/European League Against Rheumatism (EULAR) classification criteria for the diagnosis of RA were introduced in 2010 and focus on early inflammatory disease parameters, rather than late-stage features (16). As a result, anticitrullinated protein antibody

TABLE 22.1 Common Extra-Articular Manifestations of Rheumatoid Arthritis

Ocular	Keratoconjunctivitis sicca, episcleritis, scleritis
Oral	Sicca (associated with secondary Sjogren's syndrome)
Hematologic	Anemia, Felty's syndrome, thrombocytosis, thrombocytopenia, large granular lymphocyte syndrome, amyloid
Neurologic	Vasculitic neuropathy, cervical myelopathy
Cardiac	Coronary artery disease, pericarditis, myocarditis, valvular disease
Pulmonary	Interstitial lung disease, pleural effusion
Skin	Nodules, cutaneous vasculitis, pyoderma gangrenosum
Renal	Mesangial glomerulonephritis

(ACPA) has been added, as have the acute phase reactants ESR and C-reactive protein (CRP), while the concept of symmetry has been greatly minimized and erosive disease eliminated from the tree algorithm.

RA Management

RA management must include both early pharmacologic therapy and nonpharmacologic interventions. *ROM exercises* and *stretching* should be regularly practiced. *Isometric* strengthening exercises are preferred to minimize joint inflammation. *Splints,* particularly resting wrist–hand splints and knee or hindfoot splints, are helpful in reducing pain and preventing progression of deformity. A dorsal hand orthosis with an ulnar aspect MCP block and individual finger stops can be useful in the setting of ulnar deviation. Education should emphasize *avoidance of overuse* and *joint protection techniques* (e.g., decreasing activity during flare-ups, modifying activities to reduce joint stress, using splints, and maintaining strength).

Current treatment algorithms involve early institution of disease-modifying antirheumatic drugs (DMARDs) and/or biologics/small molecule therapy and allow the primary target for treatment of RA to be a state of remission (17). Although *NSAIDs, COX*-2 inhibitors, and corticosteroids may be helpful symptomatically in mild or early disease, they are currently used only as adjunctive therapy. DMARDs offer symptomatic relief, have been shown to modify disease progression, and are currently the first-line therapy in early RA, being initiated within 3 months of disease onset (18). Examples of currently used DMARDs include methotrexate (MTX), leflunomide, sulfasalazine, and hydroxychloroquine, although MTX is by far the most common and best tolerated.

TABLE 22.2 Biologics

Biologic class	Generic name	Trade name
TNF-a inhibitor	Etanercept	Enbrel
	Infliximab	Remicade
	Adalimumab	Humira
	Certolizumab	Cimzia
	Golimumab	Simponi
CTLA4-Ig	Abatacept	Orencia
B-cell depletion	Rituximab	Rituxan
IL-6 inhibitor	Tocilizumab	Actemra
IL-1 inhibitor	Anakinra	Kineret

CTLA4, cytotoxic T-lymphocyte associated protein 4; IL, interleukin; TNF, tumor necrosis factor.

Biologics

Biologics (Table 22.2) significantly inhibit joint damage and are often used in combination with DMARDs to offer the most efficient suppression of disease. They include the tumor necrosis factor-alpha (TNF-a) inhibitors, B-cell depletion, interleukin (IL)-6 and IL-1 inhibitors, and CTLA4-Ig. Adverse events, though less common, may be life-threatening, and long-term effects are still unclear.

JAK Inhibitors

Janus kinase (JAK) inhibitors are a new subclass DMARD therapy used for RA. Currently the only approved JAK inhibitor is tofacitinib (trade name: Xeljanz). Tofacitinib is a selective JAK 1/JAK3 inhibitor that has been shown to be superior to MTX in achieving disease remission (19). Tofacitinib is an oral medication while the biologics are intravenous or subcutaneous medications.

Arthroscopic *synovectomy* can be performed to reduce joint destruction and relieve symptoms not alleviated by conservative management. Arthroscopic synovectomy is not commonly used in the therapy of RA.

Juvenile Idiopathic Arthritis

Juvenile idiopathic arthritis (JIA) is a common childhood chronic illness, affecting some 70,000 to 100,000 persons younger than 16 years of age in the United States (1,20). There are seven subtypes: systemic, polyarthritis rheumatoid factor (RF) positive, polyarthritis RF negative, oligoarthritis (persistent and extended), enthesitis-related arthritis, psoriatic, and undifferentiated. JIA is discussed in Chapter 8 of this book.

SERONEGATIVE SPONDYLOARTHRITIS

Seronegative spondyloarthropathies (SpA) include ankylosing spondylitis (AS), psoriatic arthritis (PsA), arthritis associated with inflammatory bowel disease, reactive arthritis, and undifferentiated SpA. Shared clinical manifestations include inflammatory back pain (IBP) with inflammation of the sacroiliac (SI) joints and/or the spine, peripheral arthritis, enthesitis, dactylitis, and uveitis (Table 22.3). AS and PsA are discussed here. AS, a chronic inflammatory disease of SI joints and spine, may be associated with extra-spinal lesions of the eye, bowel, and heart. Patients develop progressive stiffening of spine; ankylosis (fusion) occurs in about two-thirds of patients after some years. Risk factors include HLA-B27 and male gender (male-to-female incidence is 2:1; 1). Onset is typically in late adolescence or early adulthood; however, there is an average 8- to 9-year delay in diagnosis from symptom onset. Initial symptoms include pain and stiffness in the buttock or lumbar area, which are worse with inactivity and improve with exercise or hot showers. Bilateral symmetric *sacroiliitis* is a characteristic early x-ray finding. Inflammation of the spine can lead to syndesmophyte formation and then ultimately to a kyphotic bony ankylosis ("*bamboo spine*"). Progression of spinal inflexibility can be followed by Schober's test (1). Extra-articular manifestations include peripheral large joint arthritis, uveitis, cardiac conduction abnormalities, aortic regurgitation, and pulmonary fibrosis of the upper lobes. *Uveitis* typically is painful, anterior, unilateral, and acute. It is associated with redness and photophobia and may progress to blindness.

Treatment includes *spinal extension exercises* (e.g., swimming and push-ups), expansive chest breathing, pectoral and hip flexor stretching, and prone lying. A *hard mattress*, preferably without pillows behind the head, should be recommended. NSAIDs (e.g., naproxen and indomethacin) may reduce pain and symptoms of spinal stiffness. Sulfasalazine is useful in cases of significant peripheral arthritis but

TABLE 22.3 Spectrum of Disease in Spondyloarthropathy

Inflammatory arthropathy	Predominant feature
Ankylosing spondylitis	Axial involvement
Psoriatic arthritis	Psoriasis, nail changes, enthesitis
Inflammatory bowel disease–related arthritis	Ulcerative colitis, Crohn's disease
Reactive arthritis	Conjunctivitis, uveitis, urethritis – postinfection GI/GU
Undifferentiated SpA	Characteristic symptoms without specific features

GI, gastrointestinal; GU, genitourinary; SpA, seronegative spondyloarthropathy.

this and other traditional DMARDs do not impact the spine manifestations. Biologic agents (TNF-*a* inhibitors [21] and the more recently approved drug Secukinumab, an IL-17A inhibitor, should be used for patients with axial manifestations. In the setting of ankylosing spondylitis, hip replacement surgery is often required [22]).

Patients with PsA and skin disease are often referred to as having psoriatic disease, as this has been widely accepted as a systemic illness with many extra-articular and dermatologic manifestations including uveitis and colitis as in AS. The clinical spectrum of PsA is wide because of the different targets of the disease, which include the axial skeleton, peripheral joints, peripheral entheses, and the tenosynovial sheaths (dactylitis), each of which can be involved in isolation. PsA includes the following subtypes: asymmetric oligoarthritis, predominantly DIP involvement (classic), symmetric polyarthritis, sacroiliitis and spondylitis resembling AS, arthritis mutilans with resorption of the phalanges, and enthesitis. PsA can result in significant emotional distress, loss of function, and disability. Lack of available biomarkers responsive to pharmacological intervention impedes the development of potential disease-modifying agents. In the past, PsA was considered a mild disease. In the past 20 years, evidence has accumulated that PsA is erosive and deforming in 40% to 60% of patients with joint damage in the first year of disease. Patients with inflammatory arthritis in typical joint distribution may be diagnosed with PsA if they have a personal or family history of skin psoriasis. Psoriatic disease patients have higher rates of metabolic syndrome, risk of myocardial infarction (MI), and increased BMI than age-matched cohorts without the disease (23). The care of the psoriatic patient must be comprehensive of these systemic manifestations. Treatments include traditional DMARDs, though little evidence of efficacy has been documented; however, TNF alpha inhibitors, anti-IL-17 and anti-IL 12/23 biologic agents are widely in use and effective to treat skin and joint manifestations. In addition, an oral PDE-4 inhibitor is approved as well (Table 22.4; 24).

FIBROMYALGIA

Fibromyalgia (FM) is a disorder of widespread body pain that affects women much more frequently than men. It is characterized by widespread, chronic pain and systemic symptoms (e.g., fatigue, sleep disturbance, and depression). FM patients have a hypersensitivity to pain, thought partially to be due to abnormal afferent nerve processing of the environment and an excess of neurotransmitters that cause increased CNS pain processing. These patients suffer fatigue, sleep abnormalities, and potential cognitive dysfunction. FM may be triggered by environmental factors, infections, physical trauma or injury, or life stressors (e.g., work, family, life-changing events; 25) or may develop spontaneously without an obvious inciting event.

The original ACR criteria (26) include (a) *pain and tenderness lasting for 3 months* or longer (involving bilateral sides, plus above and

TABLE 22.4 Treatments for PsA

	Peripheral arthritis	Skin and nail disease	Axial disease	Dactylitis	Enthesitis
NSAIDs	X		X		
Intra-articular steroids	X				
Topical agents		x			
Physiotherapy			x		
Psoralen UVA/ UVB		x			
Oral DMARDs (MTX, SSA, Lef)	X	x			
Biologic agents	X	x	x	x	x

DMARD, disease-modifying antirheumatic drug; Lef, leflunomide; MTX, metho-trexate; NSAID, nonsteroidal anti-inflammatory drug; PsA, psoriatic arthritis; SSA, sulfasalazine; UVA, ultraviolet A; UVB, ultraviolet B.
Source: Adapted from Ref. (24).

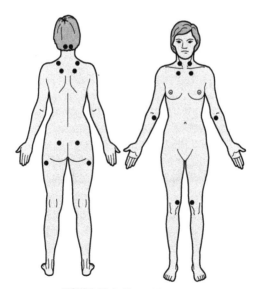

FIGURE 22.1 Fibromyalgia test areas.

below the waist; in addition, axial skeletal pain must be present) and (b) *pain in 11 or more of 18 predetermined tender points on examination* (see the following text), elicited by applying approximately 4 kg/cm pressure (enough to blanch a fingernail). More recently, a non "tender point" diagnostic criterion has been introduced, which underscores the chronic widespread nature of this pain syndrome (27). These revised criteria measure the Widespread Pain Index and the patient's Symptom Severity Score (SSS). The SSS score, with an emphasis on fatigue, nonrestorative sleep patterns, and cognitive abnormalities, is part of the diagnostic tool, but is envisioned to be useful in following the disease longitudinally (Figure 22.1; 27).

New Clinical Fibromyalgia Diagnostic Criteria - Part 1.

To answer the following questions, patients should take into consideration
• how you felt the **past week**,
• while taking your current therapies and treatments, and
• exclude your pain or symptoms from other known illnesses such as arthritis, Lupus, Sjogren's, etc.

Determining Your Widespread Pain Index (WPI)
The WPI Index score from Part 1 is between 0 and 19.

Check each area you have felt pain in over the past week.

☐ Shoulder girdle, left
☐ Shoulder girdle, right
☐ Upper arm, left
☐ Upper arm, right
☐ Lower arm, left
☐ Lower arm, right
☐ Hip (buttock) left
☐ Hip (buttock) right
☐ Upper leg left
☐ Upper leg right
☐ Lower leg left
☐ Lower leg right
☐ Jaw left
☐ Jaw right
☐ Chest
☐ Abdomen
☐ Neck
☐ Upper back
☐ Lower back
☐ None of these areas

Count up the number of areas checked and enter your Widespread Pain Index or WPI score here _____.

Symptom Severity Score (SS score) - Part 2a.

Indicate your level of symptom severity over the *past week* using the following scale.

Fatigue	Waking unrefreshed	Cognitive symptoms
☐ 0 = No problem	☐ 0 = No problem	☐ 0 = No problem
☐ 1 = Slight or mild problems; generally mild or intermittent	☐ 1 = Slight or mild problems; generally mild or intermittent	☐ 1 = Slight or mild problems; generally mild or intermittent
☐ 2 = Moderate; considerable problems; often present and/or at a moderate level	☐ 2 = Moderate; considerable problems; often present and/or at a moderate level	☐ 2 = Moderate; considerable problems; often present and/or at a moderate level
☐ 3 = Severe: pervasive, continuous, life disturbing problems	☐ 3 = Severe: pervasive, continuous, life disturbing problems	☐ 3 = Severe: pervasive, continuous, life disturbing problems

Tally your score for part 2a (not the number of checkmarks) and enter it here _____.

Source: Adapted from Fibromyalgia Network (www.fmnetnews.com).

A multidimensional approach that incorporates nonpharmacologic and pharmacologic therapies is needed for FM. Treatment should include education, sleep management, low-impact aerobic activities, and analgesia. Recently, tai chi has been demonstrated to have a positive effect on pain and function in FM (28). Pharmaceutical options include low-dose tricyclic antidepressants at bedtime, serotonin–norepinephrine reuptake inhibitors (SNRIs), selective serotonin reuptake inhibitors (SSRIs), and NSAIDs; specifically tramadol, pregabalin, duloxetine, and tender point injections are frequently successful. TENS, acupuncture, massage, and relaxation therapy are other options. Any underlying depression should be addressed.

REFERENCES

1. Klippel J, ed. *Primer on the Rheumatic Diseases*. 13th ed. Atlanta, GA: Arthritis Foundation; 2008.

2. American College of Rheumatology. Criteria for Rheumatic Diseases. http://www.rheumatology.org/practice/clinical/classification/index.asp

3. Ettinger WH. A randomized trial comparing aerobic exercise and resistance exercise with a health education program in older adults with knee OA [FAST]. *JAMA*. 1997;277:25–31.

4. Felsen DT, Zhang Y, Anthony JM, et al. Weight loss reduces the risk for symptomatic knee OA in women. The Framingham Study. *Ann Intern Med*. 1992;116:598–599.

5. Arthritis Foundation. Arthritis Foundation Self Help Program. http://www.arthritis.org/self-help-program.php

6. Vargo MM. Contralateral vs. ipsilateral cane use. Effects on muscles crossing the knee joint. *Am J Phys Med Rehabil*. 1992;71:170–176.

7. Hochberg MC, Altman RD, April KT, et al. ACR 2012 Recommendations for the use of nonpharmacologic and pharmacologic therapies in osteoarthritis of the hand, hip, and knee. *Arthritis Care Res*. 2012;64(4):465–474.

8. Chou R, Fanciullo GJ, Fine PG, et al. Clinical guidelines for the use of chronic opioid therapy in chronic noncancer pain. *J Pain*. 2009 Feb;10(2):113–130.

9. McAlindon TE, Bannuru RR, Sullivan MC, et al. OARSI guidelines for the non-surgical management of knee osteoarthritis. *Osteoarthritis Cartilage*. 2014 Mar;22(3):363–388.

10. Jevsevar D, Donnelly P, Brown GA, et al. Viscosupplementation for osteoarthritis of the knee: a systematic review of the evidence. *J Bone Joint Surg Am*. 2015 Dec 16;97(24):2047–2060.

11. Sawitzke AD, Shih H, Finco MF, et al. Clinical efficacy and safety of glucosamine, chondroitin sulphate, their combination, celecoxib or placebo taken to treat osteoarthritis of the knee: 2-year results from GAIT. *Ann Rheum Dis*. 2010;69(8):1459–1464.

12. Bailie AG, Lewis PL, Brumby SA, et al. The Unispacer knee implant: early clinical results. *J Bone Joint Surg Br*. 2008;90(4):446–450.

13. Campbell KA, Saltzman BM, Mascarenhas R, et al. Does intra-articular platelet-rich plasma injection provide clinically superior outcomes compared with other therapies in the treatment of knee osteoarthritis? A systematic review of overlapping meta-analyses. *Arthroscopy*. 2015;31(11):2213–2221.

14. Turesson L, Jacobson L, Bergsstrom U. Extra-articular rheumatoid arthritis: Prevalance and mortality. *Rheumatology*. 1999;38:668–674.

15. Richman NC, Yazdany J, Graf J, et al. Extra-articular manidestations of rheumatoid arthritis in a multiethnic cohort of predmonaintlay hispanic and Asian patients. *Medicine*. 2013;92:92–97.

16. Aletaha D. 2010 rheumatoid arthritis classification criteria. *Arthritis Rheum*. 2010;62:2569–2581.

17. Smolen JS, Aletaha D, Bijlsma JWJ, et al. Treating rheumatoid arthritis to target: recommendation of an international task force. *Ann Rheum Dis*. 2010;69:631–637.

18. Singh JA, Saag KG, Bridges Jr L, et al. American College of Rheumatology guideline for the treatment of rheumatoid arthritis. *Arthritis Care Res*. 2015;68:1–25.

19. He Y, Wong AYS, Chan EW, et al. Efficacy and safety of tofacitinib in the treatment of rheumatoid arthritis: a systematic review and meta-analysis. *BMC Musculoskelet Disord*. 2013;14:298.

20. CDC: Childhood Arthritis. http://www.cdc.gov/arthritis/basics/childhood.htm

21. Gorman JD. Treatment of AS by inhibition of TNF-*a*. *N Engl J Med*. 2002;246:1349–1356.

22. Guan M, Wang J, Zhao L, et al. Management of hip involvement in ankylosing spondylitis. *Clin Rheumatol*. 2013;32(8):1115–1120.

23. Mease, PJ. Psoriatic arthritis: update on pathophysiology, assessment and management. *Ann Rheum Dis*. 2011;70:i77–i84.

24. Miossec, P. Targeting IL-17 and TH17 cells in chronic inflammation. *Nature Rev Drug Discov*. 2012;11;763–776.

25. Mease PJ. Fibromyalgia syndrome: review of clinical presentation, pathogenesis, outcome measures, and treatment. *J Rheumatol*. 2005;32(suppl 75):6–21.

26. Wolfe F, Smythe HA, Yunus MB, et al. The ACR 1990 criteria for the classification of fibromyalgia. *Arthritis Rheum*. 1990;33:160–172.

27. Wolfe F, Clauw DJ, Fitzcharles MA, et al. The American College of Rheumatology preliminary diagnostic criteria for fibromyalgia and measurement of symptom severity. *Arthritis Care Res*. 2010;62:600–610.

28. Wang C. A randomized trial of tai chi for fibromyalgia. *N Engl J Med*. 2010;365:743–754.

SUGGESTED READING

Sulzbacker, I. Osteoarthritis: histology and pathogenesis. *Wien Med Wochenschr*. 2013;163(9):212–219.

CHAPTER 23

OSTEOPOROSIS

Osteoporosis (OP) is a systemic skeletal disease characterized by low bone mass, caused by an imbalance between bone resorption and bone formation. Peak bone mass is reached between 30 and 35 years of age, after which bone remodeling leads to bone loss. The imbalance between resorption and formation causes microarchitectural deterioration of bone tissue, increasing bone fragility. *Risk factors for OP* include age >50 years, female gender, Caucasian race, positive family history, excessive thinness, sedentary lifestyle, immobility (e.g., spinal cord injury), excessive alcohol use, smoking, history of prior fractures, calcium deficiency, decreased estrogen, hyperthyroidism, diabetes, anticonvulsant use, and glucocorticoid use (generally for at least 3 months; 1–3).

Bone mineral density (BMD), measured using dual-energy x-ray absorptiometry (DXA) scan, is a well-established predictor of future fracture risk. BMD is reported using T-scores and Z-scores, which are expressed in standard deviations from the means of reference populations. T-scores use a reference population of young, healthy adults matched for gender. Z-scores use age-, gender-, and ethnicity-matched reference populations. WHO BMD criteria (which use T-scores at the lumbar spine and femoral neck) are recommended for diagnosis of OP in postmenopausal women and men aged ≥50 years (2,3), see Table 23.1.

Besides BMD testing, diagnosis of OP can also be made clinically by history of hip or vertebral fracture during adulthood in the absence of major trauma such as a motor vehicle accident or multistory fall (2,3). WHO BMD criteria should not be used for diagnosing OP in children, premenopausal women, or men aged <50 years. In these groups, the diagnosis of OP should not generally be made by BMD criteria alone, and only Z-scores should be reported, not t-scores (2,3). A Z-score greater than -2.0 is interpreted as within the expected range for age, and a Z-score of -2.0 or below is interpreted as below the expected range for age. Low Z-scores typically alert clinicians to the presence of secondary OP.

TABLE 23.1 WHO Criteria for Diagnosis of OP	
Normal BMD	T-score -1 or greater
Osteopenia	T-score between -1 and -2.5
Osteoporosis	T-score -2.5 or less
Severe osteoporosis	T-score -2.5 or less, with fracture

BMD, bone mineral density.

SCREENING

The National Osteoporosis Foundation (NOF) recommends BMD testing for all women aged ≥65 years and all men aged ≥70 years, regardless of clinical risk factors; as well as for postmenopausal women and men aged 50 to 69 years based on risk factor profile (2,3). Postmenopausal women and men aged ≥50 years who have had an adulthood fracture should also be tested to diagnose and determine the degree of OP (2,3).

SUPPLEMENTS AND PHARMACOTHERAPY

NOF treatment guidelines are recommended for use in all individuals with or at risk for OP, but are primarily directed for use in postmenopausal women and men >50 years of age. Per current NOF guidelines, men aged 50 to 70 years are advised to consume 1,000 mg/day of calcium. Women aged >50 years and men aged >70 years are advised to consume 1,200 mg/day of calcium. Intake of higher amounts of calcium has not been shown to confer additional benefit but may increase the risk of kidney stones, cardiovascular disease, and stroke (2,3). Adults aged >50 years are recommended to consume 800 to 1,000 IU/day of vitamin D (2,3).

Pharmacotherapy is recommended for use in postmenopausal women and men >50 years with any of the following: (a) *t*-score less than -2.5 at the femoral neck, total hip, or lumbar spine; (b) hip/vertebral fracture; (c) *t*-score between -1.0 and -2.5 at the femoral neck, hip, or spine, a 10-year probability of a hip fracture ≥3%, or a 10-year probability of a major OP-related fracture ≥20% (2,3).

Bisphosphonates such as alendronate and risedronate are considered first-line treatment for OP. These can increase the BMD 5% to 10% within the first 2 years of treatment (4), and vertebral fracture risk is reduced by 30% to 50% (5). Use of unopposed estrogen for the treatment of OP fell out of favor when the Women's Health Initiative study found that hormone replacement therapy can increase the risk of cancer, stroke, and venous thromboembolism (4). The goal of selective estrogen receptor modulators (raloxifene) is to maximize the beneficial effect of estrogen on bone while minimizing the deleterious effects on breast and endometrium. Raloxifene has reduced vertebral fracture risk by 36% in large clinical trials (5). *Salmon calcitonin* (100 IU IM/SQ qd) improves BMD and reduces vertebral fracture risk at the lumbar spine, but not at the hip (6). Nasal calcitonin (200 IU qd) has similar benefits, but is not as effective in treating bone pain as the injectable (5). Denosumab (60 mg subcutaneous [SC] q 6 months) is a RANK ligand inhibitor that inhibits osteoclast development and thus mitigates bone resorption. Repeat BMD testing should be performed 1 to 2 years after starting any pharmacologic agent and every 2 years thereafter (2,3).

EXERCISE AND REHABILITATION

The NOF recommends an exercise prevention program, focusing on weight-bearing exercises for a total of 30 minutes 5 to 7 days per week and muscle strengthening 2 to 3 days per week (7). Interventions to reduce the risk and/or impact of falls (e.g., appropriate assistive mobility devices, exercise programs, hip padding, and avoidance of medications affecting the CNS) may reduce hip fracture incidence. Poor back extensor strength has been reported to correlate with a higher incidence of vertebral fractures (8).

Acute vertebral fractures can be painful and are often managed with *bed rest, orthotic immobilization,* and *analgesics* (e.g., narcotics). NSAIDs should be used with caution. Rigid orthoses to limit spinal flexion (e.g., cruciform anterior spinal hyperextension [CASH] and Jewett) may reduce the risk of additional vertebral body fractures. *Postural training, back extensor exercises, pectoral stretching, walking,* or other weight-bearing exercises are the mainstays of rehabilitation.

Percutaneous vertebral augmentation interventions (i.e., vertebroplasty and balloon kyphoplasty) are minimally invasive and have been shown in case series to provide excellent short-term analgesic relief, although long-term benefits with respect to pain or function have only rarely been noted (9). These interventions, which involve the injection of polymethyl methacrylate to provide a rigid vertebral reinforcement, may increase the risk of new vertebral fractures, particularly at adjacent vertebrae (9). Absolute contraindications include discitis, osteomyelitis, and sepsis. Relative contraindications include significant spinal canal compromise due to bone fragments, fractures older than 2 years, >75% collapse of the vertebral body, fractures above T5, and traumatic compression fractures or disruption of the posterior vertebral body wall. In clinical practice, many physicians limit the use of these procedures to fractures that are less than 6 months old. Spine surgery is reserved for rare cases involving neurologic deficits or an unstable spine.

REFERENCES

1. Dawson-Hughes B, Looker AC, Tosteson AN, et al. The potential impact of new National Osteoporosis Foundation guidance on treatment patterns. *Osteoporos Int.* 2010;21:41–52.
2. Cosman F, de Beur SJ, LeBoff MS, et al. Clinician's guide to prevention and treatment of osteoporosis. *Osteoporos Int.* 2014;25(10):2359–2381.
3. Cosman F, de Beur SJ, LeBoff MS, et al. Erratum to: Clinician's guide to prevention and treatment of osteoporosis. *Osteoporos Int.* 2015;26:2045–2047.
4. Sinaki M. Osteoporosis. In Cifu DX, ed. *Braddom's Physical Medicine & Rehabilitation.* 5th ed. Philadelphia, PA: Elsevier, 2016. 747–768.
5. Osteoporosis Prevention, Diagnosis, and Therapy. NIH Consensus Statement March 27–29. 2000;17:1–36.
6. Ahmed SF, Elmantaser M. Secondary osteoporosis. *Endocr Dev.* 2009;16:170–190.

7. Exercise for Your Bone Health. National Osteoporosis Foundation. 2013.

8. Sinaki M. Can strong back extensors prevent vertebral fractures in women with osteoporosis? *Mayo Clin Proc.* 1996;71:951–956.

9. Lamy O, Uebelhart B, Aubry-Rozier B. Risks and benefits of percutaneous vertebroplasty or kyphoplasty in the management of osteoporotic vertebral fractures. *Osteoporos Int.* 2014;25(3):807–819.

SUGGESTED READING

Abramson AS. Influence of weight-bearing and muscle contraction in disuse osteoporosis. *Arch Phys Med Rehabil.* 1961;42:147–151.

International Society for Clinical Densitometry Official Positions. www.iscd.org.

CHAPTER 24

MULTIPLE SCLEROSIS

INTRODUCTION AND EPIDEMIOLOGY (1,2)

Multiple sclerosis (MS) is a chronic inflammatory demyelinating disease of unknown etiology (thought to be immune-mediated) characterized by areas of CNS demyelination that is disseminated in time and space. Prevalence is about 2.5 million people worldwide, and about 400,000 in the United States (2). There is a female-to-male ratio of 2:1, and it is most common in Caucasians. The onset of MS is typically between 20 and 40 years of age, with a mean onset of 30. Incidence and death rates are higher in the northern latitudes, although this differential appears to be decreasing. Significant factors that increase risk of developing MS include population genetics, association between genes and environment, and socioeconomic status. The strongest genetic predictor is HLA-DRB1*1501, which has a two- to fourfold increased risk (2).

DIAGNOSIS AND CLINICAL FEATURES

A clinical attack (relapse or exacerbation) is defined as a subjective (current or historic) *or* objectively observed event (the latter is typical of an acute inflammatory demyelinating event) that lasts 24 hours or more, in the absence of fever or infection. Signs and symptoms will vary, depending on lesion location. Common presenting symptoms include visual, sensory, and motor changes. Common clinical features include paresthesias, weakness, spasticity, fatigue (may be worsened by heat, i.e., Uhthoff's phenomenon), vertigo, bladder dysfunction, sexual dysfunction, cognitive changes, depression, dysphagia, neuropathic pain, and L'hermitte sign (neck flexion causing electric shock sensation down spine/limbs). Diagnosis may be made clinically; however, corroboration with objective testing (e.g., MRI and visual evoked potentials) is recommended.

MS is formally diagnosed using McDonald's criteria (see Table 24.1), which were revised in 2010 for simplification (3). A diagnosis of MS requires demonstration of CNS demyelinating lesions disseminated in space and time, and exclusion of other diagnoses. T2 lesions in at least two of four MS-typical regions (periventricular, juxtacortical, infratentorial, or spinal cord) qualify as dissemination in space (DIS). An additional new lesion not seen on prior imaging, or asymptomatic gadolinium-enhancing and nonenhancing lesions seen on a single scan, qualifies as dissemination in time (DIT). CSF analysis is not required for diagnosis, but may be helpful to rule out other pathologies in equivocal cases. Presence of increased protein and oligoclonal bands (IgG>IgM and IgA) is consistent with MS.

TABLE 24.1 Summary of 2010 Revised McDonald Criteria for Diagnosis of MS

Clinical presentation or signs	Additional requirements for diagnosis
– Two or more attacks – Two or more lesions – One lesion, evidence of prior attack	None; clinical evidence alone will suffice; additional evidence desirable but must be consistent with MS
– Two or more attacks – One lesion	DIS: *or* await a further clinical attack suggesting a different CNS site
– One attack – Two or more lesions	DIT or second clinical attack
– One attack – One lesion	DIS or DIT *or* second clinical attack
Zero (insidious neurological progression)	Disease progression for 1 year (retrospective or prospective) and at least two of the following: 1. DIS (≥1 T2 lesion) in the brain 2. DIS (≥2 T2 lesions) in the spinal cord 3. Positive CSF

Source: Adapted from Ref. (3).

CLINICAL CATEGORIES AND TREATMENT

Clinically isolated syndrome is the first attack compatible with MS (optic neuritis, brainstem syndromes, transverse myelitis), but full diagnostic criteria are not fully met (4). Relapsing-remitting MS (RRMS)—approximately 85% of cases—is defined by acute attacks (<1 per month), followed by spontaneous recovery with little or no residual neurologic deficit.

Due to accumulation of damaged tissue over time (10–20 years), most RRMS patients eventually develop a secondary progressive course (SPMS), which includes remissions and plateaus and gradual worsening with or without relapses. Interferon beta-1b may delay progression of disability in SPMS (e.g., wheelchair dependence).

Primary progressive MS (PPMS)—approximately 10% to 15% of cases—is characterized by an insidious onset with gradual worsening and progressive accumulation of disability. Over 60% present after age 40. Male and female prevalence are equal. For patients with PPMS or SPMS, annual assessments (independent of relapses) are recommended to detect/follow disease progression. Further delineation may include active with or without progression, or not-active with or without progression. Progressive relapsing MS (<5%) is a progressive disease from the onset, with superimposed acute relapses with or without some recovery. IV steroids, which are a mainstay of acute treatment (e.g., methylprednisolone IV 500 mg qd × 5 days or 1 g qd

× 3 days followed by oral prednisone taper), shorten the exacerbation period, but do not change the ultimate extent of recovery.

Disease-modifying therapy (DMT) modulates immune response, with the goal of preventing relapses, slowing brain lesion accumulation, and reducing disease burden. However, DMTs are FDA approved only for relapsing forms of MS (5). The response to DMT, moreover, declines over time. Injectables include interferon beta-1a (Avonex [IM], Rebif [SC]), interferon beta-1b (Betaseron, Extavia), and glatiramer acetate (Copaxone). Orals include fingolimod (Gilenya)—a sphingosine-1-phosphate modulator (monitor for cardiac side effects); teriflunomide (Aubagio)—inhibits T-cell activation and cytokine production (is highly teratogenic); and dimethyl fumarate (Tecfidera)—mechanism of action is unknown, although likely related to nuclear factor Nrf2 (monitor for lymphopenia). Intravenous treatment includes natalizumab (Tysabri)—a monoclonal antibody that targets the VLA-4 cellular adhesion molecule (monitor for PML if administered with IFN beta-1a).

Rehabilitation management includes focus on cognitive impairments, bladder/bowel/sexual dysfunction, visual impairment, spasticity, mobility, balance, pain, and mood (6). Fatigue can be addressed with energy-conservation techniques and/or pharmaceuticals (e.g., amantadine, pemoline, modafinil, and methylphenidate). Weakness may be targeted with physical and occupational therapies. Four-aminopyridine (Ampyra) has been shown to improve walking ability in MS patients as measured by the timed-25-foot walk tests, 6-minute walk test, and 12-item MS walking scale (7,8). Recent randomized controlled trials (RCTs) have produced class II evidence for good tolerability, long-term safety, and efficacy of dalfampiridine with improved walking speed for up to 5 years; the efficacy of the medications were lost after the medications were discontinued (8,9). Exercise, once considered contraindicated in MS, is safe and should be prescribed to maintain health and help delay secondary disability. At least some of the disability associated with MS may be due to deconditioning.

PROGNOSIS

Classically, some factors are reported to have favorable prognosis. For example, presentation with sensory symptoms and optic neuritis are favorable prognostically. Unfavorable factors include pyramidal or brainstem lesions, male gender, and older age at onset. These factors, however, are limited in reliability and accuracy and none has been confirmed as independent prognostic factors. Although commonly accepted that higher lesion load at initial diagnosis correlates with worse prognosis, some studies suggest MRI lesion load does not necessarily correlate to disease burden (10). Bowel and/or bladder impairment correlates with poor prognosis. A relapsing course where there is an incomplete recovery from the first attack, followed by a short interval before the second attack, typically augurs a poorer prognosis

(11). A relapsing course, nevertheless, generally has a better prognosis than a progressive course. Tools including the Kurtzke disability scale, Disability Status Scale (DSS, Expanded-DSS), or Patient-Determined Disease Steps (PDDS) may be used clinically as measures of disability affecting persons with MS.

Fertility is not affected by MS. There are fewer MS exacerbations during pregnancy, but exacerbation risk is increased early postpartum.

REFERENCES

1. Dendrou CA, Fugger L, Friese MA. Immunopathology of multiple sclerosis. *Nat Rev Immunol*. 2015;15:545–558.

2. Tullman MJ. Overview of the epidemiology, diagnosis, and disease progression associated with multiple sclerosis. *Am J Manag Care*. 2013;19:S15–S20.

3. Polman CH, Reingold SC, Banwell B, et al. Diagnostic criteria for multiple sclerosis: 2010 Revision to the McDonald criteria. *Ann Neurol*. 2011;69(2):292–302.

4. Lublin FD, Reingold SC, Cohen JA, et al. Defining the clinical course of multiple sclerosis: the 2013 revision. *Neurology*. 2014;83(3):278–286.

5. Thomas RH, Wakefield RA. Oral disease-modifying therapies for relapsing-remitting multiple sclerosis. *Am J Health Syst. Pharm*. 2015;72(1):25–38.

6. Burks JS, Bigley GK, Hill HH. Rehabilitation challenges in multiple sclerosis. *Ann Indian Acad Neurol*. 2009;12(4):296–306.

7. Goodman AD, Brown TR, Edwards KR, et al. A phase 3 trial of extended release oral dalfampridine in multiple sclerosis. *Ann Neurol*. 2010;68(4):494–502.

8. Filli L, Zörner B, Kapitza S, et al. Monitoring long-term efficacy of fampridine in gait-impaired patients with multiple sclerosis. *Neurology*. 2017;88(9):832–841.

9. Goodman AD, Behoux F, Brown TR, et al. Long-term safety and efficacy of dalfampridine for walking impairment in patients with multiple sclerosis: results of open-label extension of two Phase 3 clinical trials. *Mult Scler*. 2015;21(10):1322–13s31.

10. Li DK, Held U, Petkau J, et al. MRI T2 lesion burden in multiple sclerosis: a plateauing relationship with clinical disability. *Neurology*. 2006;66(9):1384.

11. Langer-Gould A, Popat RA, Huang SM, et al. Clinical and demographic predictors of long-term disability in patients with relapsing-remitting multiple sclerosis: a systematic review. *Arch Neurol*. 2006;63(12):1686–1691.

CHAPTER 25

MOVEMENT DISORDERS

Definition – A group of central nervous system (CNS) degenerative diseases associated with involuntary movements or abnormalities of skeletal muscle tone and posture. They can be broadly classified as hypokinetic (too little) or hyperkinetic (too much) movement disorders.

HYPOKINETIC MOVEMENT DISORDERS (PARKINSON'S DISEASE)

Pathophysiology of Parkinson's Disease (PD; Hypokinetic Movement Disorder) – The predominant area of involvement is the basal ganglia, which are primarily inhibitory in function. Affects the dopamine-producing cells (substantia nigra and locus coeruleus) of the basal ganglia, resulting in degeneration of the nigrostriatal pathway and thereby causing decreased dopamine in the corpus striatum. This results in loss of inhibitory input to the cholinergic system, allowing excessive excitatory output.

Epidemiology – PD is the most common movement disorder, affecting 1% of the population over 50 years of age. Incidence is 20/100,000 per year. Male: female ratio is 3:2. Associated with pesticide and herbicide use; 5% to 10% is hereditary.

Clinical Presentation

- The most common initial symptom is resting tremor (pill-rolling tremor) in the hands, 3 to 5 Hz
- Characterized by a triad of resting tremor, bradykinesia, and cogwheel rigidity
- Features of advanced disease include masked facies, festinating gait (shuffling), and postural instability due to loss of postural reflexes, resulting in fall to side or backward
- Freezing phenomenon (transient inability to perform or restart certain tasks)
- Depression and psychosis
- Dementia (40%)
- Orthostatic hypotension

Treatment – Medical or surgical. The goal of medical treatment is to increase dopamine action and decrease cholinergic effect. A guiding principle is to start treatment when symptoms interfere with performing ADLs.

1. L-dopa: Precursor of dopamine. Given with carbidopa (a dopa decarboxylase inhibitor), which prevents systemic metabolism of L-dopa (e.g., Sinemet)

2. Dopaminergic agonists: Pramipexole (Mirapex, ropinirole (Requip), and rotigotine (Neupro patch), a once-daily transdermal (skin) patch that is changed every 24 hours

   a. Ergot derivatives – Bromocriptine (stimulates D2 receptors) and pergolide (stimulates D1 and D2 receptors)

   b. Non-ergot derivatives (possible neuroprotective) – Ropinirole (Requip) and pramipexole (Mirapex)

3. Amantadine: An antiviral that potentiates release of endogenous dopamine and has mild anticholinergic activity

4. Anticholinergics: Effective in relieving tremor. Includes trihexiphenidyl (Artane), benztropine (Cogentin), procyclidine, and orphenadrine

5. Inhibitors of dopamine metabolism: Inhibits monoamine oxidase (MAO)-B that is predominant in the striatum

   a. Selegiline and Rasagiline – Decrease oxidative damage in substantia nigra and slow disease progression

   b. Tolcapone – Catechol-O-methyltransferase inhibitor, inhibits metabolism of dopamine in the liver, gastrointestinal (GI) tract, and other organs

Surgical treatment is indicated in patients with advanced disease in whom medical treatment is ineffective or poorly tolerated. Mostly effective in relief of tremor. Complications include brain hemorrhage, infection, and device failure.

1. Destructive surgery – Thalamotomy or pallidotomy

2. Deep brain stimulator – Electrode placed into the subthalamic nucleus or ventral intermediate nucleus of the thalamus

Causes for Disability

1. Social isolation

2. Manual dexterity (inability to perform ADLs such as dressing, cutting food, writing, and fine motor skills)

3. Stooped posture, resulting in loss of balance and increased risk of falls

4. Slowness of gait, resulting in retropulsion (staggering backward) or propulsion (stumbling forward)

5. Speech impairment

6. Dysphagia, resulting in silent aspiration

7. Drooling due to decreased frequency of spontaneous swallowing

8. Psychiatric dysfunction: Psychosis can be treated with quetiapine (Seroquel), clozapine (Clozaril), or pimavanserin (Nuplazid), the only FDA-approved medication

Rationale for Rehabilitation – Functionally based, that is, objectively assessed using unified Parkinson's disease rating scale (UPDRS), which includes assessment of walking speed, distance, backward and forward stepping, ability to navigate obstacles, fine motor tasks, equilibrium, and simultaneous and sequential tasks.

Rehabilitation Strategies

Physical therapy

- Posture training (hip extension, pelvic tilt, and standing)
- Postural reflexes
- ROM (passive/active and relaxation techniques)
- Ambulation: Use of walker with wheels. Sometimes may use weighted walker to prevent retropulsion
- Conditioning (quadriceps and hip extensor strengthening)
- Frenkel's exercises for coordination of foot placement
- Wobble board or balance feedback trainers to improve body alignment and postural reflexes
- Fall prevention; home assessment, modification of environment

Occupational therapy

- Adaptive equipment such as plate guards, cups/utensils with large handles, and swivel forks and spoons
- Replace buttons on clothing with Velcro/zipper closures

Other strategies

- Swallow evaluation
- Diaphragmatic breathing exercises to improve dysarthria

HYPERKINETIC MOVEMENT DISORDERS

Include tremors, tics, Tourette's syndrome, dystonia (generalized and focal), dyskinesia, chorea, hemiballismus, myoclonus, and asterixis.

Tremor – Rhythmic oscillation of a body part. Occurs in 6% of the population. Treatment of essential tremor includes propranolol, primidone, benzodiazepines (BZDs; alprazolam), anticonvulsants (gabapentin and topiramate), and Botox.

Tics – Sustained nonrhythmic muscle contractions that are rapid and stereotyped and often occurring in the same extremity or body part during stress.

Tourette's Syndrome – Involuntary use of obscenities (coprolalia) and obscene gestures (copropraxia). Treated using neuroleptics (pimozide and haloperidol).

Dystonia – Slow sustained contractions of muscles, which frequently cause twisting movements or abnormal postures.

- Idiopathic
- Focal (torticollis, blepharospasm, oromandibular dystonia, and writer's cramp)

- Generalized (Wilson's disease and lipid storage disorders)
- Neurodegenerative diseases such as PD and Huntington's disease
- Acquired with perinatal brain injury, CO poisoning, and encephalitis

Treatment includes anticholinergics, baclofen, carbamazepine, clonazepam, and Botox for focal dystonias.

Tardive Dyskinesia – Involuntary choreiform movements of face and tongue such as chewing, sucking, licking, puckering, and smacking due to hypersensitivity of dopamine receptors due to long-term blockade.

- Associated with long-term neuroleptic medication use (20%)
- Decreased since the advent of atypical neuroleptics such as clozapine, risperidone, and olanzapine
- Treatment includes BZDs

Ataxia – Usually associated with cerebellar disease.

- Causes include stroke, multiple sclerosis (MS), acute/chronic alcohol toxicity, and hereditary (slowly progressive) Friedreich's ataxia
- Treatment includes compensatory techniques, gait training, and assistive devices

Athetosis – Slow, writhing, and repetitive movements affecting face and upper extremities, seen in Huntington's disease.

Chorea – Nonstereotyped, unpredictable, jerky movements involving oral structures.

Hemiballismus – Extremely violent flinging of unilateral arm and leg secondary to infarct or bleeding in subthalamic nuclei.

Myoclonus – Sudden jerky irregular contraction of muscle.

- Can be physiological (sleep jerks and hiccups)
- Essential (increasing with activity)
- Epileptic
- Symptomatic (part of underlying encephalopathy or stroke)
- Spinal myoclonus (group of muscles innervated by spinal segments). Occurs in spinal cord disorders such as tumor, trauma, or MS
- Treatment includes clonazepam, valproate, and Keppra

SUGGESTED READING

Cifu DX. *Braddom's Physical Medicine and Rehabilitation.* 5th ed. Philadelphia, PA: Elsevier; 2016.

Cuccurullo SJ. *Physical Medicine and Rehabilitation Board Review.* 3rd ed. New York, NY: Demos Medical Publishing; 2015.

CHAPTER 26

ACUTE INFLAMMATORY DEMYELINATING POLYNEUROPATHY

Acute inflammatory demyelinating polyneuropathy (AIDP, Guillain-Barré syndrome) is an acquired disease of autoimmune etiology characterized by ascending paresthesias and weakness that can progress to total body paralysis, autonomic disturbances, and respiratory failure. *Campylobacter jejuni,* mycoplasma pneumoniae, cytomegalovirus, Epstein-Barr virus, and *Haemophilus influenzae* are pathogens commonly associated with AIDP. The global incidence is about 0.4 to 1.7/100,000; a mild flu-like illness precedes ~60% of cases by 1 to 4 weeks. More than 50% of patients will complain of pain that is initially described as muscular aching; this may transition to neuropathic pain as disease progresses. Extraocular muscles and sphincter function are typically spared. Diagnosis is supported by areflexia, progressive weakness in all limbs, relative symmetry of involvement, cerebrospinal fluid (CSF) cytoalbuminologic dissociation (elevated protein, <10 mononuclear cells/mm³), and electrodiagnostic findings.

The electrodiagnostic findings will depend on which structure is most affected. Most cases of AIDP are demyelinating. As such, the electrodiagnostic tests show prolonged latency, slowed conduction velocity, conduction block, and temporal dispersion. F- waves are useful as they assess long segments of the nerve, and the inflammatory process frequently begins at the nerve roots. Absent or prolonged F-waves are usually the earliest electrodiagnostic findings. If there is an axonal component to the disease, motor unit action potentials may have low amplitudes, and there may be denervation on needle testing.

Patients should be admitted to a monitored bed. Respiratory complications occur in 10% to 30% of patients and may require ventilator support. Tachycardia, urinary retention, hypertension, hypotension, orthostatic hypotension, arrhythmias, ileus, and bradycardia can occur. *Plasmapheresis* or *IV Ig* (400 mg/kg/day × 5 days) given during the evolution of symptoms (within 2 weeks of onset) is effective and has proven to decrease the overall recovery time. Glucocorticoids are *not* effective. Early rehabilitation should emphasize *stretching* and *gradual strengthening*; aggressive therapies may cause overwork weakness. A *tilt table* may be useful in patients with autonomic instability. Prescription of appropriate assistive mobility devices and lower limb orthotics is often indicated. Pain occurs in about 66% of patients. Most patients reach a clinical nadir about 4 weeks after the onset of symptoms, and then improvement begins.

Mortality is about 3% to 5%, usually due to respiratory or cardiovascular causes from autonomic dysfunction. Most patients recover completely or nearly completely. Recovery time can be weeks to months, or up to 6 to 18 months if axonal damage has occurred. About 10% have a pronounced residual disability, most often lower leg weakness and numbness of the feet; ~5% to 10% may suffer one or more recurrences of acute polyneuropathy and some cases may evolve into a chronic, progressive inflammatory polyneuropathy.

CHRONIC INFLAMMATORY DEMYELINATING POLYNEUROPATHY (CIDP)

Chronic inflammatory demyelinating polyneuropathy (CIDP) is pathologically similar to AIDP, but tends to have a slower onset of at least 2 months and may recur multiple times. Weakness is symmetrical, with more distal than proximal muscle involvement. Differentiation between AIDP and CIDP is based primarily on temporal presentation. Treatment is the same as with AIDP, but CIDP patients with both sensory and motor involvement will respond to high-dose corticosteroids (usual regimen is 80 mg prednisone qd, tapered over months to the lowest effective dose). As with AIDP, diagnosis is supported by electrodiagnostics, CSF findings, and nerve biopsy (if indicated).

SUGGESTED READING

Cuccurullo SJ. *Physical Medicine & Rehabilitation Board Review*. 3rd ed. New York, NY: Demos Medical Publishing; 2015.

Victor M. *Adams & Victor's Principles of Neurology*. 7th ed. New York, NY: McGraw Hill; 2001.

Weiss J, Weiss L, Silver J. *Easy EMG*. 2nd ed. London, UK: Elsevier; 2016.

CHAPTER 27

SPASTICITY

Spasticity is a disorder characterized by a velocity-dependent increased resistance to passive stretch, associated with exaggerated tendon jerks, resulting from hyperexcitability of the stretch reflex. Spasticity is part of the *upper motor neuron (UMN) syndrome,* which includes the *positive* symptoms of spasticity and uninhibited flexor reflexes in the lower limbs and the *negative* symptoms of weakness and poor dexterity. It is an important disorder to treat, as spasticity can impair function within and outside of therapy, including positioning, transfers, and hygiene and produce a cycle of symptoms that can make management more complex as depicted in Figure 27.1. Commonly used clinical scales are listed in Table 27.1.

TREATMENT

Indications for treating spasticity include pain, decreased function, poor hygiene, skin breakdown, poor cosmesis, and poor positioning. Potential factors that may be exacerbating spasticity (e.g., pressure ulcers, urinary tract infections [UTIs], bowel impaction, ingrown toenails, and selective serotonin reuptake inhibitors [SSRIs]) should be addressed. Care should be taken before treating any spasticity that

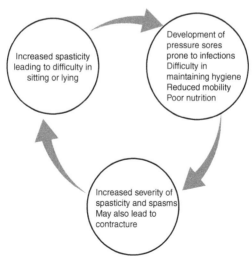

FIGURE 27.1 Vicious cycle of spasticity.
Source: Adapted from Ref. (1).

TABLE 27.1 Commonly Used Clinical Scales

Modified Ashworth Scale

0	No increase in tone
1	Slightly increased tone, with a catch/release or minimal resistance at terminal ROM
1 +	Slightly increased tone, with a catch, followed by minimal resistance throughout the remainder (less than half) of the ROM
2	Increased tone through most of the ROM, but affected part easily moved
3	Considerably increased tone; passive movement difficult
4	Affected part rigid in flexion or extension

Spasm Frequency Score*

0	No spasms
1	Spasms induced by stimulation
2	Infrequent spontaneous spasms (<1/hr)
3	Spontaneous spasms (>1/hr)
4	Spontaneous spasms (>10/hr)

*By subject self-report.
Source: Adapted from Refs. (2,3).

may be utilized functionally (e.g., hypertonia in the lower limbs assisting transfers or gait). One algorithm for treating spasticity may be as per Figure 27.2.

PHYSICAL MODALITIES

A *stretching program* should be the cornerstone for most spasticity treatment programs. *Splints, casting,* or *bracing* can help preserve ROM by "resetting the muscle spindles." Contractures can be reduced by serially casting a joint (i.e., increasing the stretch stepwise for 1 to 2 days at a time), although this technique is not always well tolerated and may lead to skin breakdown. *Cryotherapy* (>15 min) may be helpful transiently by reducing the hyperexcitability of the muscle stretch reflex and reducing nerve conduction velocities. *Functional electrical stimulation* (>15 min) can improve function and reduce tone for hours after the stimulation (thought to be due to neurotransmitter modulation at the spinal cord level). Hippotherapy, which involves rhythmic movements, is found useful in spasticity reduction in lower limbs. Other modalities include application of tendon pressure, cold, warmth, vibration, massage, low-power laser, and acupuncture (5).

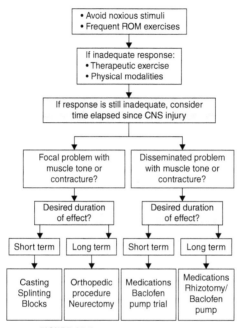

FIGURE 27.2 Algorithm for treating spasticity.
CNS, central nervous system.
Source: Adapted from Ref. (4).

PHARMACEUTICAL OPTIONS

Oral Medications – These may be indicated for *nonfocal* spasticity. Efficacy is often limited by side effects. FDA–approved medications include baclofen, diazepam, dantrolene (*clonidine*), and tizanidine. Off-label use of *gabapentin* has shown promising results in the treatment of spasticity in a small group of multiple sclerosis (MS) patients undergoing a crossover study (6). Cannabinoids have recently been investigated for potential therapeutic efficacy in the treatment of spasticity, especially in MS patients otherwise refractory to treatment (7,8).

Botulinum Toxin-A (BTX-A) – BTX irreversibly blocks neuromuscular junction (NMJ) transmission by inhibiting presynaptic acetylcholine (ACh) release. BTX-A (Figure 27.3; Botox and Allergan) is FDA approved for blepharospasm, strabismus, cervical dystonia, overactive bladder including urinary incontinence caused by detrusor

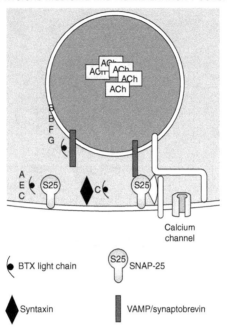

FIGURE 27.3 There are seven distinct BTX subtypes. The BTX heavy chain binds to the presynaptic end plate and the receptor–BTX complex is internalized by endocytosis. The light chain of BTX-A lyses SNAP-25, a protein needed for fusion of ACh vesicles with the presynaptic membrane.

Ach, acetylcholine; BTX, botulinum toxin.
Source: Adapted from Refs. (6,9).

overactivity as in spinal cord injury (SCI) and MS patients, severe glabellar (between the eyebrows) frown lines, chronic migraine, severe axillary hyperhidrosis, upper limb spasticity, and most recently, lower limb spasticity. Prior to the updated FDA approval, BTX-A was widely used for spasticity and myofascial pain with favorable results. Onset of effect is typically 24 to 72 hours. Peak effect is at 2 to 6 weeks. Clinical efficacy is typically up to 3 to 4 months. Recovery is due to axonal sprouting.

The theoretical parenteral median lethal dose (LD50) for a 75-kg adult is 3,000 U; the recommended maximum dose is 10 U/kg IM (up to 400 U) per visit. At least 3 months of interval between sessions is recommended to decrease the potential for antibody formation. BTX-A is contraindicated in pregnancy, lactation, NMJ disease, social and psychological instability, local skin or muscle infection, history of adverse effect, concomitant aminoglycoside use, and for those with human albumin USP allergy. Relative contraindication includes fixed contracture of the joint to be injected (10). BTX-A should be stored at -5°C to -20°C and should be reconstituted with 0.9% preservative-free saline only. It is available for use for up to 4 hours if refrigerated (2°C–8°C).

Advantages of BTX-A over phenol include ready diffusion into the injected area (up to 3 to 4 cm), making injections technically easier, and the absence of dysesthesias (since it is selective for the NMJ; see Table 27.2 for suggested BTX-A dosing).

TABLE 27.2 Suggested BTX-A Dosing (in Units)

Clinical pattern	Potential muscles involved	Avg starting dose	Range, per visit	Injection sites, #
Adducted/ internally rotated shoulder	Pectoralis complex	100	75 to 100	4
	Latissimus dorsi	100	50 to 150	4
	Teres major	50	27 to 75	1
	Subscapularis	50	25 to 75	1
Flexed elbow	Brachioradialis	50	75	1
	Biceps	100	50 to 200	4
	Brachialis	50	25 to 75	2
Pronated forearm	Pronator quadratus	25	10 to 50	1
	Pronator teres	40	25 to 75	1
Flexed wrist	Flexor carpi radialis	50	25 to 100	2
	Flexor carpi ulnaris	40	10 to 50	2
Thumb in palm	Flexor pollicis longus	15	5 to 25	1
	Adductor pollicis	10	5 to 25	1
	Opponens pollicis	10	5 to 25	1
Clenched fist	Flexor digitorum superficialis	50	25 to 75	4
	Flexor digitorum profundus	15	25 to 100	2
Intrinsic-plus hand	Lumbricals interossei	15	10 to 50/ hand	3
Flexed hip	Iliacus	100	50 to 150	2
	Psoas	100	50 to 200	2
	Rectus femoris	100	75 to 200	3

(continued)

TABLE 27.2 Suggested BTX-A Dosing (in Units) *(continued)*

Clinical pattern	Potential muscles involved	Avg starting dose	Range, per visit	Injection sites, #
Flexed knee	Medial hamstrings	100	50 to 150	3
	Gastrocnemius	150	50 to 150	4
	Lateral hamstrings	100	100 to 200	3
Adducted thighs	Adductor brev/long/ magnus	200/leg	75 to 300	6/leg
Extended knee	Quadriceps femoris	100	50 to 200	4
Equinovarus foot	Gastrocnemius medial/ lateral	100	50 to 200	4
	Soleus	75	50 to 100	2
	Tibialis posterior	50	50 to 200	2
	Tibialis anterior	75	50 to 150	3
	Flexor digitorum long/ brevis	75	50 to 100	4
	Flexor hallucis longus	50	25 to 75	2
Striatal toe	Extensor hallucis longus	50	20 to 100	2
Neck	Sternocleidomastoid*	40	15 to 75	2
	Scalenus complex	30	15 to 50	3
	Trapezius	60	50 to 150	3
	Levator scapulae	80	25 to 100	3

*The dose should be reduced by half if both SCMs are being injected.
Dosing guidelines: The recommended maximum dose per visit is 10 U/kg, not to exceed 400 U. The maximum dose per injection site is 50 U. The maximum volume per site is typically 0.5 mL. Reinjection should occur no more frequently than every 3 months. Consider lowering the dosing if patient's Ashworth scores are in the low range, if patient's weight or muscle bulk is low, or if the likely duration of treatment is chronic.
Brev, brevis; BTX-A, botulinum toxin-A; long, longus; SCM, sternocleidomastoid.
Source: Adapted from Ref. (11).

BTX-B (Myobloc) – BTX-B was FDA approved in 2000 for cervical dystonia. Clinically, it is used for similar indications as BTX-A, although the units are markedly different (initially, 2,500 to 5,000 U of BTX-B divided among the affected muscles). BTX-B may be effective in patients who have developed resistance to BTX-A due to repeated use. It may be stored at room temperature for up to 9 months, or 21 months if refrigerated (2°C–8°C). It does not need to be reconstituted, but may be diluted with normal saline, in which case it must be used within 4 hours.

Phenol (Carboxylic Acid) – Phenol destroys nerves in a dose-dependent manner, with onset within 1 hour and a duration that can last years (duration varies widely in the literature). Target nerves are localized with a nerve stimulator and destroyed by direct perineural injection (with subsequent Wallerian degeneration). Alternatively, the motor point area (located by nerve stimulator) can be injected (e.g., 1–10 mL of 3%–5% solution intramuscular [IM]; max: 10 mL of 5%). Recovery with either option occurs by nerve fiber regeneration.

Phenol injections can be combined with BTX injections during a single session, which may be especially useful when there are BTX dosage concerns (i.e., phenol for large, proximal muscles and BTX for smaller, distal muscles). Advantages over BTX include low cost, lack of antibody formation, and longer duration of effect. Disadvantages versus BTX include the greater technical skill involved and potential for dysesthesias, although the latter can be reduced by limiting injections to relatively accessible motor branches of nerves (e.g., pectoral, musculocutaneous, obturator, inferior gluteal, and branches to hamstrings, gastroc-soleus, and tibialis anterior) and avoiding mixed nerve injections (main tibial or median nerve). A trial with a local anesthetic (e.g., marcaine, 0.25%–0.5%) prior to phenol neurolysis can be helpful in predicting the potential effects.

Intrathecal Baclofen (ITB) – ITB is indicated for severe spasticity (Ashworth grade ≥3) due to SCI (FDA approved in 1992) and severe spasticity of cerebral origin (FDA approved in 1996). It is also used with fair-to-good success off-label for severe muscle spasms in chronic back pain and radicular pain. Patients should have a history of poor response to conservative treatments and be older than 4 years or have adequate body weight (>40 lb.). A trial of epidural baclofen or a subarachnoid catheter with external pump is often given before implantation of an internal pump. A screening trial of epidural baclofen might be as follows: 50 µg epidural bolus on day 1; if not efficacious, 75 µg on day 2; if prior doses not successful, 100 µg on day 3. A drop in spasticity of ≈2 Ashworth grades during the trial may roughly predict efficacy of the implanted pump. Patients with no response to the 100 µg dose should not be considered as candidates for chronic ITB infusion according to the FDA (12).

The pump is typically placed in the left lower quadrant of the abdomen (LLQ) to be away from the appendix. The pump is typically refilled every 4 to 12 weeks depending on the dosage being administered and the size of the pump. The patient must be committed to being compliant with seeing the physician for refills of the medication. The battery lasts about 5 years (the pump must be removed to replace the battery). Advantages of ITB include reduced CNS side effects (e.g., sedations) versus oral medications. Potential problems with the implanted system include infection, catheter kinking or dislodgment, and headaches due to CSF leak out of the catheter site. A typical infusion rate for a lumbar pump may be about 600 µg/day. Increased spasticity should be worked up and treated before adjusting the ITB dose.

SURGICAL OPTIONS

Numerous procedures exist, including tendon transfer, tendon/muscle lengthening, and neurosurgical (brain/spinal cord) lesioning (Figure 27.4). The *split anterior tibial tendon transfer (SPLATT; right)* procedure can be an effective treatment for the spastic equinovarus foot. The lateral portion of the split distal anterior tibialis tendon is reattached to the third cuneiform and cuboid bones. *Achilles tendon lengthening* usually accompanies the SPLATT.

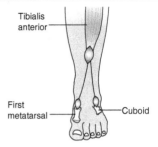

FIGURE 27.4 Tendons in lower leg.
Source: Adapted from Ref. (13).

Selective dorsal rhizotomy may be of some benefit in cerebral palsy (CP). The procedure involves laminectomy and exposure of the cauda equina. The dorsal rootlets are stimulated individually, and rootlets that produce abnormal EMG responses in limb musculature (believed to be contributing to spasticity) are then severed. Anterior rootlet lesions are undesirable as denervation atrophy may follow, with resultant skin breakdown. Favorable selection criteria for rhizotomy include spastic CP (without athetosis), age between 3 and 8 years, heterotopic ossification (HO) prematurity, good truncal balance, and a supportive family.

REFERENCES

1. Ghai A. Spasticity – Pathogenesis, prevention and treatment strategies. *Saudi J Anaesth.* 2013;7(4):453–460.
2. Bohannon RW. Interrater reliability on a modified Ashworth scale of muscle spasticity. *Phys Ther.* 1987;67:206–207.
3. Penn RD. Intrathecal baclofen for severe spasticity. *Ann N Y Acad Sci.* 1988;531:15–66.
4. Katz R. Spasticity. In: O'Young BJ, ed. *Physical Medicine & Rehabilitation Secrets.* 2nd ed. Philadelphia, PA: Hanley & Belfus; 2002:144.
5. Grades JM. Physical modalities other than stretch in spastic hypertonia. *Phys Med Rehabil Clin North Am.* 2001;12:747–768.
6. Cutter NC. Gabapentin effect on spasticity in MS: a placebo-controlled, randomized trial. *Arch Phys Med Rehabil.* 2000;81:164–169.
7. Ashton JC. Emerging treatment options for spasticity in multiple sclerosis–clinical utility of cannabinoids. *Degener Neurol Neuromuscul Dis.* 2011;1:15–23.
8. Chang E. A Review of Spasticity Treatments: Pharmacological and Interventional Approaches. *Crit Rev Phys Rehabil Med.* 2013; 25(1–2): 11–22.
9. Brin MF, ed. *Muscle & Nerve. Spasticity: Etiology, Evaluation, Management, and the Role of BTX-A* (Vol. 6, Suppl). New York, NY: John Wiley & Sons; 1997:S151.

10. Marco O. Botulinum Neurotoxin Type A in Neurology: Update. *Neurol Int*. 2015;7(2):5886.

11. Brin MF. Dosing, administration, and a treatment algorithm for use of BTX-A for adult-onset spasticity. *Muscle Nerve*. 1997;6(Suppl):S214.

12. Lioresal® Intrathecal. Access Data Document. U.S. Food and Drug Administration. http://www.accessdata.fda.gov/drugsatfda_docs/label/2011/020075s021lbl.pdf

13. Keenan MA. *Manual of Orthopaedic Surgery for Spasticity*. Philadelphia, PA: Raven Press; 1993.

CHAPTER 28

NEUROGENIC BLADDER

Neurophysiology – Bladder distension activates detrusor muscle stretch (δ) receptors, which provides feedback to the *sacral micturition center* at spinal segments S2 to S4 via afferent nerves. An intact cerebral cortex, however, inhibits the sacral micturition center and reflex bladder contraction. Furthermore, *sympathetic efferents* (arising from T10 to L2, hypogastric nerve) stimulate fundal δ-receptors (relaxation) and trigonal/bladder neck a-receptors (contraction) via the neurotransmitter norepinephrine, with an overall result of bladder storage without leakage. Bladder filling is typically initially sensed at ≈100 mL. A feeling of fullness is typically appreciated at ≈300 to 400 mL, with urge to void. Voluntary continence is maintained via *somatic efferents* (Onuf's nucleus, S2–S4, pudendal nerve), which innervate the external urethral sphincter (Figure 28.1).

During physiological voiding, the sacral micturition center stimulates detrusor contraction via *parasympathetic fibers* traveling in the pelvic nerves, which release acetylcholine that targets cholinergic (muscarinic M2) receptors in the bladder. The *pontine micturition center* (PMC) coordinates a synergic interaction between the contracting detrusor and a relaxing urethral sphincter, allowing urine to be excreted (Figure 28.2; mnemonic: *s*ympathetic is for *s*torage; *p*arasympathetic is for *p*eeing).

Neurogenic Bladder (Table 28.1) – A *suprapontine* lesion (e.g., traumatic brain injury [TBI] or stroke) compromises cerebral inhibition of the micturition reflex. Clinically, this typically manifests as frequency and incontinence due to detrusor hyperreflexia. Detrusor-sphincter dyssynergia (DSD) is not seen because the PMC's synergic control of the bladder and sphincter is intact. *Treatment* options include timed voids (e.g., toileting q2h), urinary collection devices (e.g., condom catheter), and oral anticholinergics to decrease bladder tone and suppress bladder contractions.

A *suprasacral* (subpontine) spinal cord injury (SCI) disrupts the transmission of cerebral signals inhibiting the micturition reflex, and, importantly, also compromises the Pontine Micturation Center's synergic control of the detrusor and sphincter, resulting in DSD. In DSD, the sphincter does not relax during bladder contraction, causing incomplete (or absence of) voiding despite high bladder contraction pressures. Complications of DSD (due to frequently or persistently elevated bladder pressures) include bladder diverticula, vesicoureteral reflux, hydronephrosis, acute kidney injury, pyelonephritis, or nephrolithiasis. Clinical presentation of these conditions may be atypical in patients with SCI due to sensory impairment. Chronic detrusor hyperactivity results in reflexive bladder contractions with emptying of low bladder volumes, which, over time, can lead to diminished bladder capacity.

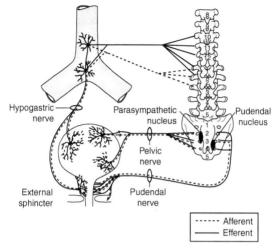

FIGURE 28.1 Bladder innervation.
Source: Adapted from Ref. (1).

There are multiple options for the management of neurogenic bladder in the setting of suprasacral SCI, which should be determined on an individual basis, given anatomical considerations, history of complications, abilities, goals, motivations, and resources. To date, there is a lack of conclusive data in the literature to broadly support one single method over other forms of management. The Consortium for Spinal Cord Medicine's clinical practice guideline on neurogenic bladder management in SCI discusses the indications, advantages, and disadvantages of the various options in detail (3).

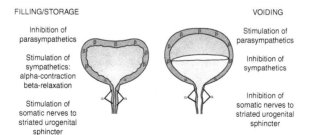

FIGURE 28.2 Bladder filling and emptying.

TABLE 28.1 Classification of Neurogenic Bladder

Type of failure	Bladder factors	Outlet factors
Failurs to store	Hyperactivity	
	Decreased compliance	Denervated pelvic floor
		Bladder neck descent
		Intrinsic bladder neck sphincter failure
Failure to empty	Areflexia	
	Hypocontractility	Detrusor–sphincter dyssynergia (striated sphincter and bladder neck)
		Nonrelaxing voluntary sphincter
		Mechanical obstruction (benign prostatic hypertrophy or stricture)

Source: Adapted from Ref. (2).

Intermittent catheterization (IC) is recommended when an individual has sufficient hand skills or a willing caregiver to perform IC. Body habitus, spasticity, gender, and urethral anatomical abnormalities may be factors that preclude an effective IC program. Alternatives to IC should be considered when bladder capacity is <200 mL or bladder volumes consistently exceed 500 mL despite adjustments in fluid intake or IC frequency. A tendency for autonomic dysreflexia may make IC a less appropriate option. Clean IC (CIC) consists of reusing catheters that are washed with mild soap and water, rinsed thoroughly, air-dried, and stored in a clean, dry towel or bag. Catheters may be reused until brittle or visibly defective (e.g., cracked), or if there is buildup of sediment. Catheters for CIC are generally replaced every 2 to 4 weeks or more often if needed. Sterile IC should be considered if CIC results in recurrent symptomatic infections. Single-use hydrophilic catheters are an option if urethral irritation is suspected to be a cause of recurrent urinary tract infections (UTIs). Touchless catheters are an option if hygienic facilities are unavailable (e.g., during travel or sports activities).

Reflex voiding with a condom catheter is an option in males. This option sometimes requires an endourethral stent, transurethral surgical sphincterotomy, or pharmacological measures (e.g., sphincter botulinum toxin injection or oral alpha-adrenergic blockers [ephedrine or phenylpropanolamine]) to facilitate urine flow.

Indwelling catheters are considered when an individual has poor hand skills, there are limitations in caregiver availability or willingness, when less invasive methods have been unsuccessful, or in the setting of elevated risk of nephric or urologic complications due to persistently elevated detrusor pressures. The primary disadvantages of an indwelling catheter over properly performed IC are increased risks of infection, autonomic dysreflexia, urolithiasis, and bladder neoplasm, as well as lifestyle issues (e.g., wearing a urinary collection bag). Routine irrigation with normal saline or sterile water is not generally recommended due to denuding of the uroepithelium. Indwelling urethral catheters increase the risk for urethral strictures, hypospadias, prostatitis, and epididymitis. Anchoring the catheter to the thigh or abdomen is recommended to minimize urethral erosion. Suprapubic catheters (#22 or #24 Fr size preferred) should be considered in the setting of urethral abnormalities or complications, difficulty with urethral catheterization, recurrent urethral catheter obstruction, psychological considerations (e.g., body image or personal preference), or to improve sexual function. Suprapubic catheters should generally be changed every 4 weeks, or every 1 to 2 weeks in the setting of catheter encrustation or stones.

Other treatment options in the setting of suprasacral SCI aim to enhance storage or to facilitate/enhance emptying. Options to enhance storage include oral anticholinergics (e.g., oxybutynin or tolterodine), intravesical anticholinergics (e.g., capsaicin or resiniferatoxin), intravesical botulinum toxin injection, and bladder augmentation surgery. Options to facilitate/enhance emptying include oral alpha-adrenergic blockers, cutaneous ileovesicostomy, Mitrofanoff appendicovesicostomy (i.e., using the appendix to create a conduit from the bladder to the abdominal skin with a catheterizable stoma, usually at the umbilicus), or neurostimulation with implanted sacral nerve modulators (often combined with posterior sacral rhizotomy). Alpha-adrenergic blockers must be used with care due to the risk of hypotension.

A *sacral or peripheral nerve lesion* can cause detrusor areflexia, which may manifest as retention, with or without overflow incontinence. Treatment options may include Valsalva maneuver, suprapubic pressure (Crede maneuver) or percussion, cholinergic agonists (e.g., bethanechol), which enhance the emptying of a hypotonic bladder, CIC, or indwelling catheter.

The overall goals of treatment for neurogenic bladder are to preserve renal function, avoid high bladder pressures, incontinence, urinary retention, and infections, and optimize lifestyle and social considerations. Regular monitoring of the upper and lower urinary tracts is necessary for guiding management, although there is no consensus, based on the available scientifically rigorous evidence, on the optimal battery of investigations or the frequency of testing. In practice, many centers perform routine monitoring annually. Renal scans, CT scans, and intravenous pyelograms are options to monitor the upper tract. Urodynamics, cystograms, and cystoscopy are used to monitor the lower tract.

REFERENCES

1. Blaivas JG, Management of bladder dysfunction in multiple sclerosis. *Neurology*. 1980;30:12–18.
2. Lance L. Goetz, Adam P, Klausner, Diana D. Cardenas; Neurogenic bladder. In Cifu DX, ed. *Braddom's Physical Medicine and Rehabilitation*. 5th ed. Philadelphia, PA: Elsevier; 2016:427–447.
3. Consortium for Spinal Cord Medicine. Bladder management for adults with spinal cord injury: a clinical practice guideline for health-care providers. *J Spinal Cord Med*. 2006;29(5):527–573.

SUGGESTED READING

Burns AS, Rivas DA, Ditunno JF. The management of neurogenic bladder and sexual dysfunction after spinal cord injury. *Spine*. 2001;26(24 Suppl):S129.

Chiodo AE, Scelza WM, Kirshblum SC, et al. Spinal cord injury medicine. Long-term medical issues and health maintenance. *Arch Phys Med Rehabil*. 2007;88(3 Suppl 1):S76.

McKinley WO, Jackson AB, Cardenas DD, DeVivo MJ. Long-term medical complications after traumatic spinal cord injury: a regional model systems analysis. *Arch Phys Med Rehabil*. 1999;80(11):1402.

Thomas B. Spinal cord injury–Genitourinary system. In Cifu DX, ed. *Braddom's Physical Medicine and Rehabilitation*. 5th ed. Philadelphia, PA: Elsevier; 2016: 1126–1127.

CHAPTER 29

LANGUAGE, SPEECH, AND SWALLOWING

APHASIA

Aphasia is an acquired communication disorder caused by brain damage that impairs an individual's ability to produce and/or understand written and/or spoken language. Ischemic stroke is the most common cause of aphasia (1). Other etiologies include, but are not limited to, hemorrhagic stroke, neoplasm, and central nervous system infections.

Aphasia can be classified as fluent or nonfluent. Individuals with nonfluent aphasia have difficulty producing words, and sentences are lacking in content. In contrast, individuals with fluent aphasia easily produce connected speech and have difficulty understanding the meaning of words. Deficits in nonfluent and fluent aphasia reflect errors in expressive language (repetition skills, naming skills, and writing) and receptive language (oral comprehension and reading comprehension). It is important to remember that an individual's symptoms may not fit into a single aphasia type. Additionally, aphasia symptoms can co-occur with speech impairments such as dysarthria and apraxia of speech (AOS). Table 29.1 summarizes the types of aphasia syndromes, corresponding site of lesions, and associated language characteristics.

Nonfluent Aphasias

Broca's aphasia is associated with damage to "Broca's area or Brodmann's area 44 in the posterior inferior frontal gyrus" (1) of the left hemisphere. Broca's aphasia can be associated with right hemiparesis and oral apraxia (1). Language is agrammatic and often limited to nouns and verbs, and verbal output is limited to short phrases and sentences. Naming is often impaired. Repetition skills may be limited to single words or short phrases. Writing skills are impaired (notable for spelling errors and letter omissions). Auditory comprehension is relatively intact; however, an individual may have difficulty with syntactically complex speech.

Transcortical motor aphasia is associated with lesions in the "anterior cerebral artery and/or the anterior middle cerebral artery watershed that damage the supplementary motor area and/or connections to the frontal perisylvian speech area" (1). Echolalia and perseveration are common (1). Naming, auditory comprehension, and repetition skills remain relatively intact, while reading and writing are deficient.

TABLE 29.1 Types of Aphasia Syndromes

Aphasia syndrome	Site of lesion	Language characteristics
Broca's aphasia	Broca's area. Left, frontal lobe	Nonfluent; impaired naming skills and writing skills; limited repetition; auditory comprehension is good for simple material
Transcortical motor aphasia	Anterior cerebral artery and/or the anterior middle cerebral artery, supplementary motor area	Nonfluent; echolalia; relatively intact naming skills and repetition skills; difficulty initiating speech and completing a thought; auditory comprehension good for conversational interaction; deficits are seen in reading and writing skills
Transcortical mixed aphasia	Anterior and posterior watershed area, multifocal cerebral emboli	Nonfluent; little-to-no spontaneous verbal speech; echolalia; severely impaired auditory comprehension, reading comprehension, and writing skills
Global aphasia	Extensive damage to the language centers in the left hemisphere	Nonfluent; deficits across all modes of communication
Wernicke's aphasia	Posterior superior temporal gyrus of the left hemisphere of the brain.	Fluent; severe anomia with paraphasic errors and neologisms; significantly impaired repetition skills and auditory comprehension
Anomic aphasia	Basal temporal lobe; anterior inferior temporal lobe; temporo-parieto-occipital junction; inferior parietal lobe.	Fluent; notable for circumlocutions; normal utterance length; impaired naming skills, intact repetition skills; auditory comprehension good for everyday conversation; intact oral reading and reading comprehension
Conduction aphasia	Left hemisphere supramarginal gyrus and the arcuate fasciculus	Fluent; phonemic paraphasias and word-finding errors common; repetition skills are impaired; relatively intact auditory comprehension; deficits in writing skills are seen
Transcortical sensory aphasia	Temporal-occipital or parietal-occipital areas	Fluent with paraphasic errors; significantly impaired naming skills; intact repetition skills; impaired reading comprehension

A salient feature of transcortical motor aphasia is difficulty initiating speech and completing a thought (1).

Transcortical mixed aphasia is associated with damage to the "anterior and posterior watershed area or multifocal cerebral emboli" (1). Individuals have little-to-no spontaneous verbal speech and may present with severe echolalia. Auditory comprehension is severely impaired as well as reading, reading comprehension, and writing. Visual field deficits may be present.

Global aphasia is a severe form of nonfluent aphasia with deficits across all modes of communication. It results from extensive damage to the language centers of the left hemisphere. Naming, repetition, and auditory comprehension are significantly impaired. Individuals may respond to intonation of the voice (1). Right-sided hemiparesis and right visual field deficits are common in people with global aphasia.

Fluent Aphasias

Wernicke's aphasia is associated with insults "in the posterior superior temporal gyrus" (1) of the left hemisphere of the brain. Language is notable for severe anomia as evidenced by paraphasic errors and neologisms. In general, an individual with Wernicke's aphasia does not attempt to self-correct or demonstrate awareness of errors. Repetition skills can be significantly impaired as well as auditory comprehension, reading, and writing. Motor deficits are not typically associated with Wernicke's aphasia; however, right visual field deficits may be present (1).

Anomic aphasia is associated with lesions in the "basal temporal lobe, anterior inferior temporal lobe, the temporo-parieto-occipital junction, and the inferior parietal lobe" (2). Individuals with anomic aphasia will typically have normal utterance length; however, circumlocutions may occur. Naming is always impaired, repetition skills are relatively intact, and auditory comprehension is typically functional for everyday conversation. Oral reading and reading comprehension skills are not impaired.

Conduction aphasia is a fluent aphasia often associated with lesions "in the left hemisphere supramarginal gyrus and the arcuate fasciculus" (2). Auditory comprehension is relatively intact. Spontaneous speech is notable for phonemic paraphasias and word-finding errors. Repetition skills are impaired, especially with the repetition of longer words, phrases, and sentences. Individuals are typically aware of errors; however, they have significant difficulty self-correcting. Deficits in writing are seen in most cases of conduction aphasia (1).

Transcortical sensory aphasia is linked with lesions "adjacent to Wernicke's area in the temporal-occipital or parietal occipital areas" (1). Language is fluent and paraphasic errors are typically found. Repetition skills are relatively intact. Individuals are able to read aloud often without comprehension. Naming skills are often significantly impaired.

Subcortical Aphasias

The aforementioned aphasias are associated with damage to the cortical areas of the brain. Subcortical aphasia may be associated with damage to the "basal ganglia, internal capsule and left thalamus" (1). Speech is fluent with relatively intact repetition skills. Auditory comprehension is good for everyday conversation; however, an individual may have difficulty with more complex material. Articulation errors and word-finding problems are common.

Aphasia Prognosis and Treatment

Aphasia outcomes will vary from person to person and are generally influenced by site of lesion and severity of brain injury. "Most improvement occurs within the first few months and plateaus after 1 year" (1). Consulting a speech–language pathologist to assist in recovering linguistic ability and training family members on the use of communication strategies will maximize a person's quality of life and communication success. Table 29.2 provides a description of various behavioral treatments for individuals with aphasia (3).

RIGHT HEMISPHERE DAMAGE

The right hemisphere of the brain is also susceptible to similar types of neuropathology, such as stroke and tumors. Individuals with right hemisphere damage (RHD) typically have little or no difficulty with

TABLE 29.2 Types of Therapy for Aphasia	
Treatment	**Description**
Melodic Intonation Therapy (MIT)	Uses intonation patterns such as melody, rhythm, and stress to increase the length of phrases and sentences. MIT targets improvement in spoken language
Visual Action Therapy	Recommended for individuals with global aphasia. A person is trained to use hand gestures to indicate specific items
Promoting Aphasics' Communication Effectiveness	Designed to improve conversational skills. The clinician and patient take turns sending new information to each other, and the clinician responds to the patient based on whether the patient's message was understood
Oral Reading for Language in Aphasia	Treatment using auditory, visual, and written cues to assist the person with aphasia in reading sentences aloud
Augmentative and Alternative Communication	Involves using picture and symbol communication boards and electronic devices

basic language comprehension and expression. Characteristics of RHD include deficits in organization, reasoning, sequencing, problem solving, attention, and pragmatic skills. Anosognosia (denial of illness) "may occur in up to 40% of individuals with RHD" (2).

Dysarthria

Dysarthria is an impairment of the motor functions necessary for speech production resulting in reduced speech intelligibility. "The articulatory movements of patients suffering from dysarthria are characterized by weakness, reduction in speed, malcoordination, altered muscle tone or by dyskinetic symptoms" (4). Table 29.3 summarizes the dysarthria types, areas of lesion, and speech characteristics.

Spastic dysarthria is linked to lesions of the upper motor neuron (5). The speech characteristics of spastic dysarthria include a strained and harsh voice quality, hypernasality, and slow, monotonous speech. "Spastic dysarthria is the most common type of dysarthria resulting from closed head trauma" (4). Bilateral facial weakness may be present as well as a hyperactive gag (6). Neuromuscular deficits include hypertonia, weakness, and reduced range and speed of movement. Spastic dysarthria can be associated with pseudobulbar palsy, stroke, encephalitis, and spastic cerebral palsy.

TABLE 29.3 Categories of Dysarthria

Type of dysarthria	Site of lesion	Speech characteristics
Spastic dysarthria	Upper motor neuron	Strained and harsh vocal quality; hypernasality; slow, monotonous speech
Hypokinetic dysarthria	Basal ganglia	Reduced loudness; monotone voice; rapid rate of speech; imprecise articulation
Ataxic dysarthria	Cerebellum	Excess and equal stress; monotone pitch; monoloudness; reduced rate of speech; irregular articulatory breakdowns
Flaccid dysarthria	Lower motor neuron	Weak, breathy voice; reduced rate of speech; hypernasality
Hyperkinetic dysarthria	Basal ganglia	Varying impairments in voice quality; interruptions in speech flow; involuntary vocal output
Mixed dysarthria	Variable; upper and lower motor neurons; cerebellar	Harsh vocal quality; monopitch; hypernasality; slow rate of speech

Hypokinetic dysarthria is associated with damage to the basal ganglia (5). Rigidity and reduced range and speed of movement account for the reduced loudness, monotone voice, imprecise articulation, and rapid speech rate, which make up the speech characteristics of hypokinetic dysarthria (5). Individuals with Parkinson's disease will typically present with hypokinetic dysarthria.

Ataxic dysarthria is caused by damage to the cerebellum (5). Ataxic dysarthria is "most commonly the result of inflammatory and degenerative diseases of the cerebellum" (4). Hypotonia and slow and inaccurate movements of the oral musculature lead to a reduced rate of speech. Excess and equal stress, monotone pitch, monoloudness, and irregular articulatory breakdowns are also characteristics of this type of dysarthria (5). Ataxic dysarthria is often linked to stroke, tumors, and alcohol abuse.

Flaccid dysarthria is caused by damage to the lower motor neuron, most frequently due to damage in the brain stem; however, peripheral nerve damage may also lead to symptoms of flaccid dysarthria (4). Neuromuscular deficits including weakness, hypotonia, and fasciculations result in a weak, breathy voice, hypernasality, and a reduced rate of speech (4). Myasthenia gravis and bulbar palsy are associated with flaccid dysarthria.

Hyperkinetic dysarthria is a motor speech disorder associated with damage to the basal ganglia (5). Neuromuscular deficits include "abnormal rhythmic or irregular and unpredictable, rapid or slow involuntary movements" (5) leading to "varying impairments of voice quality, interruptions in speech flow or to involuntary vocal output" (4). Huntington's disease, athetosis, spasmodic dysphonia, tremor, and myoclonus are associated with hyperkinetic dysarthria (5).

The aforementioned dysarthrias reflect damage to a "localized or centralized area of the motor speech system" (5). Mixed dysarthria occurs when there is damage from more than one neurologic event, for example, multiple strokes. The speech characteristics of mixed dysarthria include harsh vocal quality, hypernasality, slow rate of speech, and monopitch (5). Toxic metabolic conditions, infectious processes, tumors of the brain stem, closed head injuries, neurodegenerative diseases, and multiple cerebral infarcts are associated with mixed dysarthria (5).

Treatment of dysarthria may include a combination of medical intervention, behavioral treatment, and prosthetic management (5). Treatment goals include modification of respiratory, phonatory, articulatory, and prosodic problems to improve the naturalness of communication (6).

Apraxia of Speech

Apraxia is impairment in the programming of movements. AOS is impairment in the ability to plan and execute the motor movements responsible for speech. AOS is unrelated to errors of articulation due to musculature weakness and is independent of impairments in language. Speech production errors include sound substitutions and distortions, groping, and struggling with attempts at speech (5). Individuals with AOS present with a slower rate of speech, with difficulty in increasing or changing the rate when requested, impaired intonation, and fluency problems (5). While AOS has been long associated with damage to Broca's area, research also indicates "the lateral premotor cortex (BA6), anterior insula, supplementary motor area, somatosensory cortex, supramarginal gyrus and basal ganglia implicating a distributed neural network underpinning speech production" (7). Etiologies include vascular disturbances, trauma, and tumors. Evaluation of AOS encompasses assessment of apraxic speech symptoms in a natural context (i.e., conversation) and in structured speech tasks (i.e., repetition of words with varying length and syllable complexity).

Oral apraxia is a "disorder of orofacial movements for non-speech gestures" (8). Assessment of oral apraxia involves examination of the oral musculature during volitional, non-speech oral–facial movement. Individuals typically do not have difficulty in natural contexts, such as giving a loved one a kiss; however, they will have difficulty puckering the lips on command.

Treatment of apraxia should be "sequenced to move from more automatic speech to less automatic speech and eventually spontaneous speech" (6). Depending on the severity of symptoms, individuals with apraxia may benefit from using all modalities of communication (verbal expression combined with gestures, writing, or augmentative communication devices).

Neurogenic Stuttering

Neurogenic stuttering is a type of dysfluency associated with neuropathology. Etiologies include stroke, extrapyramidal disease, and drug toxicity. Neurogenic stuttering may be classified as persistent (associated with bilateral brain damage) or transient (associated with multiple lesions of a single hemisphere; 6). Treatment of neurogenic stuttering may involve teaching individuals to reduce their rate of speech, use of delayed auditory feedback, pacing boards, relaxation techniques, and/or biofeedback (6).

Dysphagia

Dysphagia involves impairment in the oral, pharyngeal, and/or esophageal stage of swallowing. The cranial nerves responsible for a functional swallow sequence are the trigeminal (CN V), facial (CN VII), glossopharyngeal (CN IX), vagus (CN X), accessory (CN XI), and hypoglossal (CN XII). Dysphagia in the oral preparatory/oral stages of swallow will manifest itself with pocketing of food/liquid material in the oral cavity; reduced mastication; or reduced management of oral secretions. Symptoms of a pharyngeal-stage dysphagia include reduced management of pharyngeal secretions; immediate or delayed coughing or clearing of the throat before or after the swallow; a wet vocal quality; a delayed or absent swallow reflex; and changes in respiration and/or respiratory rate. Coughing while eating or drinking may be indicative of aspiration (food or liquid falling below the level of the vocal cords and entering the trachea); however, detection of silent aspiration (food or liquid entering the trachea with no immediate signs) may not be evident upon clinical evaluation. Ruling out silent aspiration requires an instrumental swallow study. A diminished or absent gag reflex does not determine a person's ability to safely swallow, and individuals who aspirate may have an intact gag reflex. Individuals may report a globus sensation (feeling of a lump or foreign body in the throat) or endorse episodes of regurgitation during or after meals, chest pain upon swallowing, or an acidic taste in the mouth, which are suggestive of dysphagia related to the esophageal stage of swallow.

Etiologies can be due to adverse neurological events; degenerative disease; infectious processes; metabolic disorders; and myopathic conditions. Structural etiologies such as a cricopharyngeal bar, Zenker's diverticulum, oropharyngeal tumor, or skeletal abnormality are often associated with dysphagia. Trauma to the larynx related to intubation can also manifest itself in difficulty swallowing.

While the most common cause of dysphagia may be neurologic in nature (9), medication-related dysphagia is a known cause. "Drug-induced dysphagia is far more common than reports in medical literature suggest, and it is one of the most readily corrected causes of dysphagia" (10). Symptoms of drug-related dysphagia can be classified as dysphagia as a side effect of the drug, dysphagia as a complication of the drug's therapeutic action, and medication-induced esophageal injury (10).

Dysphagia as a Side Effect of Drugs

Medications that affect the smooth and striated muscles of the esophagus (anticholinergic or antimuscarinic effects) may cause symptoms of dysphagia (10). Ace inhibitors and diuretics can result in xerostomia (dry mouth) impairing the swallow mechanism (10). Antipsychotic or neuroleptic medications may affect swallowing as they can cause xerostomia and movement disorders that impact the muscles of the face, tongue, and pharynx, which are involved in swallowing (10).

Dysphagia as a Complication of Therapeutic Action

Medications that are given to depress the central nervous system (such as narcotics for pain relief or benzodiazepines for antianxiety) may reduce awareness and voluntary control, causing dysphagia (10).

Dysphagia Caused by Esophageal Injury

Medications can cause injury to the esophagus due to irritation. When an inadequate amount of fluid is taken with the medication and it remains in the esophagus too long, damage can occur. "Chemotherapeutic (anti-cancer) preparations may cause muscle wasting or damage to the esophagus and may suppress the immune system making the person susceptible to infection" (10).

A speech–language pathologist will complete a clinical evaluation of swallowing, which consists of obtaining a comprehensive history of an individual's past medical and surgical history, current medications, and symptoms and risk factors for dysphagia. Varying consistencies of food and liquid are administered to establish the presence of dysphagia, evaluate the severity, and determine if modifications in diet will eliminate or reduce dysphagia symptoms. If further assessment of the swallow mechanism is warranted, instrumental testing will then be recommended. An individual's cognitive status, such as alertness level, and awareness of and orientation to feeding should be assessed, as reduced cognition can increase the risk for and consequences of aspiration.

Instrumental Assessment of the Swallow Mechanism

A modified barium swallow (MBS) is a videofluoroscopic exam where an individual ingests barium-impregnated foods and liquids. It allows for visualization of the sequences that make up the oral, pharyngeal, and upper esophageal stages of the swallow. An MBS allows the speech pathologist to assess the type and degree of dysfunction and severity of aspiration.

Fiberoptic Endoscopic Evaluation of Swallowing With Sensory Testing (FEESST) is an exam in which a flexible fiberoptic endoscope is passed transnasally, giving a direct visualization of the laryngeal and pharyngeal structures of the swallow. Sensory testing can be "performed by administering pulses of air at sequentially increased pressures to elicit the laryngeal adductor reflex" (9). Varying consistencies of foods and liquids are administered to assess structure and function of the swallow mechanism. A FEESST provides visualization of secretions and vocal fold pathology that cannot be detected during an MBS. Assessment for the presence of laryngo–pharyngo reflux can be determined.

When there is a concern for esophageal dysphagia, the speech–language pathologist will refer to a gastroenterologist for possible diagnostic imaging (such as a barium swallow or esophagram) for a complete evaluation of the structure and function of the esophagus.

Management and Treatment of Dysphagia

Consideration of food preferences, patient and family wishes regarding oral versus non-oral means of nutrition, and cultural background should be taken into account when developing a treatment plan for dysphagia. Diet or texture modification (e.g., the use of thickened fluids or pureed foods) to improve oral intake and reduce the potential for aspiration may be included in an individual's dysphagia management. For patients with "structural disorders, treatment of the underlying disorder may require surgery (e.g., oropharyngeal tumors) or endoscopic dilation (e.g., esophageal webs or strictures)" (9). Rehabilitation of the disordered swallow mechanism may involve exercises to improve or increase strength and function and/or postural adjustments to improve airway protection. Neuromuscular electrical stimulation is a treatment for dysphagia, which involves eliciting muscular contractions utilizing electrical impulses to improve muscle strength.

Once the treatment plan for dysphagia has been established, families and caregivers should be educated and trained to carry over the specific airway protection strategies and/or changes in diet to reinforce safe swallowing in the home.

REFERENCES

1. Clark DG. Approach to the patient with Aphasia. *UpToDate*. Up to Date. 2014. Web. 23 May 2016.

2. LaPointe, Leonard L. *Aphasia and related neurogenic language disorders*. Thieme, 2005.

3. Aphasia. *American Speech-Language Hearing Association*. Web, 23 May 2016.

4. Schröter-Morasch, Heidrun, and Wolfram Ziegler. "Rehabilitation of impaired speech function (dysarthria, dysglossia)." *GMS current topics in otorhinolaryngology, head and neck surgery* 4 (2005).

5. Duffy JR. *Motor Speech Disorders: Substrates, Differential Diagnosis, and Management*. Elsevier Health Sciences, 2013.

6. Roseberry-McKibbin C, Mahabalagiri NH. *An Advanced Review of Speech-Language Pathology: Preparation for Praxis and Comprehensive Examination*. Austin, TX: PRO-ED, Inc; 2006.

7. Ballard KJ, Tourville JA, Robin DA. Behavioral, computational, and neuroimaging studies of acquired apraxia of speech. *Front Hum Neurosci.* 2014;8:892.

8. Yadegari F, Azimian M, Rahgozar M, Shekarchi B. Brain areas impaired in oral and verbal apraxic patients. *Iran J Neurol.* 2014;13(2):77–82.

9. Lembo AJ. *Oropharyngeal Dysphagia: Clinical Features, Diagnosis, and Management*; 2014.

10. Balzer KM. Drug-induced dysphagia. *Int J MS Care.* 2000;2(1):40–50.

SUGGESTED READING

Hemphill III, JC. Traumatic brain injury: epidemiology, classification, and pathophysiology. *UpToDate*. UpToDate;2012;21.

Watts CR. A retrospective study of long-term treatment outcomes for reduced vocal intensity in hypokinetic dysarthria. *BMC Ear, Nose and Throat Disorders.* 2016;16(1):1.

CHAPTER 30

HETEROTOPIC OSSIFICATION

Heterotopic ossification (HO) is the formation of lamellar bone at an abnormal anatomical site, usually in soft tissue, due to the metaplasia of mesenchymal cells into osteoblasts. Precipitating factors include musculoskeletal trauma (e.g., fracture, burn injury, or joint replacement surgery) and neurological pathology (e.g., spinal cord injury [SCI], stroke, and traumatic brain injury [TBI]). Risk factors for HO include prolonged immobilization and degree of spasticity (1). Reports of incidence in the literature vary, depending on the methodology used and whether clinically silent HO is included. With burn injury, common HO sites include the elbow (the most common site; posterior > anterior), shoulder (adults), and hip (children). HO locations do not necessarily coincide with the area of the burn. Burns involving >20% of the body have a higher risk for HO (1). In SCI and TBI, HO is seen at the hip (anterior > posterior) > knee > elbow > shoulder > feet. With SCI, injuries to the thoracic and cervical spine result in a higher risk of HO (1). Hip HO is commonly seen following total hip arthroplasty (THA). HO may occur at the distal end of amputated limbs. Overall, HO is typically seen around large joints and below levels of neurologic injury.

Symptoms of HO may include edema, pain, and loss of joint mobility (in later stages). If HO is suspected, a plain x-ray or three-phase bone scan may be obtained. The bone scan may be positive at least 1 week before the x-ray is positive; phases 1 and 2 of the bone scan are highly sensitive. Some complications of HO include peripheral nerve entrapment, pressure ulcers, and functional impairment if joint ankylosis develops.

TREATMENT

Resting the acutely involved joint for up to 2 weeks is recommended to reduce inflammation and microscopic hemorrhage (2). Ice may also be helpful. While still an area of controversy, gentle and painless (passive and/or active) ROM exercises are recommended to maintain joint mobility (3). More aggressive ROM may be initiated after the first 2 weeks, but must be curtailed if erythema or swelling increases (2). Immobilization in a functional position is prudent if ankylosis is inevitable.

Medical options include (NSAIDs, e.g., indomethacin, 25 mg po tid × ≥6 weeks) or etidronate (e.g., 20 mg/kg po qd × 2 weeks, then 10 mg/kg po qd × 10 weeks; other regimens exist). NSAIDs inhibit prostaglandin E2, a major contributor of HO formation. Etidronate is thought to reduce further HO formation by reducing osteoblastic/clastic activity and calcium phosphate precipitation (2). Etidronate does not treat HO that has already formed.

Radiation therapy has been used with success to prevent and/or treat HO in post-THA patients, although it is infrequently used (3).

Surgical resection may be indicated to address significant functional limitations. The ideal surgical candidate has no joint pain or swelling; a normal alkaline phosphatase level (which tends to normalize with maturity); and a three-phase bone scan demonstrating mature HO. It is important to ensure that the HO has reached maturity before resection, because resection of immature HO leads to recurrence rates of nearly 100%. Gentle, early (within 48 hours) postoperative ROM is recommended (2).

REFERENCES

1. Ranganathan K, Loder S, Agarwal S, et al. Heterotopic ossification: basic-science principles and clinical correlates. *J Bone Joint Surg Am*. 2015;97(13):1101–1111.

2. Subbarao J. Heterotopic ossification. In: O'Young BJ, Young MA, Steins SA, eds. *Physical Medicine & Rehabilitation Secrets*. 2nd ed. Philadelphia, PA: Hanley & Belfus; 2002:456–459.

3. Shehab D, Elgazzar A, Collier D. Heterotopic ossification. *J Nucl Med*. 2002;43:346–353.

CHAPTER 31

DEEP VENOUS THROMBOSIS

Risk factors for DVT include prior history of venous thromboembolism (VTE), major trauma, immobility, surgery lasting >2 hours, cancer, long-distance travel, paralysis, spinal cord injury (SCI), prolonged hospitalization, smoking, congestive heart failure, central venous access devices, increased estrogen states, pregnancy, brain injury, stroke, obesity, chronic obstructive pulmonary disease, and inherited coagulopathies (1). A majority of DVTs (greater than 90%) occur in the lower limbs. Approximately 25% of distal DVTs do propagate to proximal veins. Most pulmonary embolisms are associated with proximal DVTs of the lower limbs (above the knee). Despite the fact that VTE is recognized to be a common preventable cause of hospital-related death, studies have shown that many hospitalized patients do not receive appropriate preventive care. For instance, Amin et al. (2008) noted that only 33% of inpatients in U.S. hospitals were receiving appropriate VTE prevention (2).

SELECTED PROPHYLAXIS OPTIONS

Low-Dose Unfractionated Heparin (LDUH) – LDUH binds with antithrombin III to inhibit factor IIa (thrombin) and factor Xa (intrinsic clotting pathway).

Low-Molecular-Weight Heparin (LMWH) – Mechanism of action is similar to LDUH, but the reduced binding with plasma proteins results in a longer and more predictable half-life. LMWH is contraindicated in heparin-induced thrombocytopenia (HIT). Enoxaparin (Lovenox), 30 mg subcutaneous (SC) bid or 40 mg qd, is approved by the FDA for s/p total hip arthroplasty (THA); 30 mg bid is approved for s/p total knee arthroplasty (TKA). Dalteparin (Fragmin), 5,000 U SC qd, is approved by the FDA for s/p THA.

Vitamin K antagonists (VKAs or Warfarin) Inhibit the Vitamin K – mediated production of procoagulant factors X, IX, VII, and II (extrinsic pathway) and anticoagulant proteins C and S. There is an initial paradoxical procoagulant effect since proteins C and S are depleted first (thus, initiating therapy with "loading" doses >5 mg qd is not usually recommended). To reverse, for international normalized ratios (INRs) 5 to 9 without significant bleeding, give 1 to 2.5 mg po vitamin K or follow INRs without vitamin K. For INRs >9 without significant bleeding, give 3 to 5 mg po vitamin K and monitor INRs (repeat vitamin K if necessary). For elevated INRs with serious bleeding, give 10 mg vitamin K by slow IV infusion (repeat q12h if necessary) and supplement with plasma or prothrombin complex concentrate.

Fondaparinux (Arixtra), 2.5 mg SC qd, is a heparin derivative that selectively inhibits factor Xa and is approved by the FDA for s/p hip fracture surgery (HFS), THA, and TKA.

Select Direct Oral Anticoagulants (DOACs) – Compared to heparin and warfarin, DOACs provide the advantage of lower bleeding risk (3), less need for laboratory monitoring (due to wider therapeutic windows), and improved pharmacokinetic profiles. However, they are generally contraindicated in settings of prosthetic heart valves, pregnancy, renal impairment, and antiphospholipid syndrome. DOACs are also more expensive than warfarin. *Dabigatran* (Pradaxa) is an active direct thrombin inhibitor, which inhibits clot-bound and circulating thrombin (4). For VTE prophylaxis in surgical patients, dosing is 110 mg given 1 to 4 hours after surgery followed by 220 mg daily for 28 to 35 days (hip replacement) or 10 days (knee replacement). For treatment and secondary prevention of VTE, dosing is 150 mg BID. *Rivaroxaban* (Xarelto) is a direct factor Xa inhibitor, with a half-life of 7 to 17 hours. For VTE prophylaxis in surgical patients, dosing is 10 mg daily for 35 days (hip replacement) or 10 days (knee replacement). For treatment and secondary prevention of VTE, dosing is 15 mg BID with food for 21 days, followed by 20 mg daily with food (5). *Apixaban* (Eliquis) is a factor Xa inhibitor, with a half-life of 5 to 9 hours. For VTE prophylaxis in surgical patients, dosing is 2.5 mg BID for 35 days (hip replacement) or 12 days (knee replacement). For treatment and secondary prevention of VTE, dosing is 10 mg BID for 7 days, followed by 5 mg BID.

Aspirin inhibits platelet aggregation. Low-dose ASA is now a recommended option as a primary thromboprophylactic agent in primary arthroplasty per the ninth edition (2012) of the American College of Chest Physicians (ACCP) clinical practice guideline and multiple recent reviews in the orthopedic literature (e.g., Ogonda L, et al., 2016). ASA was not generally recommended as a thromboprophylactic agent in the eighth edition (2008) of the ACCP clinical practice guideline.

Other – *Hirudins* (e.g., lepirudin, 15 mg SC BID) are direct thrombin inhibitors indicated in the setting of HIT. *Inferior vena cava filters* are used for pulmonary embolism (*not* DVT) prophylaxis.

DVT PROPHYLAXIS IN SELECTED CONDITIONS

Major Orthopedic Surgery (6): THA or TKA – The recommended options are LMWH, fondaparinux, adjusted-dose VKA, dabigatran, rivaroxaban, apixaban, low-dose ASA, or intermittent pneumatic compression device (IPCD).

Hip Fracture Surgery (HFS) – LMWH, fondaparinux, LDUH, adjusted-dose VKA, ASA, or an IPCD. LMWH is the preferred choice for THA, TKA, and HFS. Dual prophylaxis with an antithrombotic agent and an IPCD is recommended during the hospitalization following major orthopedic surgery. Newer generation portable IPCDs that record and report wear compliance are recommended, to be worn 18 hours/day, for both inpatient and outpatient use.

Duration – The recommended duration of prophylaxis after major orthopedic surgery is a minimum of 10 to 14 days, for up to 35 days.

Medical Patients (7) – LMWH, LDUH (BID or TID dosing), or fondaparinux is recommended for acutely ill hospitalized patients at increased risk of thrombosis, with duration of prophylaxis not recommended to extend beyond the period of immobilization or acute hospital stay.

SCI – Mechanical and anticoagulation treatment should be initiated as early as possible, provided there is no active bleeding, coagulopathy, or other contraindication (8). Intermittent pneumatic devices with or without graduated compression stockings plus LMWH are the prophylactic options of choice during the acute care phase following SCI. UH and warfarin are not recommended, unless there is a contraindication for LMWH. Inferior vena cava filters are not recommended for primary prophylaxis. It is not necessary to routinely screen for DVTs with Doppler ultrasonography.

During the rehabilitation phase, the following are all recommended options: LMWH, warfarin, or DOACs. Suggested duration of chemoprophylaxis is based upon American Spinal Injury Association (ASIA) grading:

ASIA A or ASIA B, with other risk factors*	At least 12 weeks
ASIA A or ASIA B, without other risk factors*	At least 8 weeks
ASIA C	Up to 8 weeks
ASIA D	During hospitalization

*Other risk factors = lower limb fracture, cancer, previous DVT, heart failure, obesity, age >70 years

DVT TREATMENT

In the absence of contraindications, initial treatment is typically *IV heparin*. *Warfarin* is usually started within 24 hours of DVT diagnosis, once the heparin is therapeutic. A 5-mg initial dose of warfarin is preferred over a 10-mg dose due to early paradoxical hypercoagulability. Heparin is discontinued when the INR has been ≥2 for 2 consecutive days. Warfarin is typically instituted for 3 to 6 months. For the outpatient treatment of uncomplicated DVT, warfarin can be started with a weight-based, therapeutic-dose LMWH bridge instead of IV heparin (e.g., enoxaparin, 1 mg/kg SC bid, or dalteparin, 200 U/kg SC qd); the LMWH can be discontinued after 5 days and when INR >2 (9). *Thrombolytics* may have a role in patients with extensive proximal DVT and low bleed risk.

The treatment of isolated calf DVT remains controversial. The risks of proximal propagation and life-threatening embolization must be balanced with the generally more benign natural history of isolated calf thrombi and the individual patient's risk factors for propagation and complications from anticoagulation (10).

REFERENCES

1. Snow V, Qaseem A, Barry P, et al. Management of venous thromboembolism: a clinical practice guideline from the American College of Physicians and the American Academy of Family Physicians. *Ann Intern Med.* 2007;146(3):204–210.

2. Amin AN, Stemkowski S, Lin J, Yang G. Preventing venous thromboembolism in US hospitals: are surgical patients receiving appropriate prophylaxis? *Thromb Haemost.* 2008;99(4):796–797.

3. Chai-Adisaksopha C, Hillis C, Isayama T, et al. Mortality outcomes in patients receiving direct oral anticoagulants: a systematic review and meta-analysis of randomized controlled trials. *J Thromb Haemost.* 2015;13:2012.

4. Hauel NH, Nar H, Priepke H, et al. Structure-based design of novel potent nonpeptide thrombin inhibitors. *J Med Chem.* 2002;45:1757.

5. Beyer-Westendorf J, Siegert G. Of men and meals. *J Thromb Haemost.* 2015;13:943.

6. Falck-Ytter Y, Francis CW, Johanson NA, et al. Prevention of VTE in orthopedic surgery patients: Antithrombotic therapy and prevention of thrombosis, 9th ed: American College of Chest Physicians Evidence-Based Clinical Practice Guidelines. *Chest.* 2012;141(2 Suppl):e278S–e325S.

7. Kahn SR, Lim W, Dunn AS, et al. Prevention of VTE in nonsurgical patients: Antithrombotic therapy and prevention of thrombosis, 9th ed: American College of Chest Physicians Evidence-Based Clinical Practice Guidelines. *Chest.* 2012;141(2 Suppl):e195S–e226S.

8. Consortium for Spinal Cord Medicine. *Clinical Practice Guideline. Thromboembolism.* 3rd ed. Washington, DC: Paralyzed Veterans of America; 2016.

9. Levine M. A comparison of home LMWH vs. hospital UH for proximal DVT, *N Engl J Med.* 1996;334:677–681.

10. Kitchen L, Lawrence M, Speicher M, et al. Emergency department management of suspected calf-vein deep venous thrombosis: A diagnostic algorithm. *West J Emerg Med.* 2016;17(4):384–390.

SUGGESTED READING

Ogonda L, Hill J, Doran E, et al. Aspirin for thromboprophylaxis after primary lower limb arthroplasty: early thromboembolic events and 90 day mortality in 11,459 patients. *Bone Joint J.* 2016;98-B(3):341–348.

CHAPTER 32

PRESSURE INJURY

In 1961, Kosiak reported that just 70 mmHg of pressure applied continuously over 2 hours produced moderate histologic changes in rat muscle (1). In 1974, Dinsdale reported that shear can significantly reduce the amount of pressure necessary to disrupt blood flow facilitating the development of pressure injuries (2). From 1992 to 1995, the Agency for Health Care Policy and Research (AHCPR; now Agency for Healthcare Research and Quality [AHRQ]) published landmark guidelines on pressure ulcer prevention and treatment. In 2014, a collaboration between the National Pressure Ulcer Advisory Panel (NPUAP) and other international agencies published a comprehensive clinical practice guideline with 575 evidence-based recommendations (available for purchase at www.npuap.org).

In April 2016, the NPUAP replaced the general term *pressure ulcer* with *pressure injury*, because stage 1 injuries were described as "ulcers" in the prior staging system. A pressure injury is defined by NPUAP as (3):

> localized damage to the skin and/or underlying soft tissue usually over a bony prominence or related to a medical or other device. The injury can present as intact skin or an open ulcer and may be painful. The injury occurs as a result of intense and/or prolonged pressure or pressure in combination with shear. The tolerance of soft tissue for pressure and shear may also be affected by microclimate, nutrition, perfusion, co-morbidities and condition of the soft tissue.

Pressure injury is currently staged according to NPUAP guidelines (now with Arabic numbers instead of Roman numerals) as follows:

Stage 1 Pressure Injury: Non-blanchable erythema of intact skin – Intact skin with a localized area of non-blanchable erythema, which may appear differently in darkly pigmented skin. Presence of blanchable erythema or changes in sensation, temperature, or firmness may precede visual changes. Color changes do not include purple or maroon discoloration; these may indicate deep tissue pressure injury (Figure 32.1A).

Stage 2 Pressure Injury: Partial-thickness skin loss with exposed dermis – Partial-thickness loss of skin with exposed dermis. The wound bed is viable, pink or red, moist, and may also present as an intact or ruptured serum-filled blister. Adipose (fat) is not visible and deeper tissues are not visible. Granulation tissue, slough and eschar are not present. These injuries commonly result from adverse microclimate and shear in the skin over the pelvis and shear in the heel. This stage should not be used to describe moisture associated skin damage (MASD) including incontinence associated dermatitis (IAD), intertriginous dermatitis

(ITD), medical adhesive related skin injury (MARSI), or traumatic wounds (skin tears, burns, abrasions) (Figure 32.1B).

Stage 3 Pressure Injury: Full-thickness skin loss – Full-thickness loss of skin, in which adipose (fat) is visible in the ulcer and granulation tissue and epibole (rolled wound edges) are often present. Slough and/or eschar may be visible. The depth of tissue damage varies by anatomical location; areas of significant adiposity can develop deep

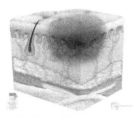

(A) STAGE 1,
Non-blanchable erythema of
intact skin

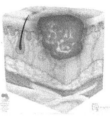

(B) STAGE 2,
Partial-thickness skin loss with
exposed dermis

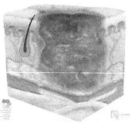

(C) STAGE 3,
Full-thickness skin loss

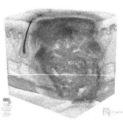

(D) STAGE 4,
Full-thickness skin and tissue loss

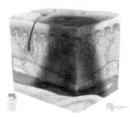

(E) Deep tissue pressure injury

FIGURE 32.1 Stages of a pressure ulcer: (A) Stage 1; (B) Stage 2; (C) Stage 3; and (D) Stage 4. (E) Deep tissue injury. **See the inside back cover for a color version of this figure.**
Source: From Ref. (3), with permission from National Pressure Ulcer Advisory Panel (www.npuap.org).

wounds. Undermining and tunneling may occur. Fascia, muscle, tendon, ligament, cartilage and/or bone are not exposed. If slough or eschar obscures the extent of tissue loss this is an Unstageable Pressure Injury (Figure 32.1C).

Stage 4 Pressure Injury: Full-thickness skin and tissue loss – Full-thickness skin and tissue loss with exposed or directly palpable fascia, muscle, tendon, ligament, cartilage or bone in the ulcer. Slough and/or eschar may be visible. Epibole (rolled edges), undermining and/or tunneling often occur. Depth varies by anatomical location. If slough or eschar obscures the extent of tissue loss this is an Unstageable Pressure Injury (Figure 32.1D).

Unstageable Pressure Injury: Obscured full-thickness skin and tissue loss – Full-thickness skin and tissue loss in which the extent of tissue damage within the ulcer cannot be confirmed because it is obscured by slough or eschar. If slough or eschar is removed, a Stage 3 or Stage 4 pressure injury will be revealed. Stable eschar (i.e., dry, adherent, intact without erythema or fluctuance) on the heel or ischemic limb should not be softened or removed.

Deep Tissue Pressure Injury: Persistent non-blanchable deep red, maroon or purple discoloration – Intact or non-intact skin with localized area of persistent non-blanchable deep red, maroon, purple discoloration or epidermal separation revealing a dark wound bed or blood filled blister. Pain and temperature change often precede skin color changes. Discoloration may appear differently in darkly pigmented skin. This injury results from intense and/or prolonged pressure and shear forces at the bone-muscle interface. The wound may evolve rapidly to reveal the actual extent of tissue injury, or may resolve without tissue loss. If necrotic tissue, subcutaneous tissue, granulation tissue, fascia, muscle or other underlying structures are visible, this indicates a full thickness pressure injury (Unstageable, Stage 3 or Stage 4). Do not use DTPI to describe vascular, traumatic, neuropathic, or dermatologic conditions (Figure 32.1E).

Additional pressure injury definitions:

Medical Device Related Pressure Injury – This describes an etiology. Medical device related pressure injuries result from the use of devices designed and applied for diagnostic or therapeutic purposes. The resultant pressure injury generally conforms to the pattern or shape of the device. The injury should be staged using the staging system.

Mucosal Membrane Pressure Injury – Mucosal membrane pressure injury is found on mucous membranes with a history of a medical device in use at the location of the injury. Due to the anatomy of the tissue these injuries cannot be staged.

PREVENTION AND TREATMENT

Pressure injury prevention should include appropriate seating/bed equipment, proper positioning, education about pressure relief (e.g., weight shifting every 15–20 min for ≥30 sec while sitting; turning in bed q2 hr), and proper skin monitoring. Other issues that may need to be addressed include nutrition, tissue perfusion, oxygenation, local body heat management, and skin moisture management.

Treatment of pressure injuries includes pressure relief, addressing other etiologic factors, treatment of infections, debridement of necrotic tissue (sharp, mechanical, enzymatic, or autolytic), regular wound cleansing, and use of appropriate wound dressings. A trial of topical antibiotics (e.g., silver sulfadiazine) may be helpful in wounds not healing with optimal debridement and cleansing. Wound cultures are *not* generally thought to be helpful because most wounds are colonized with bacteria. Systemic antibiotics should be reserved for cases with evidence of osteomyelitis, infectious cellulitis, or systemic infection.

Modalities such as electrical stimulation (ES), ultrasound (US), ultraviolet (UV) light, laser radiation, and hyperbaric O_2 have been utilized clinically to accelerate wound repair. ES has been shown to have beneficial effects in various phases of acute and chronic wound healing. ES may reduce infection, improve cellular immunity, increase perfusion, and accelerate cutaneous wound healing (4,5). US may facilitate healing through cavitation and microstreaming. Cavitation is the production and vibration of tiny, micron-sized bubbles within underlying soft tissues. Applying pressure to these bubbles is thought to produce cellular changes. US also concurrently produces microstreaming, which is the movement of underlying fluid due to mechanical pressure. These properties of US in combination can produce cellular activity alterations, which may be capable of facilitating wound healing (5). US may also be used to assess and visualize wound beds. More recently, low-intensity vibration (LIV) at various frequencies and amplitudes has also been employed for wound healing, with an aim of enhancing blood flow and healing through macro- and microcirculation (5).

Surgical flaps may expedite the healing of noninfected deep ulcers by filling the void with well-vascularized healthy tissue. The flaps, however, are themselves still vulnerable to pressure injury, particularly during the early healing stages.

REFERENCES

1. Kosiak M. Etiology of decubitus ulcers. *Arch Phys Med Rehabil.* 1961;42:19–29.
2. Dinsdale SN. Decubitus ulcers: role of pressure and friction in causation. *Arch Phys Med Rehabil.* 1974;55:147–154.
3. The National Pressure Ulcer Advisory Panel. Stages of a Pressure Ulcer from the National Pressure Ulcer Advisory Panel (NPUAP) announces a change in terminology from pressure ulcer to pressure injury and updates the stages of pressure injury. www.npuap.org

4. Ennis WJ, Lee C, Gellada K, et al. Advanced technologies to improve wound healing: electrical stimulation, vibration therapy, and ultrasound-what is the evidence? *Plast Reconstr Surg*. 2016;138(3 Suppl):94S–104S.

5. Ud-Din S, Bayat A. Electrical stimulation and cutaneous wound healing: a review of clinical evidence. *Healthcare (Basel)*. 2014;2(4):445–467.

CHAPTER 33

QUALITY IMPROVEMENT

INTRODUCTION (1–5)

Quality in health care can be defined as the "direct correlation between the level of improved health services and the desired health outcomes of individuals and populations" (2). This quality is centered around the goal of making health care safe, effective, patient centered, efficient, timely, and equitable.

Quality improvement (QI) as defined by the U.S. Health and Human Services "includes systematic and continuous actions that lead to measurable improvement in health care services and the health status of targeted patient groups" (2). In 2001, the Institute of Medicine (IOM) released a report *Crossing the Quality Chasm: A New Health System for the 21st Century*, which outlined the "chasm" between the health care presently offered and what health care can be with a focus on how to reinvent the health care system to "foster innovation and improve the delivery of care." The report outlined six aims that must be addressed in order to meet the needs of patients, improve function, and reduce health care–associated burden and disability. These aims include safe, effective, patient-centered, timely, efficient, and equitable health care. The system must be both responsive to current health care needs and anticipate future needs (3).

The implementation of QI projects can lead to improved patient health, efficiency of processes, decrease of waste, improving communication, and proactively solving problems. In order to improve quality, change must be implemented within both current microsystems and systems at large.

In order to achieve this change, four key principles must be incorporated: (a) *QI works on systems and processes*—this includes changes, which improve performance and are individualized to specific needs; (b) *the primary focus of QI is the patient's well-being*—the health care must be safe, delivered by competent clinicians, coordinated, and culturally sensitive; (c) *QI utilizes a multidisciplinary approach*—it incorporates each team member's skill set and ideas, creating effective leadership, policies, and procedures; (d) *QI is data driven*—it uses quantitative and qualitative measures to understand how current systems are working, barriers, implemented interventions, and their level of success.

Patients undergoing rehabilitation are at increased risk for injury as they move through the rehabilitation continuum of care. This continuum of care includes care in the acute inpatient rehabilitation, subacute, outpatient, and home settings. In the acute inpatient rehabilitation setting, injuries can include infections, blood clots, pressure ulcers, adverse effects of medications, and falls. In the outpatient setting, injuries can include trauma from interventional procedures, burns from heat modalities, and falls.

A systems-based approach to identifying and studying the risks for these injuries using QI methodology can serve as the foundation for implementing interventions to minimize their occurrence.

In addition, there is increased interest in safety and quality in rehabilitation medicine. The Centers for Medicare and Medicaid Services (CMS) requires the reporting of data on quality metrics such as infections and falls. Accrediting organizations such as the Commission on Accreditation of Rehabilitation Facilities (CARF) require the collection of outcomes data and engagement in QI activities based on the analysis of this data. For practicing physiatrists, the American Board of Physical Medicine and Rehabilitation (ABPMR) requires the completion of a practice improvement project (PIP) for maintenance of the ABPMR certificate. One project per cycle is required for those with certificates issued before 2012 and two projects per cycle if issued in 2012 or beyond (5).

HOW TO PERFORM A QI PROJECT (6)

Implementation of an effective QI project requires changing the culture and infrastructure of an organization in order to break down traditional barriers and work toward a common goal. The steps typically involved in a QI project include

(a) *Identifying the team*, which may include a day-to-day leader, data entry person, provider champion, operations coordinator, and data specialist. A diverse team brings unique perspectives, experiences, and backgrounds; staff engagement is paramount for successful implementation of a program
(b) *Delineating the problem(s)* or areas in need of improvement. Team members also perform a literature search for relevant materials and references
(c) *Identifying variables and benchmarks* to assess the outcome
(d) *Defining the steps* in the current process
(e) *Identifying barriers and bottlenecks to the current process* in need of improvement
(f) *Brainstorming* for possible interventions
(g) *Implementing* the interventions
(h) *Collecting outcomes' data after the interventions have been initiated*
(i) *Analyzing the data* to confirm that all relevant issues have been addressed and that the intervention was successful
(j) *Communicating* the "lessons learned" to stakeholders

A selected list of QI models include the Care Model (high-quality disease and prevention management); the Learn Model (cost and time efficiency); Model for Improvement (see PDSA cycle section); FADE (focus, analyze, develop, execute); and Six Sigma (measurement-based strategy for process improvement and problem reduction). Finally, *tracking performance over time* is necessary for the immediate and long-term application of the study; this can be done in a setting of formal and informal communication/meetings, newsletters, and so forth.

Plan-Do-Study-Act Cycle (6,7)

The Institute for Healthcare Improvement (IHI) advocates for the use of the Model for Improvement as a tool to accelerate improvement. The Plan-Do-Study-Act (PDSA) cycle aims to test the change in a real work setting, implement the change on a larger scale (pilot population or unit), and finally spread the change (6). This model is composed of three fundamental questions followed by the PDSA cycle

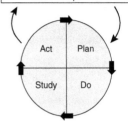

Model for Improvement

| What are we trying to accomplish? |
| How will we know that a change is an improvement? |
| What change can we make that will result in improvement? |

FIGURE 33.1 The PDSA Cycle and Model for Improvement developed by Associates in Process Improvement: a quality improvement tool to test an idea and measure the impact.
Source: Adapted from Ref. (8).

itself (Figure 33.1). The questions involve setting time-specific aims, establishing and using quantitative measures to determine successful improvement, and selecting changes. Each component of the PDSA cycle has a specific goal; the "Plan" phase identifies the question to be answered/changes to be implemented, the people responsible for the project, timeline, and resources/data necessary. The "Do" phase entails carrying out the test on a small scale and appropriate data. The "Study" phase includes the results and data analysis compared with what was predicted during the planning phase, identifying successes, failures, and unintended consequences. The "Act" phase describes changes that must be made based on the data; the project may be adapted (modifying the change and repeating the cycle), adopted (instituting the change on a larger scale), or abandoned (restarting the cycle with a new question; 7).

TOOLKIT (7,9)

A wide array of tools can be used as part of performing a QI project. These tools can be divided into improvement situations including working with numbers, working with ideas, or working in teams. A selected list of tools that can be implemented as part of the QI project include:

- A *fishbone diagram (cause and effect;* Figure 33.2A) is an example of working with ideas and allows for a team to identify and graphically display potential (root) causes for a problem or effect. It is especially useful if limited quantitative data is available. In order to construct a fishbone diagram, frame the problem as a "why" question, which is placed in the head of the diagram, with the aim of each root cause to answer the question. The branches are formed by different categories, which contribute to the problem/effect. Some sample categories include people, processes, plant, and equipment causes contributing to the problem.

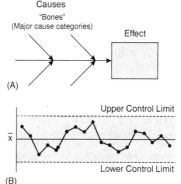

FIGURE 33.2 Examples of a fishbone diagram (A) and control chart (B); two essential components of the quality improvement toolkit.
Source: Adapted from Ref. (9).

- A *control chart* (Figure 33.2B) is an example of working with numbers and is used to graphically track a process over time in order to recognize and study sources of variation and improve performance.
- A *tree diagram* is an example of working as a team and is used to break down a broad goal into smaller, detailed levels of action, which can or should be done to achieve the goal.
- *Brainstorming* is an example of working with ideas and involves a group working together to creatively and efficiently amass a large number of ideas on a specific topic. Brainstorming may be performed in a structured (taking turns) or unstructured environment, silently or out loud.

ROOT CAUSE ANALYSIS (6,10)

A root cause analysis (RCA) is a retrospective tool that can be used to identify the causes of an adverse event and the specific failures, which can be modified in order to prevent the error from occurring again. The goal of the RCA is to focus on causes of the flaw, not blame. It calls into question "What circumstances led a reasonable person to make reasonable decisions that resulted in an undesirable outcome?" (3). The team is formed by four to six individuals from a variety of disciplines and may also include patients and family members. Six steps are followed to perform an RCA: (a) identify what happened accurately and completely, (b) determine what should have happened in an ideal situation, (c) determine causes and factors that contributed to the event,

(d) generate the causal statement (cause, effect, and event), (e) provide recommendations to prevent similar future situations, and (f) share the findings and summary with other involved members.

FAILURE MODE AND EFFECTS ANALYSIS (6,9)

The Failure Mode and Effects Analysis (FMEA) is a tool that focuses on identifying potential failures in process and taking proactive measures to avoid such failures, thereby reducing adverse events and potential harms. FMEA involves describing the steps in the process, what could go wrong, why something would go wrong, and what the consequence of the failure would be. Therefore, in contrast to an RCA (reactive), an FMEA is a proactive process, which seeks to identify potential failures and their effects before the events actually occur.

TRANSITION POINTS/HANDOFFS

Transitions in care refer to a patient leaving one medical setting and moving to another (e.g., hospital, skilled nursing facility, inpatient rehabilitation facility, home health care, primary care physician). During these transitions, effective communication is necessary to avoid confusion about the patient's condition and medication profile. Errors during this process can lead to harm/adverse events, duplicative testing, inconsistent monitoring, and generalized medication errors. These errors create concerns for patient safety, quality of care and health outcomes, and, ultimately, dissatisfaction with health care (7). Key information passed between treatment teams should include hospital course and complications, past medical and surgical history, relevant results (laboratory, radiology), operative and procedure reports, medication reconciliation, allergies, advanced directives, and contact information (next of kin). Improved communication and verbal discussion of the key elements between providers, patients, and family members is crucial to ensure safe transitions of care (11).

REFERENCES

1. Health and Medicine Division of the National Academies of Sciences, Engineering, and Medicine. http://www.nationalacademies.org/hmd
2. Quality Improvement U.S. Department of Health and Human Services Health Resources and Services Administration. April 2011.
3. IOM. Shaping the Future for Health. The National Academy of Sciences; March 2001
4. Kalra L, Yu G, Wilson K, Roots P. Medical complications during stroke rehabilitation. *Stroke*. 1995;26:990–994.
5. The American Board of Physical Medicine and Rehabilitation Maintenance of Certification Booklet of Information 2015–2016.
6. Institute for Health Care Improvement. http://www.ihi.org
7. Centers for Medicare and Medicaid Services. PDSA Cycle Template. www.CMS.gov

8. How to Improve. http://www.ihi.org/resources/Pages/HowtoImprove/default.aspx

9. Six Sigma Quality. www.SixSigma.com

10. Cristian A, Batmangelich S. *Physical Medicine and Rehabilitation Patient Centered Care: Mastering the Competencies*. New York, NY: Demos Medical Publishing; 2015.

11. National Transitions of Care Coalition. *Improving Transitional Communications*. September 2010.

SUGGESTED READING

CARF International. http://www.carf.org/home

Brassard, M, Ritter D. *The Memory Jogger II Healthcare Edition*. Salem, NH: GOAL/QPC. 2008.

ABBREVIATIONS

2D	two-dimensional
6MWT	6-minute walk test
AAPM&R	American Academy of Physical Medicine and Rehabilitation
ABI	ankle-brachial index
ABPMR	American Board of Physical Medicine and Rehabilitation
AC	acromioclavicular
ACC	American College of Cardiology
ACCP	American College of Chest Physicians
ACL	anterior cruciate ligament
ACPA	anticitrullinated protein antibody
ACSM	American College of Sports Medicine
ADL	activities of daily living
ADM	abductor digiti minimi
AFO	ankle–foot orthosis
AHA	American Heart Association
AHCPR	Agency for Health Care Policy and Research
AHRQ	Agency for Healthcare Research and Quality
AIDP	acute inflammatory demyelinating polyradiculoneuropathy
AKA	above-knee amputation
ALARA	As Low As Reasonably Achievable
ALND	axillary lymph node dissection
ALS	amyotrophic lateral sclerosis
ALT	alanine transaminase
ANA	antinuclear antibody
AOS	apraxia of speech
AP	action potential
APB	abductor pollicis brevis
APL	abductor pollicis longus
AS	ankylosing spondylitis
ASA	acetylsalicylic acid; American Stroke Association

ASIA	American Spinal Injury Association
AST	aspartate transaminase
AT	anaerobic threshold
ATFL	anterior talofibular ligament
AVERT	A Very Early Rehabilitation Trial
AVM	arteriovenous malformation
AVN	avascular necrosis
BESS	Balance Error Scoring System
BKA	below-knee amputation
BMD	Becker muscular dystrophy; bone mineral density
BTX-A	botulinum toxin-A
BW	birth weight
BZD	benzodiazepine
CABG	coronary artery bypass graft
CAD	coronary artery disease
CARF	Commission on Accreditation of Rehabilitation Facilities
CASH	cruciform anterior spinal hyperextension
CBPP	congenital brachial plexus palsy
CC	coracoclavicular
CDT	complete decongestive therapy
CEA	carotid endarterectomy
CF	cystic fibrosis
CFL	calcaneofibular ligament
CHF	congestive heart failure
CIC	clean IC
CIDP	chronic inflammatory demyelinating polyneuropathy
CIMT	constraint-induced movement therapy
CIPN	chemotherapy-induced peripheral neuropathy
CK	creatine kinase
CMAP	compound motor action potential
CMS	Centers for Medicare and Medicaid Services
CMV	cytomegalovirus
CNS	central nervous system
CO	cardiac output
COG	center of gravity
COPD	chronic obstructive pulmonary disease

COX-2	cyclooxygenase-2
CP	cerebral palsy
CPP	cerebral perfusion pressure
CPU	central processing unit
CR	cardiac rehabilitation
CRD	complex repetitive discharge
CRP	C-reactive protein
CRPS	complex regional pain syndrome
CRS-R	JFK Coma Recovery Scale-Revised
CSF	cerebrospinal fluid
CSW	cerebral salt wasting
CTS	carpal tunnel syndrome
CV	conduction velocity
CVA	cerebrovascular accident
DAI	diffuse axonal injury
DAPRE	Daily Adjusted Progressive Resistance Exercise
DBP	diastolic blood pressure
DF	dorsiflexion
DI	diabetes insipidus
DIP	distal interphalangeal
DJD	degenerative joint disease
DMOAD	disease-modifying osteoarthritis drug
DOAC	direct oral anticoagulant
DRG	dorsal root ganglion
DRS	Disability Rating Scale
DSD	detrusor-sphincter dyssynergia
DVT	deep venous thrombosis
DXA	dual-energy x-ray absorptiometry
EBV	Epstein-Barr virus
ECF	extracellular fluid
ECM	extracellular matrix
ECOG	Eastern Cooperative Oncology Group
ECRB	extensor carpi radialis brevis
ECRL	extensor carpi radialis longus
EDB	extensor digitorum brevis
EMD	Emery-Dreifuss muscular dystrophy

EPB	extensor pollicis brevis
EPP	end plate potential
ES	electrical stimulation
ESI	epidural steroid injection
ESR	erythrocyte sedimentation rate
EULAR	European League Against Rheumatism
FAST	Fitness Arthritis and Seniors Trial
FCU	flexor carpi ulnaris
FEESST	Fiberoptic Endoscopic Evaluation of Swallowing With Sensory Testing
FES	functional electrical stimulation
fib	fibrillation
FIM	Functional Independent Measure
FM	fibromyalgia
FMEA	Failure Mode and Effects Analysis
FRC	functional residual capacity
FSH	follicle-stimulating hormone
FSHD	facioscapulohumeral muscular dystrophy
FVC	forced vital capacity
GBM	glioblastoma multiforme
GBS	Guillain-Barré syndrome
GCS	Glasgow Coma Scale
GERD	gastroesophageal reflux disease
GFR	glomerular filtration rate
GGT	gamma-glutamyl transferase
GH	glenohumeral
GI	gastrointestinal
GOAT	Galveston Orientation Amnesia Test
GRF	ground reactive force
H&P	history and physical examination
HA	headache
HDL	high-density lipoprotein
HFS	hip fracture surgery
HIT	heparin-induced thrombocytopenia
HLA	human leukocyte antigen
HMSN	hereditary motor sensory neuropathy

HO	heterotopic ossification
HR	heart rate
HTN	hypertension
IADL	instrumental activities of daily living
IAPV	intermittent abdominal pressure ventilation
IASP	International Association for the Study of Pain
IBP	inflammatory back pain
IC	intermittent catheterization; internal capsule
ICP	intracranial pressure
IGF-1	insulin-like growth factor-1
IHI	Institute for Healthcare Improvement
INR	international normalized ratio
IOM	Institute of Medicine
IP	interphalangeal
IPCD	intermittent pneumatic compression device
IPPV	intermittent positive pressure ventilation
ITB	iliotibial band; intrathecal baclofen
IVH	intraventricular hemorrhage
IVIG	intravenous immunoglobulin
JAK	janus kinase
JIA	juvenile idiopathic arthritis
KAFO	knee ankle foot orthosis
KF	knee flexion
KPS	Karnofsky Performance Scale
LBP	low back pain
LDL	low-density lipoprotein
LDUH	low-dose unfractionated heparin
LEAP	Lower Extremity Assessment Project
LEMS	Lambert-Eaton myasthenic syndrome
LH	luteinizing hormone
LIV	low-intensity vibration
LLQ	left lower quadrant of the abdomen
LMN	lower motor neuron
LMWH	low-molecular-weight heparin
LOC	loss of consciousness
LT	light touch

MAC	manually assisted cough
MAO	monoamine oxidase
MBS	modified barium swallow
MCA	middle cerebral artery
MCL	medial collateral ligament
MCP	metacarpophalangeal
MCS	minimally conscious state
MEPP	miniature end plate potential
MG	myasthenia gravis
MI	myocardial infarction
MLD	manual lymphatic drainage
MPZ	myelin protein zero
MS	multiple sclerosis
MSC	mesenchymal stem cell
MTX	methotrexate
MU	motor unit
MUAP	motor unit action potential
mV	millivolt
MVA	motor vehicle accident
MWD	microwave diathermy
NASCET	North American Symptomatic Carotid Endarterectomy Trial
NCS	nerve conduction study
NCV	nerve conduction velocity
NDT	neurodevelopmental treatment
NIH	National Institutes of Health
NMES	neuromuscular electrical stimulation
NMJ	neuromuscular junction
NOAC	novel oral anticoagulant
NOF	National Osteoporosis Foundation
NPUAP	National Pressure Ulcer Advisory Panel
NSAID	nonsteroidal anti-inflammatory drug
NT	not testable
NTD	neural tube defect
NYHA	New York Heart Association
OA	osteoarthritis

O-Log	Orientation Log
OP	osteoporosis
ORIF	open reduction internal fixation
OT	occupational therapy
PAID	paroxysmal autonomic instability with dystonia
PAS	periodic acid–Schiff
PCF	peak cough flow
PCI	percutaneous coronary intervention
PCL	posterior cruciate ligament
PD	Parkinson's disease
PDSA	Plan-Do-Study-Act
PE	pulmonary embolism
PF	plantar flexion
PFO	patent foramen ovale
PIP	practice improvement project; proximal interphalangeal
PLS	primary lateral sclerosis
PLSO	posterior leaf spring orthosis
PMC	pontine micturition center
PMPS	post-mastectomy pain syndrome
PNF	proprioceptive neuromuscular facilitation
PNS	peripheral nervous system
PP	pinprick
PPE	preparticipation evaluation
PPS	post-polio syndrome
PR	pulmonary rehabilitation
PRP	platelet-rich plasma
PsA	psoriatic arthritis
PSW	positive sharp wave
PT	physical therapy; protime
PTA	post-traumatic amnesia
PTFL	posterior talofibular ligament
PTPS	post-thoracotomy pain syndrome
PVL	periventricular leukomalacia
PWB	partial weight bearing
QI	quality improvement
QSART	Quantitative Sudomotor Axon Reflex Testing

RA	rheumatoid arthritis
RAS	reticular activating system
RCA	root cause analysis
RCT	randomized controlled trial
RF	rheumatoid factor
RFS	radiation fibrosis syndrome
RHD	right hemisphere damage
RICE	rest, ice, compression, and elevation
RM	repetition maximum
RNS	repetitive nerve stimulation
RPE	Rating of Perceived Exertion
RSD	reflex sympathetic dystrophy
RV	residual volume
SACH	solid ankle cushioned heel
SAH	subarachnoid hemorrhage
SBP	systolic blood pressure
SCAT5	Sport Concussion Assessment Tool 5th edition
SCI	spinal cord injury
SCIWORA	SCI without radiographic abnormality
SCS	spinal cord stimulator
SDHs	subdural hemorrhage
SEP	somatosensory evoked potential
SFEMG	single-fiber EMG
SGA	small for gestational age
SI	sacroiliac
SIADH	syndrome of inappropriate antidiuretic hormone
SIJ	sacroiliac joint
SIS	second impact syndrome
SLAP	superior labral tear from anterior to posterior
SMA	spinal muscular atrophy
SNAP	sensory nerve action potential
SNRB	selective nerve root block
SNRI	serotonin–norepinephrine reuptake inhibitor
SpA	seronegative spondyloarthropathy
SPLATT	split anterior tibial tendon transfer
SSA	sulfasalazine

SSRI	selective serotonin reuptake inhibitor
STIR	short T1 inversion recovery
SV	stroke volume
SWD	shortwave diathermy
TBI	traumatic brain injury
TCM	Traditional Chinese Medicine
TD	terminal device
TF	transfemoral
TG	triglyceride
TH	transhumeral
THA	total hip arthroplasty
TKA	total knee arthroplasty
TLC	total lung capacity
TLSO	thoracolumbosacral orthosis
TMJ	temporomandibular joint
TNF	tumor necrosis factor
TNF-α	tumor necrosis factor-alpha
tPA	tissue plasminogen activator
TR	transradial
TSBA	total body surface area
TSF	tibial stress fracture
TT	transtibial
TUG	Timed Up and Go
TV	tidal volume
UMN	upper motor neuron
UPDRS	unified Parkinson's disease rating scale
US	ultrasound
UTI	urinary tract infection
UV	ultraviolet
UVA	ultraviolet A
UVB	ultraviolet B
VATS	video-assisted thoracoscopic surgery
VC	vital capacity
V_{CO_2}	carbon dioxide production
VCUG	voiding cysto-urethrogram
V_E	pulmonary ventilation

VKA	vitamin K antagonist
VMO	vastus medialis oblique
VTE	venous thromboembolism
WB	weight bearing
WBAT	weight bearing as tolerated
WBC	white blood cell
XRT	radiation therapy

INDEX

CPSIA information can be obtained
at www.ICGtesting.com
Printed in the USA
BVHW051930200522
637659BV00003B/20

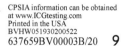

9 781620 701164